MINIMALLY INVASIVE TREATMENT, ARREST, AND CONTROL OF PERIODONTAL DISEASES, VOL 5

THE AXELSSON SERIES
ON PREVENTIVE DENTISTRY

The world-renowned authority on preventive and community dentistry presents his life's work in this six-volume series of clinical atlases focusing on risk prediction of dental caries and periodontal disease and on needs-related preventive and maintenance programs.

Volume 1 An Introduction to Risk Prediction and Preventive Dentistry

Provides a general overview of current and future trends in risk prediction, control, and nonaggressive management of caries and periodontal disease; preventive dentistry methods and programs; and quality control.

Volume 2 Diagnosis and Risk Prediction of Dental Caries

Includes a comprehensive discussion of the etiology, pathogenesis, diagnosis, risk indicators and factors, individual risk profiles, and epidemiology of caries.

Volume 3 Diagnosis and Risk Prediction of Periodontal Diseases

Presents a comprehensive discussion of the etiology, pathogenesis, diagnosis, risk indicators and factors, individual risk profiles, and epidemiology of periodontal diseases. Considers periodontal diseases as a possible risk factor for systemic diseases and presents current and future trends in the management of periodontal diseases, including nonaggressive debridement and preservation of the root cementum.

Volume 4 Preventive Materials, Methods, and Programs

Discusses self-care and professional methods of mechanical and chemical plaque control, use of fluorides and fissure sealants, and integrated caries prevention. Addresses needs-related preventive programs based on risk prediction and computer-aided epidemiology analysis for quality control and outcome.

Volume 5 Minimally Invasive Treatment, Arrest, and Control of Periodontal Diseases

Details current and future trends in minimally invasive treatment to preserve the root cementum and promote successful healing of infectious inflamed periodontal tissues as well as repair and regeneration of lost periodontal support. Provides recommendations for needs-related maintenance care to ensure the long-term success of treatment and prevent recurrence of periodontal disease.

Volume 6 Minimally Invasive Treatment, Arrest, and Control of Caries and Erosions

Describes current and future aspects of prevention and control of caries and erosions as well as arrest and remineralization of noncavitated lesions. Focuses on minimally invasive preparations, esthetic and hygienic restorations, and needs-related supportive programs to prevent recurrence of caries and erosions.

MINIMALLY INVASIVE TREATMENT, ARREST, AND
CONTROL OF PERIODONTAL DISEASES, VOL 5

Per Axelsson, DDS, Odont Dr

Professor of Preventive Dentistry
Axelsson Oral Health Promotion

Stockholm, Sweden

Quintessence Publishing Co, Inc
Chicago, Berlin, Tokyo, London, Paris, Milan, Barcelona,
Istanbul, Moscow, New Delhi, Prague, São Paulo, and Warsaw

To my wife Ingrid, my daughter Eva, and my son Torbjörn

Library of Congress Cataloging-in-Publication Data

Axelsson, Per, D.D.S.
  Minimally invasive treatment, arrest, and control of periodontal diseases / Per Axelsson.
     p. ; cm. — (Axelsson series on preventive dentistry ; v. 5)
  Includes bibliographical references and index.
    ISBN 978-0-86715-365-1
  1. Periodontal disease–Treatment. I. Title. II. Series: Axelsson, Per, D.D.S. Axelsson series on preventive
  dentistry ; v. 5.
  [DNLM: 1. Periodontal Diseases–therapy. 2. Periodontal Diseases–prevention & control. WU 240 A969m 2009]
  RK361.A97 2009
  617.6'32–dc22
                        2009014951

©2009 Quintessence Publishing Co, Inc

Quintessence Publishing Co Inc
4350 Chandler Drive
Hanover Park, IL 60133
www.quintpub.com

Questions and lecture or course requests may be directed to the author by e-mail at p.axelsson@comhem.se or by mail to Professor Per Axelsson, Rålambshovsleden 44, 11219 Stockholm, Sweden.

Editor: Kathryn Funk
Production: Angelina Sanchez

Printed in Germany

CONTENTS

PREFACE

According to the principles of *lege artis*, all members of our profession are obliged to offer treatment based on the most current scientific and clinical knowledge available. The etiology of the periodontal diseases is well understood, and we now have developed efficient methods for prevention, treatment, arrest, and control of these diseases as well as repair and regeneration of lost periodontal tissues. For example, in our 30-year longitudinal needs-related preventive study in adults, the mean number of lost teeth was only 0.5 per subject over the 30 years, and the periodontal attachment level was maintained irrespective of age (the oldest age group was 81 to 95 years at the final examination). Large-scale implementation of the study's methods in the preventive programs for the adult population in the county of Värmland, Sweden, has led to an increase of more than 15% in the number of remaining teeth in randomized samples of 65-year-old adults, as well as a reduction of more than 20% in loss of periodontal support during the first 10 years. Thus we must concentrate our efforts on prevention, control, and arrest of the periodontal diseases using treatment methods that are as minimally invasive as possible.

The aim of this book, the fifth of a six-volume series of textbooks and atlases, is to serve as a well-illustrated clinical "cookbook" that shows step-by-step how to practice minimally invasive nonsurgical treatment, healing of infectious inflamed periodontal tissues, repair and regeneration of lost periodontal tissues, and efficient supportive programs for prevention of recurrence of periodontal disease. Because of the many clinical illustrations combined with recent evidence-based scientific documentation, this volume should be useful for general dental practitioners and dental hygienists as well as undergraduate and postgraduate dental students.

The first chapter focuses on the importance of preservation of the root cementum through minimally invasive instrumentation and elimination of subgingival plaque biofilms and plaque-retentive factors such as calculus, unplaned rough root cementum, and restoration overhangs. Advantages and disadvantages of different methods of instrumentation are discussed and illustrated together with the negative consequences of iatrogenic aggressive scaling (eg, exposed dentinal tubules, plaque-retentive grooves, roughness).

Chapter 2 describes the importance of initial intensive therapy for healing of the periodontal tissues by combinations of needs-related mechanical and chemical plaque control supplemented with the elimination of plaque-retentive factors as described in chapter 1. Materials and methods for home as well as professional gingival plaque control are illustrated and discussed.

Initial intensive therapy is not always successful in healing the periodontal tissues. Chapter 3 presents information about available supplementary therapies that can be implemented in such cases. Indications, materials, and methods for use of antibiotics are discussed. Different materials and methods for supplementary treatment of furcation-involved teeth, which are very difficult to heal because of the limited accessibility for plaque removal, are also illustrated. Finally, periodontal surgery for accessibility and reduction of deep residual pockets is described.

Repair of intrabony defects may be achieved successfully by surgical as well as nonsurgical treatment in combination with excellent gingival plaque control. However, recent evidence-based studies have shown that regeneration of all the periodontal tissues (ie, alveolar bone, periodontal ligament, and cementum) can be achieved by so-called guided tissue regeneration (the use of different types of barriers) and the use of biomaterials such as enamel matrix derivatives. Chapter 4 presents several clinical cases showing the techniques and long-term outcome of different regenerative methods.

After successful treatment of periodontal disease, efficient and needs-related secondary preventive and maintenance programs must be established in order to prevent recurrence of the disease. Materials and methods for such programs are discussed in detail in chapter 5. Also presented is a computer-aided analytic epidemiologic system with relevant variables, which must be established for quality control and evaluation of the long-term outcome of the periodontal therapy.

The next and final volume in this series, *Minimally Invasive Treatment, Arrest, and Control of Caries and Erosions*, will follow this same clinical cookbook style, presenting similar information on the topic of dental caries rather than periodontal diseases.

This project could not have been completed without the support of my family, friends, and colleagues. I am grateful to all my colleagues around the world as well as several companies and publishers (including Blackwell Munksgaard and The American Academy of Periodontology), who have generously permitted me to use their illustrations (about 30% of the total). Last but not least, the excellent cooperation of the publisher is gratefully acknowledged.

CHAPTER 1

MINIMALLY INVASIVE SCALING, ROOT PLANING, AND DEBRIDEMENT

For successful treatment of periodontitis, not only supragingival plaque but also the subgingival microbiota has to be removed and controlled. The subgingival microbiota in a diseased, "true" periodontal pocket consists of an attached, well-organized plaque biofilm as well as nonattaching motile bacteria, mainly localized apically and outside the apical third of the plaque biofilm (Fig 1). The bacteria in the biofilm are inaccessible and protected from phagocytizing polymorphonuclear leukocytes, antibiotics, and other antimicrobial agents. Therefore, mechanical removal and disruption of the subgingival biofilm is the first precondition for successful healing of diseased periodontal pockets.

DEVELOPMENT OF PLAQUE BIOFILMS

A classic study of gingivitis by Löe et al (1965) established that free plaque accumulation along the gingival margin results in gingivitis within 2 to 3 weeks and that motile microbes invade the gingival sulcus within 1 to 2 weeks. Figure 2 shows the microflora in the gingival sulcus during experimental gingivitis, after 2 to 3 weeks without oral hygiene (Listgarten et al, 1975, 1976). Attached microbes are located to the left and apically, indicating the presence of a plaque biofilm.

Periodontitis is always preceded by gingivitis. If undisturbed, the gingival biofilm elicits in the gingival margin a typical inflammatory response (gingivitis), ie, edema, which deepens the gingival sulcus by formation of a pseudopocket in which the relatively anaerobic conditions favor the establishment of an anaerobic microbiota. Eventually, loss of periodontal support (periodontal ligament and alveolar bone) may occur, resulting in the development of a "true" periodontal pocket. Figure 3 shows the close correlation among the remaining periodontal ligament, the junctional epithelium, and the pattern of the attached subgingival biofilm.

Unlike the supragingival biofilm, the subgingival biofilm is protected from self-care methods of mechanical toothcleaning, intraoral abrasion, and salivary host defense components. As long as the subgingival biofilm is not disrupted by mechanical debridement, the microorganisms are inaccessible to antimicrobial agents and host factors. The main determinants limiting growth are physical space and the innate host defense system. Because gingival crevicular fluid is rich in nutrients, growth is unlikely to be limited by poor nutrition. In healthy periodontal tissues, the subgingival space available for bacterial growth is limited, but one effect of subgingival plaque accumulation is a continual increase in this space, resulting from a reduction of epithelial cell attachment levels and an increase in pocket depth.

The innate host defense system limits this spread by maintaining an intact epithelial cell barrier. Gingival crevicular fluid contains a potent array of antimicrobial agents. It is similar in composition to serum and contains the innate and

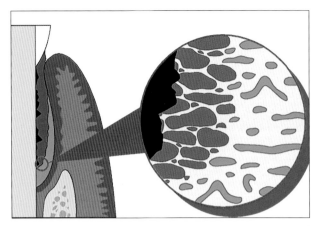

Fig 1 Diseased periodontal pocket containing attached subgingival plaque and nonattaching, motile subgingival microflora (spirochetes, vibrios, and straight rods with flagella). Note the calculus *(black)* covered by the subgingival plaque biofilm *(brown)*.

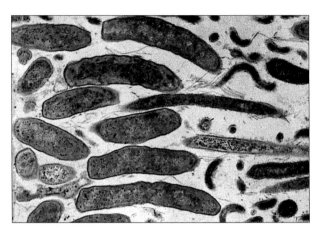

Fig 2 Cross section of gingival plaque filling the gingival sulcus while spirochetes and vibrios move around in the outer and more apical regions of the sulcus (original magnification ×12,000). (From Listgarten, 1976. Reprinted with permission.)

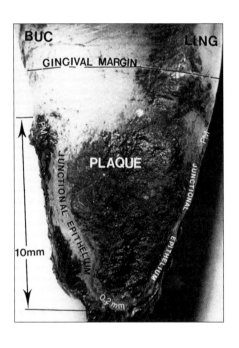

Fig 3 Autopsy material revealing the effect of subgingival plaque biofilm on root surfaces. Note the close relationship among the pattern of subgingival plaque, the junctional epithelium, and the remaining periodontal ligament. (BUC) Buccal surface; (LING) lingual surface; (PM) periodontal (membrane) ligament. (From Waerhaug, 1976. Reprinted with permission.)

adaptive components of host defense, which prevent bacteremia and systemic infection. Innate components include lysozyme, complement, and a variety of vascular permeability enhancers such as bradykinin, thrombin, and fibrinogen. Adaptive components include antibodies and lymphocytes. Of major importance is the role of the phagocytizing polymorphonuclear leukocytes, which represent the first line of nonspecific de-

fense in preventing further apical migration of the subgingival biofilm as well as motile spirochetes.

However, only nonattached bacteria and superficial species of the biofilm are accessible to polymorphonuclear leukocytes or antibiotics. Therefore, mechanical disruption and removal of the subgingival biofilm through systematic subgingival instrumentation, in combination with bactericidal irrigation, are essential for successful non-

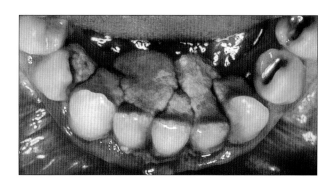

Fig 4 Extreme accumulation of supragingival calculus in the mandibular incisors in the absence of any dental care.

surgical treatment of periodontal diseases (for a more detailed discussion of the plaque biofilm concept, see volume 3 [Axelsoon, 2002]).

IMPEDIMENTS TO REMOVAL OF SUBGINGIVAL PLAQUE

Nonsurgical, systematic removal of the subgingival plaque biofilm is complicated by several factors:

1. The procedure has to be performed blindly.
2. The soft biofilm cannot be localized by tactile means. Therefore systematic, overlapping instrumentation must be carried out.
3. Plaque-retentive factors limit the accessibility to and increase the reaccumulation of plaque biofilms.

The following subgingival factors can predispose teeth to plaque retention and complicate removal of subgingival plaque biofilms: subgingival calculus; rough, unplaned root cementum surfaces; enamel pearls; root resorption defects; deep, narrow bone defects; root surface grooves; furcation involvement; vertical root fractures; iatrogenic effects of invasive scaling, such as grooves and exposed dentinal tubules on the root surfaces;

restoration overhangs; defective and ill-fitting crown margins; excess resin and other cements; unpolished restorations; recurrent caries; and root caries.

Dental calculus

Dental calculus may accumulate supragingivally as well as subgingivally. Supragingival calculus may form in the absence of dental plaque in patients with a high salivary concentration of minerals. This type of accumulation is localized lingually and approximally on the mandibular anterior teeth and buccally on the maxillary molars, where the ductal openings of the major salivary glands are located (Fig 4). Supragingival calculus is gray-yellow and relatively porous.

Subgingival calculus is composed of minerals from the gingival crevicular fluid. In contrast to supragingival calculus, subgingival calculus is very hard, homogenous, and strongly attached to the root surface. The color is brown to dark brown, and the surface is very irregular (Fig 5). Subgingival calculus may not form apically and laterally to the base of the plaque biofilm.

Such solid, rough, and sharp subgingival calculus formations not only are extremely plaque retentive but also will repeatedly cause injuries and wounds on the inner wall of the periodontal pocket, every time the free gingiva is pressed

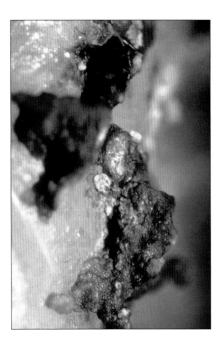

Fig 5 Sharp irregular subgingival calculus on the palatal root of an untreated and extracted maxillary first molar.

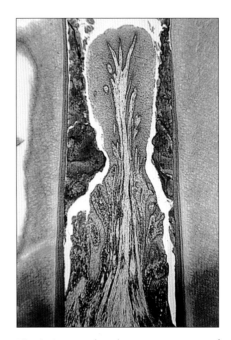

Fig 6 Autopsy histologic cross section of an interproximal space. Subgingival calculus is present on the two adjacent approximal root surfaces, and the interdental gingival papillae in the narrow space are inflamed. (From Waerhaug, 1976. Reprinted with permission.)

against the calculus during oral hygiene procedures and chewing. Because the subgingival calculus is covered by a plaque biofilm, repeated bacteremia may also be expected through the wounded inner wall of the pocket. Figure 6 shows a histologic cross section of an interproximal space with subgingival calculus on the approximal surfaces of two adjacent teeth. The space for the inflamed interdental gingival papillae is narrow. If a triangular, pointed toothpick is used for interdental cleaning in such a case without prior removal of the subgingival calculus by scaling and root planing, the papillae will be traumatized.

Most of the plaque on supragingival calculus may be removed daily by meticulous mechanical toothcleaning. However, the porous surface will never be completely clean because bacteria adhere to the calculus. Subgingival calculus is always covered by a plaque biofilm, which is inaccessible to removal by self-care and even nonsurgical professional mechanical toothcleaning (PMTC) without scaling and root planing. Dental calculus should be regarded as the most frequent and important plaque-retentive factor.

Rough, unplaned root cementum

The root cementum surface is very rough compared to the enamel surface. The cementoenamel junction is another anatomic feature with high potential for plaque retention. In particular, calculus attaches very firmly to all the irregularities of the cementum surface, including microholes resulting from the destruction of Sharpey fibers. Thus, it is obvious that nonsurgical removal of subgingival plaque biofilms, and in particular calculus, is impossible without simultaneous planing of the outer surface of the root cementum. Furthermore, subgingival plaque biofilms and calculus that have re-formed because of failing gingival plaque control are much easier to remove from a smooth surface than from the rough, intact cementum surface.

The cementum surface must be cleaned and planed as noninvasively as possible to avoid exposure of the root dentin and dentinal tubules. In addition, neither bacteria nor endotoxins penetrate the root cementum (Eide et al, 1983, 1984; Hughes and Smales, 1986; Moore et al, 1986; Nakib et al, 1982). Therefore, extensive removal of cementum may not be necessary to render the root free of bacterial endotoxins.

This question was addressed in an experimental study in dogs (Nyman et al, 1986). Plaque-accumulating floss was ligated around the necks of the mandibular premolars bilaterally, inducing breakdown of periodontal tissue to midroot level. On one side of the jaw, the root surfaces of the experimental teeth were scaled and the exposed root cementum was removed with flame-shaped diamonds. The roots of the contralateral teeth were not scaled but only polished with polishing paste in rubber cups and interdental rubber tips.

Two months after surgery, the results were evaluated histometrically. No obvious differences were found, whether or not the previously exposed root cementum had been removed. Healing had consistently resulted in the formation of a junctional epithelium with noninflamed subjacent connective tissue. Thus, removal of root cementum "to eliminate endotoxins" does not seem to be a prerequisite for periodontal healing.

This animal study was followed by a study in humans (Nyman et al, 1988). The subjects were adults with moderate to advanced periodontal disease. In a split-mouth design, the dentition of each patient was randomly allotted into test and control quadrants. Buccal and lingual mucoperiosteal flaps were elevated, and all granulation tissue was removed. In two control quadrants in each patient, the denuded root surfaces were carefully scaled and planed with hand instruments and flame-shaped diamonds to remove soft and hard deposits as well as all cementum. In the contralateral test quadrants, the roots were not scaled and planed, but soft plaque biofilms were removed from the root surfaces with polishing paste, rubber cups, and interdental rubber tips. Calculus in the test quadrants was removed carefully with curettes, avoiding removal of cementum.

Twenty-four months after treatment, the same degree of improvement in periodontal health was observed with both types of treatment. The frequency of gingival sites that bled on probing or had a Gingival Index score of 2 or 3 was low in all jaw quadrants, and the frequency of sites with shallow pockets was high. Between the baseline examination and the follow-up examinations (after 6, 12, and 24 months), there was some gain of probing attachment for both treatment modalities. This gain was most pronounced in the initially deeper pockets and was similar for both treatment modalities.

Mombelli et al (1995) investigated the effect of altering the subgingival environment on the subgingival microbiota and clinical status. The subjects were seven patients, aged 30 to 60 years, with generalized marginal periodontitis. Mucoperiosteal flaps were raised, and the bone was recontoured to eliminate angular bony defects. The control teeth were carefully debrided and thoroughly root planed. No root instrumentation was performed on the test teeth. Calculus deposits visible to the naked eye were chipped off with the tip of a scaler. Over a 1-year postoperative observation period, clinical parameters showed a similar pattern of response in the test and control sites. Probing depths and probing attachment levels were significantly reduced 1 month after surgery and remained at lower levels. A significant decrease in total anaerobic viable bacterial counts was also noted. In both groups, after treatment, the proportion of gram-negative anaerobic rods associated with periodontal diseases (eg, *Porphyromonas gingivalis*) decreased significantly.

These findings corroborate the concept that the reduction of selected subgingival microorganisms, rather than the removal of tooth substance and mineralized deposits by root instrumentation, is the key to successful periodontal therapy. Minimally invasive planing of the outer surface of the root cementum is justified, as discussed earlier, but invasive, complete removal of the cementum that results in exposed root dentin and dentinal tubules is not.

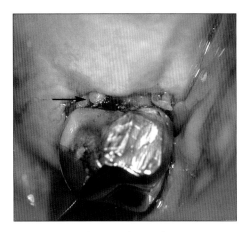

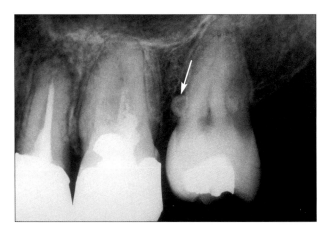

Fig 7 Enamel pearl *(arrow)*, 1.5 mm in diameter, located mesiolingually along the gingival margin of the maxillary left second molar and about 2.0 mm apical to the cementoenamel junction.

Fig 8 Typical shape and radiopacity of an enamel pearl *(arrow)*. This enamel pearl is 2.5 mm in diameter and located on the mesial root of the maxillary left second molar. There is localized loss of alveolar bone around the enamel pearl.

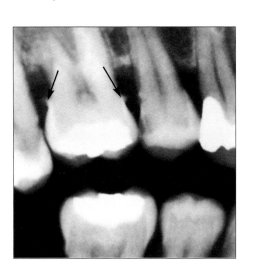

Fig 9 Typical radiographic appearance of subgingival calculus *(arrows)*. In this case, the calculus is located mesially and distally along the cementoenamel junction of the maxillary right first molar in an untreated young adult with limited chronic periodontitis.

Enamel pearls

The prevalence of enamel pearls ranges from 1% to 10%. About 75% are found on the maxillary third molars; the remainder are most frequently found on the maxillary second molars and mandibular third molars. Enamel pearls most frequently occur on the gingival third of the root.

The surface of an enamel pearl is as smooth as normal enamel on the tooth crown, and the shape is a hemisphere (Fig 7). It should be easy to distinguish its convex, smooth, and radiopaque shape on radiographs (Fig 8) from the rough, irregular, and less radiopaque subgingival calculus (Fig 9). The enamel pearl is a significant plaque-retentive factor almost comparable to subgingival calculus. A subgingival biofilm that covers an enamel pearl is inaccessible, particularly on the apical side of the enamel pearl, without mechanical removal of the pearl as well. However, the solid and hard pearl is firmly attached to the root and much more difficult to remove than calculus.

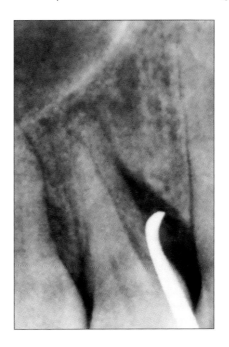

Fig 10 Subgingival microflora growing along the mesial root groove of a maxillary first premolar, resulting in a deep vertical bone defect reaching the furcation area.

A diamond-coated bur must be used as a first step before the final minimally invasive root planing.

Root resorption defects

In the presence of cementum hypoplasia and root resorption where the root dentin is not protected by cementum, bacteria may invade the dentinal tubules. The bacteria in such resorption are inaccessible to nonsurgical scaling and debridement. This condition may be one of the reasons why some diseased pockets do not respond to nonsurgical therapy.

Deep, narrow bone defects and root grooves

Deep, narrow bone defects and root surface grooves significantly limit the accessibility for removal of the plaque biofilm and calculus (Fig 10). In addition, such deep defects offer excellent anaerobic conditions that favor and maintain the growth of the anaerobic periopathogenic microflora. For successful nonsurgical instrumentation, thin, specially designed instruments are necessary. Deep root grooves sometimes must be recontoured to improve access for oral hygiene procedures and subgingival debridement.

Furcation involvement

Teeth that have lost periodontal attachment to the level of the furcation are said to exhibit *furcation involvement*. The distal and buccal surfaces of the maxillary first and second molars and the buccal and lingual surfaces of the mandibular first molars exhibit the highest prevalence of furcation involvement (Axelsson, 1978, 2002).

The anatomy of the furcation favors the retention of subgingival plaque biofilms and calculus, which are inaccessible to mechanical tooth-cleaning by self-care and very difficult to remove nonsurgically by professional scaling and debridement. In particular, furcation-involved distal surfaces of the maxillary first molars are completely inaccessible as long as the second molars remain. That is the main periodontal reason why the maxillary first molars or their distobuccal roots are lost.

Furcations vary in horizontal and vertical depth as a result of differences in features such as cervical enamel pearls, the length of the root

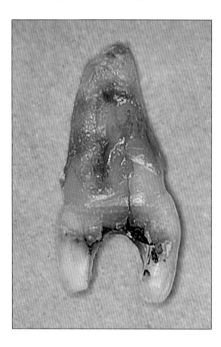

Fig 11 Partial vertical root fracture on the mesial surface of a maxillary second premolar. There is localized loss of periodontal ligament around the fracture.

trunk, the dimensions of the furcation entrance, the anatomy of the root, and the anatomy of the furcation roof. Furcation involvement must be diagnosed with a combination of good bitewing or periapical radiographs and clinical probing with a slim double-ended curette (Goldman-Fox 3) or a special curved furcation probe.

The severity of furcation involvement is highly dependent on the relationship between the amount of attachment loss and the distance from the cementoenamel junction to the furcation entrance, that is, the length of the root trunk. (For details on diagnosis and treatment of furcation involvement, see chapters 2 and 3.)

Vertical root fractures

The prognosis for teeth with vertical root fractures is very poor. The fracture will frequently continue further toward the apex, and the root segments will separate for mechanical reasons. In addition, the bacteria hiding subgingivally in the fracture are inaccessible to any mechanical cleaning or chemical agent, resulting in a localized loss of periodontal support around the fracture and a narrow, deep periodontal pocket.

Vertical root fractures are, by definition, longitudinal and confined to the root of the tooth. They may be in a mesiodistal (Fig 11) or buccolingual plane (Figs 12a and 12b) and may occur at any point along the root. The diagnosis of a vertical root fracture is difficult because several of the associated signs and symptoms are shared with other dental conditions. In some instances, a radiograph of the affected tooth may exhibit a halo appearance at the fracture site. However, unless the fractured segment has separated, radiographs are often of little use in locating the lesion, and sometimes it will simulate an apical or radicular lesion. However, a very deep, localized pocket on the buccal or lingual root surface of a nonvital tooth with a post is a typical sign of a vertical buccolingual root fracture (see Figs 12a and 12b). Almost all vertical root fractures occur in nonvital teeth with posts.

The use of transillumination and plaque-disclosing or iodine solution on the cervical part of the root is also recommended. The patient may have masticatory pain, with or without concomitant pulpal pain. The diagnosis may also be made with the use of a bite test, in which a resilient material is placed between the teeth during gentle occlusion, or exploratory surgery.

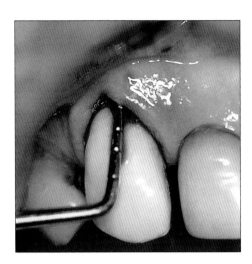

Fig 12a Very deep and narrow periodontal pocket on the buccal surface of a maxillary right lateral incisor with a post.

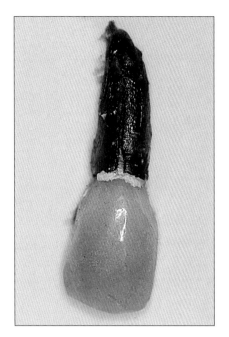

Fig 12b Vertical root fractures extending to the apex on the buccal root surface of the untreatable and extracted tooth.

If only one buccal root surface is fractured and the apical extent of the fracture is limited, an apically repositioned mini-flap can be raised to create access for mechanical and chemical treatment.

Iatrogenic effects of invasive scaling

Roughness

Successful professional instrumentation of periodontally diseased teeth should completely remove plaque biofilm, other bacterial components (endotoxins), and calculus with minimal removal of healthy tooth substance and without creation of surface roughness. Several studies have shown that invasive instrumentation results in inadequate cleaning and considerable iatrogenic effects, such as roughness, grooves that run in different directions, and exposed root dentin and dentinal tubules (Coldiron et al, 1990; Flemmig et al, 1998a, 1998b; Frentzen et al, 2002; Jacobson et al, 1994; Jotikasthira et al, 1992; Kocher and Plagmann, 1997; Kocher et al, 2001a, 2001b; Ladner et al, 1992; Leknes, 1997; Lie and Leknes, 1985; Lie and Meyer, 1977; Meyer and Lie, 1977; Ritz et al, 1991; Zappa et al, 1991).

The most invasive iatrogenic defects are caused by: diamond-coated reciprocating tips and rotating burs (Fig 13); laser instruments; sonic scalers; magnetostrictive ultrasonic scalers used at maximum power (Fig 14); hand instruments with rough sharp edges (Figs 15a and 15b) and straight angulation and used with excessive force; and air polishers used with regular abrasive powder within 3 cm from the root surface and for a lengthy time.

Figures 16a to 16e show the long-term outcome of repeated invasive scaling. Gradual, advanced loss of the tooth substance is evident on the mesial root surface of the canine and the distal surface of the maxillary right lateral incisor. Compensatory secondary dentin has formed to protect the root pulp from the invasive instrumentation and invading bacteria through the exposed dentinal tubules. In spite of this repeated invasive scaling, more alveolar bone was lost. Figure 17a shows a radiograph of a maxillary left lateral incisor exhibiting even more advanced loss of alveolar bone. In spite of frequent and extremely invasive instrumentation, all remaining alveolar bone up to the apex was lost 2 years later (Fig 17b).

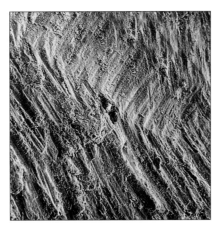

Fig 13 Results of instrumentation with a rotary diamond tip. The diamond tip has removed all the cementum and left deep gouges in the dentin. Typical undulations are traversed at right angles by regular instrumental marks (original magnification ×100). (From Meyer and Lie, 1977. Reprinted with permission.)

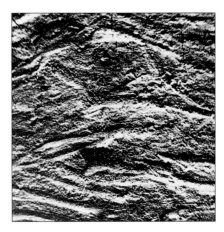

Fig 14 Extensive roughening of the root surface, partially into cementum and partially into dentin, by an ultrasonic scaler used at maximum power (original magnification ×20). (From Lie and Leknes, 1985. Reprinted with permission.)

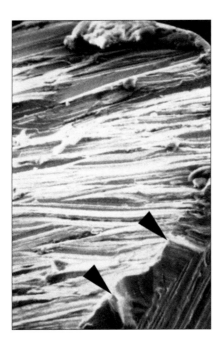

Fig 15a Curette hand instrument with an extremely rough cutting edge. There are irregularities *(arrowheads)* near the tip of the instrument (original magnification ×250). (From Tal et al, 1985. Reprinted with permission.)

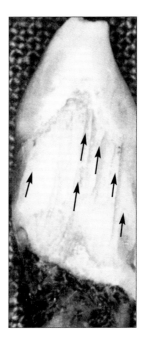

Fig 15b Effect on the root surface of instrumentation with the rough curette. Grooves and irregularities *(arrows)* have been created by instrumentation from the bottom of the pocket in a coronal direction (original magnification ×5). (From Tal et al, 1985. Reprinted with permission.)

Figs 16a to 16e Long-term outcome of repeated invasive scaling on the mesial root surface of the maxillary right canine and the distal root surface of the maxillary right lateral incisor. Note the gradually increased size of the interproximal alveolar bone loss, loss of root substance, and increased formation of secondary dentin in the root canal to protect the root pulp. (Courtesy of Dr G. Heden.)

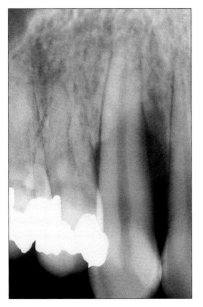

Fig 16a Pretreatment radiographic appearance.

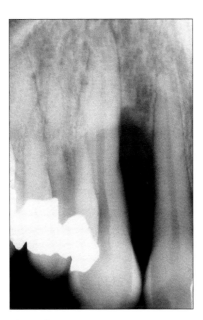

Fig 16b Six years.

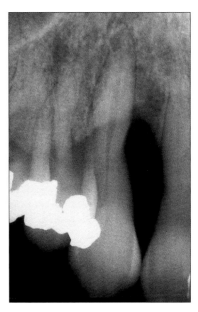

Fig 16c Twenty-two years.

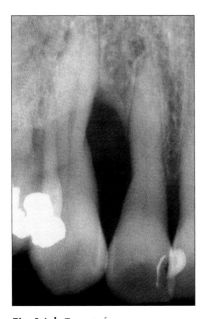

Fig 16d Twenty-five years.

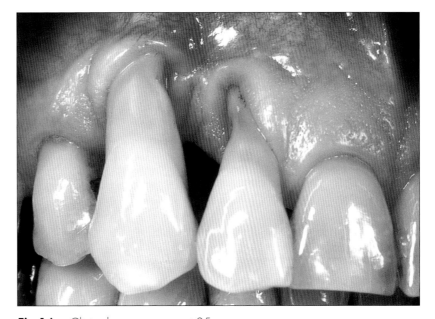

Fig 16e Clinical appearance at 25 years.

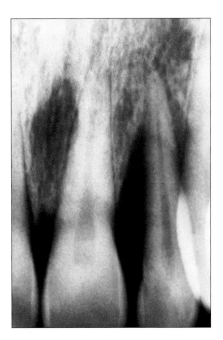 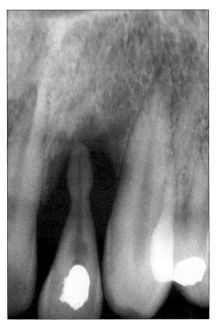

Fig 17a Radiograph of a maxillary left lateral incisor exhibiting advanced loss of alveolar bone.

Fig 17b Loss of all remaining alveolar bone up to the apex 2 years later, despite frequent and extremely invasive instrumentation.

On the other hand, examples of minimally invasive instruments suitable for debridement are: PER-IO-TOR instruments (Dentatus); piezoelectric ultrasonic scalers used at low power and with Polytetrafluoroethylene-coated tips; and blunt hand instruments used with negative angulation (about 60 degrees) and low force. PER-IO-TOR instruments are also suitable for minimally invasive root planing and final scaling.

Bacterial invasion of dentinal tubules

Iatrogenic grooves may result in lateral and apical migration of bacteria (Figs 18a and 18b). In addition, bacteria may invade exposed dentinal tubules and result in infected root canals (Fig 19) and vice versa—Bacteria from infected root canals may maintain infection of the periodontal pockets and limit the successful outcome of regenerative therapy (Adriaens et al, 1986, 1988a, 1988b).

Hypersensitivity

Exposed root dentin may result in root surface hypersensitivity. This may limit the patient's willingness to clean the exposed root surfaces properly and increase the risk for development of root caries. Aggressive use of diamond tips, in particular, as well as sonic scalers, ultrasonic scalers, and hand instruments will remove not only the plaque biofilm and calculus but also the root cementum and the superficial parts of the root dentin, exposing the dentinal tubules.

The exposed dentin and tubules will be accessible and sensitive to thermal, chemical, and mechanical stimuli in the oral environment. Such stimuli will cause sudden movements of fluid in the exposed dentinal tubules, activating the nerve fibers and causing pain. Such pain is most acute immediately after periodontal treatment but may vary in length and intensity. Without special treatment, the pain may become chronic because in some areas the dentinal tubules will remain open.

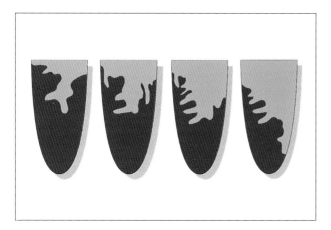

Fig 18a Iatrogenic grooves and other roughness on the root surface *(red)* may result in irregular lateral and apical migration of subgingival bacteria *(orange)*.

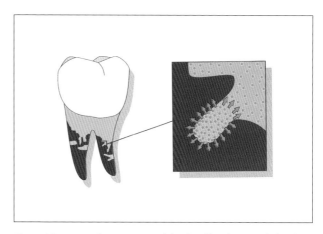

Fig 18b Lateral migration of the biofilm *(arrows)*, facilitated by iatrogenic root grooves from invasive instrumentation.

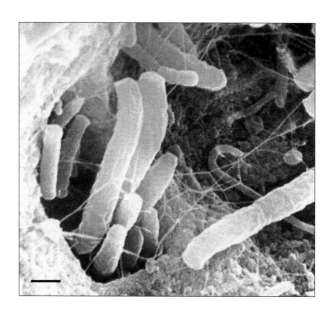

Fig 19 Invasion of bacteria in dentinal tubules via apertures denuded of cementum during invasive scaling and root planing (bar = 1 µm). (From Adriaens et al, 1988b. Reprinted with permission.)

In most cases, the tubules will eventually be obliterated, and the hypersensitivity will be reduced if the patient cleans the root surfaces daily with a fluoride toothpaste and chews fluoride chewing gum for 20 minutes after every meal. However, if the patient fails to remove the plaque daily because of hypersensitivity, the pain will worsen, and root caries may develop.

In an experimental clinical study, Tammaro et al (2000) evaluated the dental sensitivity of exposed roots. Patients reported the severity of sensitivity using a visual analog scale before and during a 3-week special oral hygiene period, as well as before and 4 weeks after scaling and root planing. The sensitivity gradually was reduced during the oral hygiene period, but there was an immediate and statistically significant increase in sensitivity as an effect of scaling and root planing. This increase remained significant during the first 3 weeks and was slightly reduced after 4 weeks.

This study indicated the importance of "noninvasive" scaling, root planing, and debridement and supplementary professional treatment of the instrumented surfaces with fluoride directly after the instrumentation. Such a protocol will reduce the sensitivity of the root surfaces and thereby increase the patient's willingness to clean them properly at least twice a day using mechanical self-care combined with application of topical fluoride agents (toothpaste and fluoride chewing gum).

Several products for professional use are available on the market for prevention and reduction

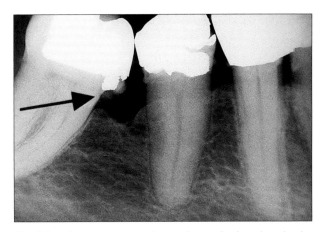

Fig 20a Restoration overhang (arrow) related to the localized loss of periodontal support.

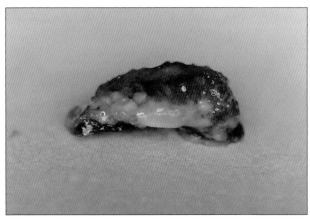

Fig 20b Subgingival calculus covering the restoration overhang in Fig 20a, removed in one piece using a curette from a lingual-approximal direction. A thick, well-matured plaque biofilm can be seen completely covering the calculus.

of root hypersensitivity. The most efficient agent seems to be Bifluorid 12 (Voco) fluoride varnish, which contains 6% sodium fluoride and 6% calcium fluoride. The high concentrations of sodium fluoride and calcium fluoride will efficiently obliterate open dentinal tubules and act as a catalyst for hypermineralization of the root surface, thereby preventing root caries (Hellwig and Attin, 1994). In a multicenter study, 92% of the subjects reported significant improvement or relief of pain after a single application (Schroers, 1994). Other slow-release fluoride agents such as Fluor Protector (Vivadent) and Duraphat (Colgate) fluoride varnishes and diluted resin-modified glass-ionomer cements may also be recommended as well as stannous fluoride gels. Special bonding materials have also been made for exposed root dentin and dentinal tubules.

Treatment failure

Comprehensive scaling and root planing should only have to be performed initially in untreated patients suffering from periodontitis. After a single session of meticulous scaling, root planing, and debridement, without invasive removal of the root cementum, the health of the periodontal tissues can be maintained through excellent gingi-

val plaque control (self-care supplemented by PMTC at needs-related intervals). The need for repeated scaling and root planing in maintenance patients must be regarded as a treatment failure.

Restoration overhangs and roughness

Several studies of bitewing radiographs have shown a strong correlation between the location and size of approximal restoration overhangs and loss of alveolar bone (Albandar, 1990; Albandar et al, 1987; Björn et al, 1969, 1970; Brunsvold and Lane, 1990; Chen et al, 1987; Eid, 1986; Gilmore and Sheiham, 1971; Hakkarainen and Ainamo, 1980; Jeffcoat and Howell, 1980; Keszthelyi and Szabo, 1984; Pack et al, 1990; Rodriguez-Ferrer et al, 1980; Tal et al, 1989). These findings confirm that overhangs are potent plaque-retentive factors. Most overhangs are located subgingivally on the approximal surfaces of the posterior teeth (Figs 20a and 20b) and therefore are difficult to remove with rotating instruments. However, the reciprocating thin double-knife–shaped Profin Lamineer diamond- and tungsten-coated tips (Dentatus) offer optimal accessibility and efficacy for removing approximal overhangs and recontouring restorations.

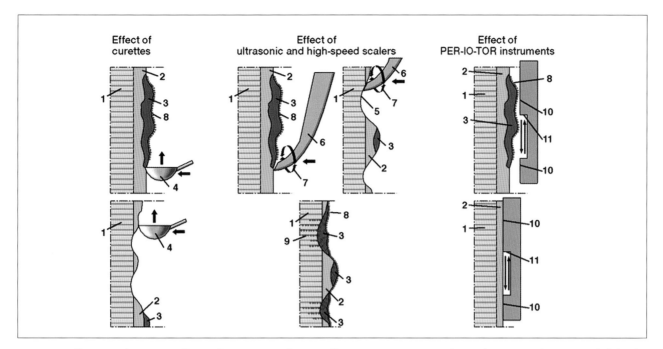

Fig 21 Differences between effects of invasive and minimally invasive instruments for scaling, root planing, and debridement. (1) Root dentin with dentinal tubules; (2) root cementum; (3) calculus; (4) curette hand instrument; (5) iatrogenic rough, exposed dentin and dentinal tubules; (6 and 7) ultrasonic or high-speed scaler; (8) subgingival plaque biofilm; (9) bacterial invasion of the dentinal tubules; (10 and 11) principal design of reciprocating PER-IO-TOR instruments.

It has been shown that removal of an overhang improves plaque control (Rodriguez-Ferrer et al, 1980) and restores gingival health (Gorzo et al, 1979). For this reason, removal of overhanging margins should be part of initial periodontal therapy. In addition, early detection of overhanging dental restorations is an important part of preventive dental care. A sensitive tactile instrument, such as a fine explorer, should be used in conjunction with radiographs to facilitate this detection.

MINIMALLY INVASIVE ALTERNATIVES FOR SCALING, ROOT PLANING, AND DEBRIDEMENT

There is a need for a new approach, based on the concept of minimally invasive subgingival instrumentation. For rational elimination of subgingival plaque-retentive factors and microflora by scaling, root planing, and debridement, and to minimize iatrogenic defects, a sharp universal curette should be used as a probe to identify calculus. Whenever located, this calculus should be carefully lifted away as a first step in previously untreated patients. A piezoelectric ultrasonic scaler also could be used for gross scaling, but for final scaling, root planing, and debridement, the instrument of choice should be as minimally invasive as possible.

Figure 21 illustrates the difference between invasive and minimally invasive instruments for scaling, root planing, and debridement. Reciprocating PER-IO-TOR instruments, designed with plane load-relieving surfaces between essentially right-angled cutting edges, are examples of a minimally invasive instrument. Once the root cementum is planed and thereby clean, no further root cementum will be removed (Axelsson, 1993).

Polytetrafluoroethylene-coated sonic scalers are specially designed for minimally invasive subgingi-

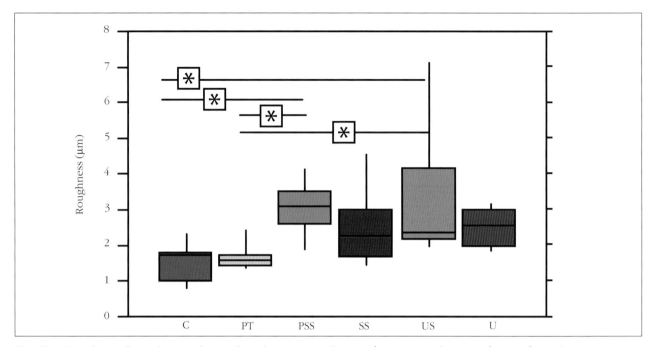

Fig 22 Boxplot, with median and quartiles, showing roughness of approximal root surfaces after subgingival instrumentation. (C) Curette; (PT) PER-IO-TOR; (PSS) polytetrafluoroethylene-coated sonic scaler; (SS) conventional sonic scaler; (US) ultrasonic scaler; (U) untreated control. *Statistically significant difference (*P* < .05). (From Kocher et al, 2001b. Reprinted with permission.)

val debridement (mainly removal of subgingival biofilms). Because of their extremely low invasiveness, these instruments are not suitable for scaling and root planing.

In an experimental clinical study, Kocher et al (2001b) used severely periodontally diseased teeth that were to be extracted to compare the roughness and topography of approximal root surfaces after subgingival instrumentation with different instruments. One approximal surface of each tooth was instrumented with *(1)* a sharp Gracey hand curette (Hu-Friedy); *(2)* PER-IO-TOR No. 3 reciprocating tip; *(3)* a sonic scaler insert coated with a heat-shrunk polytetrafluoroethylene tube (prototype, Kocher et al, 2000); *(4)* a sonic scaler (Sonicflex 2000, KaVo); or *(5)* a piezoelectric ultrasonic scaler on medium power (Perio Sonosoft Lux, KaVo). After extraction of the tooth, the instrumented approximal surface was also compared with the untreated periodontally diseased approximal surface of the same tooth, which had to be free of calculus and organic material.

The roughness values indicated that curettes and the PER-IO-TOR instrument produced the smoothest surfaces, with a mean value of about 1.5 μm (Fig 22). The other three instruments all resulted in a mean roughness value of about 3.0 μm. The untreated root surfaces exhibited a roughness value similar to those treated with conventional sonic and ultrasonic instruments. Only the curettes and the PER-IO-TOR instruments obviously smoothed the surface in comparison to an untreated control surface.

The three-dimensional topography of the five different instrumented surfaces and the untreated surfaces is shown in Fig 23. On surfaces treated with sonic scalers, ultrasonic scalers, and polytetrafluoroethylene-coated sonic scalers, peaks appeared rounded, although the valleys were still very pronounced. With the PER-IO-TOR, the peaks appeared largely flattened, and ridges consisted only of gentle undulations. On surfaces treated with curettes, grooves were observed in orderly, linear groups with unequal distances between grooves along the long axis of the tooth. Such surfaces bore no resemblance to uninstrumented topography.

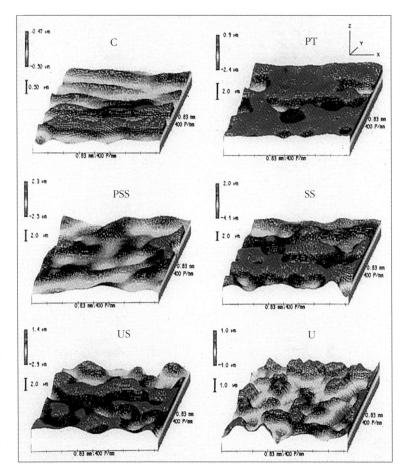

Fig 23 Surface topography after roughness has been optically removed from the structure with a 0.2 × 0.2 – mm filter. Colors are displayed from the software as a relative measure of height and cannot be directly used to compare height differences between the different instrumented surfaces in the z-axis. The colored bars show the maximum valley-to-peak distance. The area was analyzed in a field of 0.83 × 0.83 mm. (C) Curette; (PT) PER-IO-TOR; (PSS) polytetrafluoroethylene-coated sonic scaler; (SS) conventional sonic scaler; (US) ultrasonic scaler; (U) untreated control surface. (From Kocher et al, 2001b. Reprinted with permission.)

In a subsequent study, Rühling et al (2005) evaluated the amount of cementum that was removed by the aforementioned instruments: hand curette, ultrasonic scaler, sonic scaler, polytetrafluoroethylene-coated sonic scaler, and the PER-IO-TOR instrument. The results were compared to untreated cementum.

The results showed that the polytetrafluoroethylene-coated sonic scaler and the PER-IO-TOR instrument, followed by the ultrasonic scaler, removed less root cementum than the hand instrument and the sonic scaler (Figs 24a and 24b). The PER-IO-TOR instrument resulted in the smoothest surfaces (Fig 25a). While, on average,

90% to 95% of the root cementum thickness remained after instrumentation with the PER-IO-TOR and the polytetrafluoroethylene-coated sonic scaler, only about 10% remained after the use of the curette (Fig 25b).

Special plastic curettes are also available for minimally invasive subgingival debridement (removal of biofilms) of natural teeth and particularly implants in maintenance patients (Fig 26). In a short-term clinical study in maintenance patients, results achieved after a single debridement with these instruments were similar to those obtained with standard stainless steel curettes (Bardet et al, 1999).

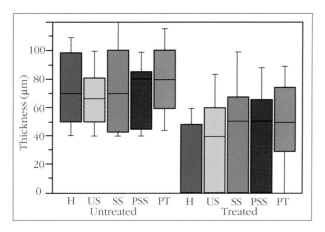

Fig 24a Box plot, with median and quartiles, showing the effects of instrumentation on the thickness of cementum on treated and untreated root surfaces. (H) Hand instrument (curette); (US) ultrasonic scaler; (SS) conventional sonic scaler; (PSS) polytetrafluoroethylene-coated sonic scaler; (PT) PER-IO-TOR. (From Rühling et al, 2005. Reprinted with permission.)

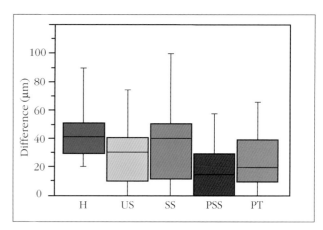

Fig 24b Box plot, with median and quartiles, showing the difference in cementum thickness between treated and untreated surfaces. For the parts in which cementum was completely removed, pretreatment cementum thickness may be underestimated because even dentin may have been removed. (H) Hand instrument (curette); (US) ultrasonic scaler; (SS) conventional sonic scaler; (PSS) polytetrafluoroethylene-coated sonic scaler; (PT) PER-IO-TOR. (From Rühling et al, 2005. Reprinted with permission.)

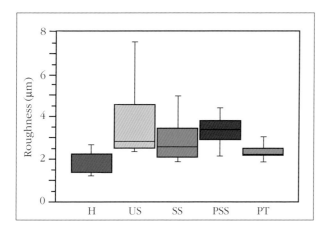

Fig 25a Box plot, with medians and quartiles, showing the effects of instrumentation on surface roughness. (H) Hand instrument (curette); (US) ultrasonic scaler; (SS) conventional sonic scaler; (PSS) polytetrafluoroethylene-coated sonic scaler; (PT) PER-IO-TOR. (From Rühling et al, 2005. Reprinted with permission.)

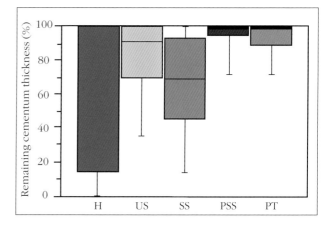

Fig 25b Box plot, with medians and quartiles, showing percentage of root cementum thickness remaining after treatment. (H) Hand instrument (curette); (US) ultrasonic scaler; (SS) conventional sonic scaler; (PSS) polytetrafluoroethylene-coated sonic scaler; (PT) PER-IO-TOR. (From Rühling et al, 2005. Reprinted with permission.)

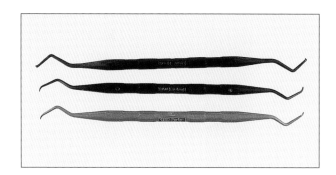

Fig 26 Plastic curette hand instruments for minimally invasive debridement (removal of plaque biofilms) of natural teeth and, in particular, implants.

METHODS AND MATERIALS FOR SCALING, ROOT PLANING, AND DEBRIDEMENT

Definition of terms

- *Scaling:* Mechanical removal of both subgingival and supragingival calculus from the tooth surfaces
- *Root planing:* Instrumentation of the root surface only until it is smooth and hard, without invasive complete removal of the root cementum
- *Debridement:* Removal of the subgingival microflora, particularly the attached nonmineralized as well as semimineralized plaque biofilms

Subgingival instrumentation can be performed nonsurgically (closed and blindly) or in combination with flap surgery (open and visible). Nonsurgically, the aforementioned types of instrumentation can successfully be carried out by dentists as well as dental hygienists.

For initial therapy in patients with untreated periodontitis, debridement as well as scaling and root planing may be necessary. However, in most maintenance patients, needs-related intervals of PMTC, supplemented with minimally invasive debridement in sites with re-formed subgingival biofilms, should be sufficient.

Goals

- Attached biofilms and nonattached microflora in the gingival sulcus and the periodontal pockets should be removed.

- Plaque-retentive factors such as calculus, restoration overhangs, and areas of cementum hypoplasia and resorption should be eliminated.
- The root surface should be rendered as smooth as possible: if the patient fails to maintain gingival plaque control, this will allow minimally invasive debridement of any reaccumulated subgingival plaque biofilm.
- To minimize the consequences of subgingival regrowth of microflora, the root cementum should be preserved; removal of the cementum will expose the dentinal tubules.
- After treatment, it is important to prevent recurrence of infection in the periodontal pocket. Meticulous gingival plaque control achieved by the patient's daily oral hygiene regimen should be supplemented, at needs-related intervals, by PMTC.

Limitations

Subgingival debridement, scaling, and root planing present the following challenges:

- When instrumentation is performed nonsurgically, it is difficult to ascertain whether all plaque biofilms and calculus have been removed; the practitioner must rely on tactile feedback and adherence to systematic procedures.
- It is necessary to reach the bottom of even very deep and narrow periodontal pockets as well as root grooves and furcation areas (see Fig 10).

In a study by Sherman et al (1990), the effectiveness of subgingival scaling and root planing in vivo was evaluated on teeth indicated for ex-

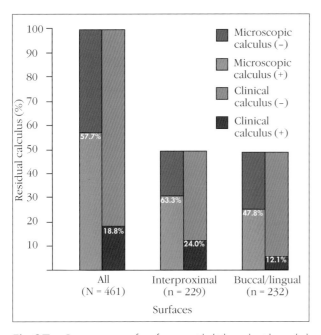

Fig 27a Percentage of surfaces with (+) and without (–) microscopically and clinically detected residual calculus after scaling and root planing, by site. (Modified from Sherman et al, 1990.)

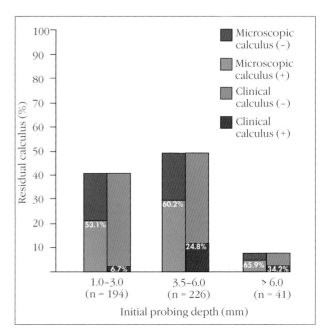

Fig 27b Percentage of surfaces with (+) and without (–) microscopically and clinically detected residual calculus after scaling and root planing, by initial probing depth. (Modified from Sherman et al, 1990.)

traction because of advanced periodontitis. The total time spent in instrumentation per tooth was 9.4 minutes, an average of 3.6 minutes with ultrasonics followed by 5.8 minutes with hand curettes.

The effect was evaluated clinically by three trained periodontists using periodontal probes and subgingival explorers. After extraction, the subgingival part of the scaled and planed root surfaces were also examined using a stereomicroscope at ×10 magnification. When examined in the stereomicroscope, 58% of a total of 461 scaled and planed root surfaces exhibited residual calculus (Fig 27a). Residual calculus was found in more than 60% of sites with initial probing depths of 3.5 mm or more (Fig 27b). The periodontists had only been able to detect calculus clinically on 19% of surfaces.

Kepic et al (1990) studied the effectiveness of total removal of all calculus from teeth scheduled for extraction because of severe periodontal disease. Fourteen teeth were treated with closed subgingival scaling and root planing with an ultrasonic instrument, and 17 others were treated with

hand instruments. Instrumentation was continued until the involved roots felt smooth to the explorer. A 45- to 60-minute appointment was allowed for each quadrant.

After a healing period of 4 to 8 weeks, the affected areas were anesthetized, and periodontal flaps were elevated to provide maximum access and visibility for instrumentation. The test tooth or teeth, along with all other affected teeth in each surgical area, were then treated with the same type of instrument (ultrasonic or hand instrument) that had been used previously. Root debridement was continued until the affected surfaces felt smooth to the explorer, approximately 10 minutes with ultrasonic tips and 20 minutes with hand instruments for each tooth. After all the teeth had been planed, the experimental tooth or teeth were extracted, and the flaps were replaced and sutured.

After extraction, the treated roots of the teeth were sectioned and evaluated using a light microscope. Retained calculus was observed on 12 of the 14 teeth treated with ultrasonic scalers and 12 of the 17 teeth treated with hand instruments.

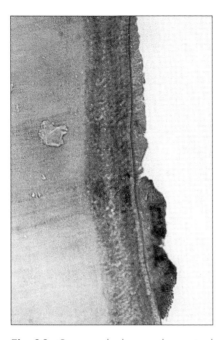

Fig 28 Gross calculus on the apical third of the furcation wall of an ultrasonically treated tooth (original magnification ×100). (From Kepic et al, 1990. Reprinted with permission.)

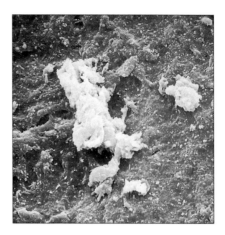

Fig 29 SEM photograph of a hand-instrumented specimen showing flecks of residual calculus (original magnification ×3,000). (From Kepic et al, 1990. Reprinted with permission.)

The results indicate that complete removal of calculus from a periodontally diseased root surface is rarely achieved (Figs 28 and 29).

Robertson (1990) summarized the results of three other studies with similar experimental designs that assessed residual calculus by microscopic examination of teeth extracted after no therapy (control), scaling and root planing alone, and scaling and root planing with surgical access (Table 1). The investigations involved experienced clinicians who spent an average of 12 to 15 minutes to complete the debridement of each tooth with a variety of hand and ultrasonic instruments.

The data were approximated from results given for nonfurcation surfaces. Taken collectively, calculus was present on about 91% of all untreated surfaces and 96% of untreated surfaces associated with deep pockets (6 mm or greater). After scaling and root planing alone, about 47% of all surfaces and 63% of surfaces associated with deep pockets showed residual calculus. Surgical access improved the results, but residual calculus

was still present on about 20% of all surfaces and 38% of surfaces adjacent to deep pockets. The frequency of residual calculus in furcation areas after scaling and root planing was much higher, and surgical access appeared to provide little additional benefit.

From these reviewed studies, it can be concluded that complete detection and absolute removal of subgingival calculus rarely are achieved. However, the original amount of calculus was reduced to 5% in the study by Kepic et al (1990) and to about 10% in the study by Sherman et al (1990).

To evaluate the potential and limitations of nonsurgical removal of subgingival calculus and plaque biofilms, Rateitschak-Plüss et al (1992) conducted an in vivo study in single-rooted teeth with advanced periodontitis. The root surfaces were cleaned and planed with fine curettes without flap reflection. The teeth were then extracted, and the root surfaces were systematically examined by scanning electron microscopy (SEM) for the presence of residual bacteria and calculus. Forty surfaces on 10 teeth were evaluated. Of

Table 1   Summary of demographics and treatments in three studies of residual calculus*

Study	Patients (No.)	Treatment[†]	Surfaces (No.)	Surfaces with calculus (%) Deep[‡]	Surfaces with calculus (%) All
Caffesse et al (1986)[§]	21	None	66	98	93
		S/RP alone	170	68	48
		S/RP + flap	168	50	24
Buchanan and Robertson (1987)[§]	10	None	88	90	82
		S/RP alone	116	40	24
		S/RP + flap	140	18	14
Fleischer et al (1989)[‖¶]	36	None	31	100	100
		S/RP alone	35	75	69
		S/RP + flap	45	45	18

* From Robertson (1990). Reprinted with permission.
[†] None = untreated control teeth; S/RP = scaling and root planing (closed); flap = flap surgery (open).
[‡] Surfaces adjacent to deep pockets (≥ 6 mm).
[§] All teeth.
[‖] Multirooted teeth.
[¶] Results from experienced operators only.

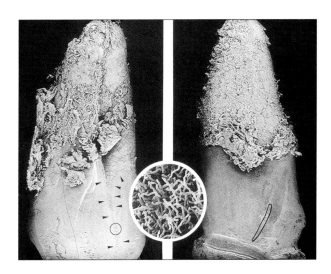

Fig 30 SEM photographs of root surfaces after nonsurgical (closed) scaling and root planing. *(left)* Distal root surface of a mandibular left first premolar after treatment. Bacterial residue *(circled area)* is present in a depression *(arrows)* caused by the fusion of two roots (original magnification ×12). *(inset)* Bacteria observed in the area of the circle (original magnification ×1,500). *(right)* Mesial root surface of a maxillary right central incisor after treatment. Bacterial residue is visible in the area of the line angle *(outlined area)* (original magnification ×10). (From Rateitschak-Plüss et al, 1992. Reprinted with permission.)

these, 29 surfaces, readily accessible to the curette, were free of all plaque and calculus. Virtually all of the residual plaque and calculus was detected in specific sites (Fig 30):

• Grooves and depressions in the root surface
• The so-called line angles, ie, the area where a

change would be made from one curette blade to another during the root planing process

In 31 of 40 treated root surfaces, the base of the pocket was not completely accessible to the curettes. Several conditions precluded instrumentation to the base of the pocket:

- *Probing depth:* The deeper the pocket, the more often the base of the pocket was not reached by the curette.
- *Probing width:* Very narrow pockets often defied access to the curette, and these root surfaces exhibited plaque and sometimes calculus.
- *Course of the base of the pocket:* Attachment loss associated with periodontitis seldom progresses evenly and on individual teeth is often very irregular (see Figs 3 and 18). The periodontal pocket may even interconnect with attachment loss apical to persistent attachment. Areas such as these could not be reached with a curette. Residual plaque and calculus were routinely detected in such areas.

Adriaens and Adriaens (2004) completed a systematic review of in vivo studies on the efficacy of nonsurgical therapy for removing the subgingival plaque biofilm and dental calculus from periodontally diseased teeth scheduled for extraction. Generally it was evident that subgingival scaling and root planing is an efficient method to reduce the bacterial biofilm and calculus attached to the subgingival root surface. However, most studies also have indicated that none of the instrumentation techniques is totally effective in eliminating all plaque biofilms and calculus from the subgingival surface of the tooth.

With increasing probing depth, the number of teeth with subgingival surfaces that are completely free of residual plaque or calculus decreases. The percentage of the treated root surfaces with residual plaque or calculus is directly related to the probing depth at the time of instrumentation. For probing depth values less than 4 mm, 4% to 43% of the root surface was still covered with remnants of plaque biofilm or calculus after thorough instrumentation. In pockets with a probing depth of 4 to 6 mm, 15% to 38% of the instrumented root surface still demonstrated the presence of calculus or plaque biofilms. In pockets deeper than 6 mm, these values varied between 19% and 66% (Adriaens and Adriaens, 2004).

Complete debridement of furcations was notably more difficult when nonsurgical techniques were used. Furthermore, repeated nonsurgical subgingival debridement comprising a first episode of no more than 10 minutes per tooth, followed 24 hours later by two additional episodes of subgingival instrumentation (each 24 hours apart) for a maximum of 5 minutes each, was not more effective in removing subgingival deposits than a single 10-minute episode of subgingival scaling and root planing for each tooth. Nonsurgical subgingival instrumentation was slightly less effective in removing subgingival plaque biofilms and calculus than access flap surgery combined with root debridement under direct visual control.

The studies reviewed by Adriaens and Adriaens (2004) demonstrated that, even with direct visual control during surgical debridement, increasing amounts of remaining calculus and plaque were found with increasing values for probing depth. This might indicate that the visualization of these surfaces during access flap surgery is not optimal because of local factors such as grooves, furcations, root resorptions, and iatrogenic defects, as discussed earlier.

When different instruments used for the subgingival debridement during nonsurgical periodontal therapy were compared, no major differences between the approaches were demonstrated. However, the experience of the operator is an important factor in the final result of the subgingival debridement. In vivo and in vitro (in mannequin heads), trained periodontists succeeded in leaving less residual plaque and calculus on the subgingival root surfaces than did periodontists in training or inexperienced dentists (Adriaens and Adriaens, 2004).

Success

Although more plaque remains in deep pockets after nonsurgical therapy than after open flap debridement, the total reduction of the subgingival microflora mostly results in improved periodontal health if excellent gingival plaque control by self-care and needs-related intervals of PMTC is maintained. The exception may be in areas with grade II and III furcation involvement.

Good long-term clinical results, even after nonsurgical therapy, are attributable to a combination of effective host response to residual microorganisms and efficient maintenance care. Within a

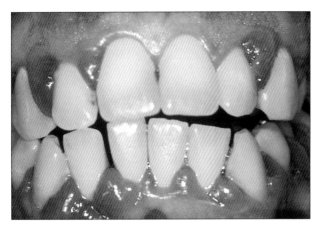

Fig 31a Facial view of a patient with advanced periodontal disease and extraordinarily inflamed gingiva.

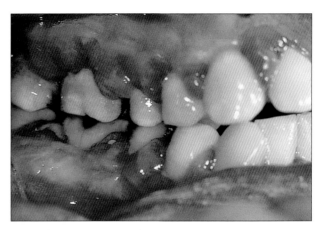

Fig 31b Buccal view of the right side. Spontaneous suppuration of purulent exudate is observed interproximally between the mandibular first and second molars.

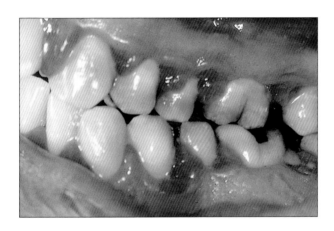

Fig 31c Buccal view of the left side. Suppuration of purulent exudate is visible between the mandibular molars.

relatively short period of time, an adult patient with very advanced marginal periodontitis can be treated successfully with nonsurgical subgingival scaling, root planing, and improved gingival plaque control. For example, the initial, very poor clinical periodontal status in a 40-year-old woman is shown in Figs 31a to 31c. The maxillary and mandibular second molars were initially extracted because of marginal-apical communication. The distobuccal roots of the maxillary first molars and the distal root of the mandibular left first molar were hemisectioned without flap surgery because

of grade III furcation involvement. The probing depth of the remaining approximal surfaces varied from 4 to 11 mm.

After a thorough initial examination and presentation of the treatment plan to the patient, treatment proceeded with scaling and root planing and the establishment of needs-related gingival plaque control by self-care and PMTC. The healing response after only 2 months is shown in Figs 31d to 31g. No pockets deeper than 3 mm persisted. Only hand curettes were used for the subgingival scaling, debridement, and root planing.

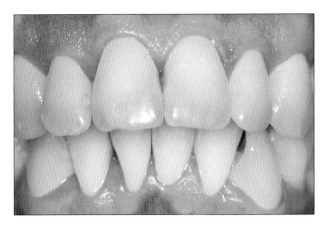

Fig 31d Anterior teeth 2 months after the initial nonsurgical therapy in combination with improved self-care and PMTC. The condition of the gingiva is excellent.

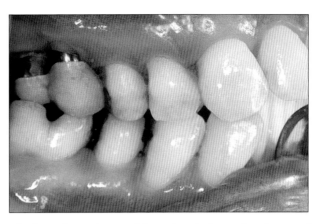

Fig 31e Buccal view of the right side 2 months after initial nonsurgical treatment.

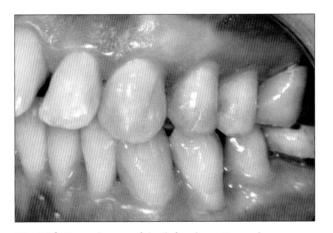

Fig 31f Buccal view of the left side at 2 months.

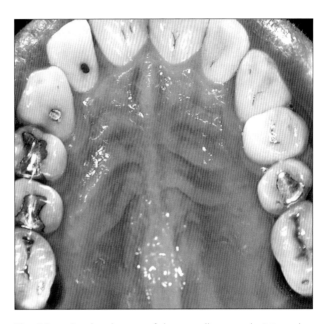

Fig 31g Occlusal view of the maxillary teeth. Note the hygienic design of the crowns placed on the maxillary first molars after hemisectioning of the distobuccal roots.

The effect of nonsurgical instrumentation may be further exemplified by some other cases. A radiograph revealed calculus on the distal root surface of the maxillary left first molar and a localized diffuse loss of alveolar bone (Fig 32a). Six months after scaling and root planing, which was followed by a combination of improved interdental self-care with a triangular-pointed toothpick, use of fluoride toothpaste, and interproximal PMTC, the periodontal tissue was healed, and some increased mineralization of the alveolar bone was observed (Fig 32b).

Figure 33a shows a mandibular right second premolar with apical-marginal communication and advanced loss of alveolar bone, particularly along the distal root surface. Figure 33b shows the same tooth 4 years after a combination of endodontic treatment and nonsurgical periodontal treatment, which was followed by a needs-related maintenance program. Alveolar bone repair is visible around the apex and along more than 5 mm of the distal root. Only curettes were used for subgingival instrumentation.

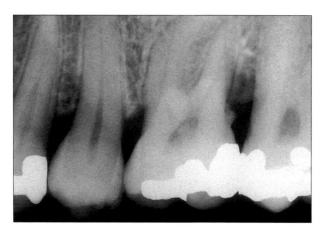

Fig 32a Radiograph showing subgingival calculus on the distal root surface of the maxillary first molar and localized interdental loss of alveolar bone.

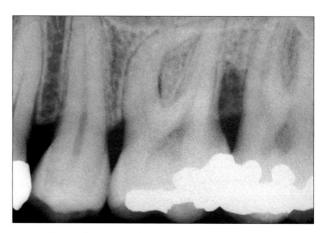

Fig 32b Radiograph of the same tooth 6 months after nonsurgical instrumentation and improved gingival plaque control. Some repair of the alveolar bone defect has been achieved.

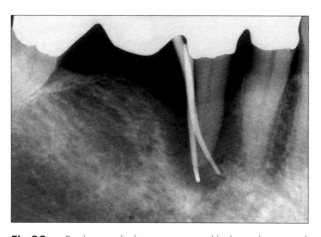

Fig 33a Radiograph showing a mandibular right second premolar with apical-marginal communication, which is visualized with two gutta-percha endodontic points placed along the distal root surface to the apex.

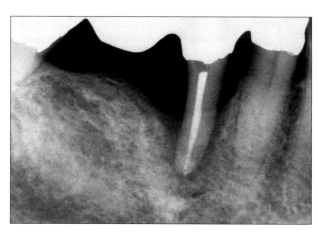

Fig 33b Radiograph of the same tooth 4 years after combined endodontic and nonsurgical periodontal treatment. Note the repair of alveolar bone around the apex and along the distal root surface.

Hand instruments

Types

Hand instruments are by far the most frequently used instruments for debridement, scaling, and root planing. Some decades ago, not only curettes and scalers but also hoes and files were used.

Today, double-ended curettes dominate the market, and double-ended scalers are used more or less as supplementary instruments for gross removal of heavy deposits of supragingival calculus, particularly approximally in anterior teeth.

The most extensive ranges of hand instruments are manufactured by Hu-Friedy and LM-Instruments, but excellent instruments are also

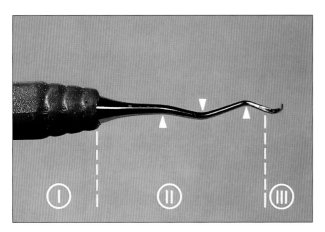

Fig 34 Parts of a curette. (I) Handle; (II) shank; (III) blade; *(arrowheads)* contra-angle curves of the instrument.

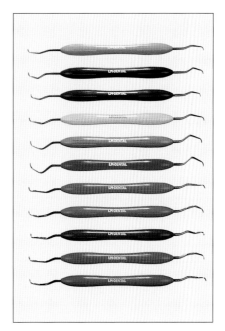

Fig 35 Assortment of curettes with soft, thick silicon grip and different colors for easy identification of the specific instrument. (Courtesy of LM-Instruments.)

made by other companies such as Star Dental and Deppeler.

Curettes are available with special shapes for optimal access to every root surface. Although many specially designed instruments are available, it is important to select a few instruments and learn to use them optimally. It is also important that the instruments be as rigid as possible for optimal tactile sensations and effectiveness, particularly during removal of calculus. For debridement in maintenance patients, less rigid but slimmer instruments may be used.

The double-ended curette consists of a handle, two shanks, and two blades (Fig 34). From an ergonomic point of view, the handles must be thick and soft with good friction for a safe and comfortable grip. In addition, color coding facilitates identification of the individual instrument (Fig 35).

There are two main groups of curettes: universal and Gracey curettes. In addition, there are some specially designed curettes, such as Syntette curettes (LM-Instruments) and Svärdström (SV) approximal curettes (LM-Instruments).

Universal curettes are designed so that one double-ended instrument is able to adapt to all tooth surfaces. Both cutting edges (A and B edges) on each blade can be used (Fig 36) because the face of the blade is at a 90-degree angle to the lower shank (Fig 37). Figure 38 shows an assortment of universal curettes. McCall 13/14

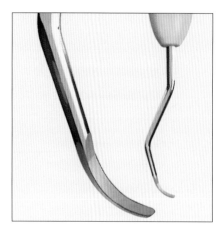

Fig 36 Typical design of the blade *(left)* and shank *(right)* of a universal curette. There are two cutting edges *(red lines)* and a rounded tip (Courtesy of LM-Instruments).

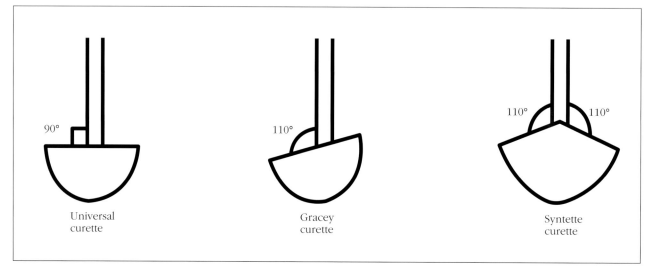

Fig 37 Angulation of the blade in relation to the shank of the universal curette (90 degrees), the Gracey curette (110 degrees), and the Syntette curette (110 degrees).

and Goldman-Fox 3 are the most useful universal curettes, particularly for approximal surfaces of posterior teeth with moderate probing depth. McCall 13S/14S has a smaller blade and thus improved accessibility in deeper pockets. McCall 17/18 and McCall 17S/18S are specially designed for molars. Therefore, the diameter of the curved blade is increased. Columbia 2R/2L is a universal curette with a long, slightly angled shank, making it excellent for use in the anterior region.

Gracey curettes are area-specific curettes, designed to adapt to specific anatomic areas of the dentition. These curettes and their modifications probably have the best accessibility among the hand instruments for debridement, scaling, and root planing in deep pockets because their size and design offer excellent adaptation to complex root anatomy. These instruments have a curved working part (blade) and only one cutting edge (Fig 39). The facial surface of the working part is offset at 110 degrees with respect to the lower part of the shank (see Fig 37) and is angled at 70 degrees to the root surface during instrumentation. This inclination makes it possible to insert the blade easily and rapidly in the gingival pocket in the correct working position with respect to the root. A specific shank angulation for the various dental surfaces enables the operator to reach areas where access is limited (Fig 40). Generally, Gracey curettes with shanks bent in several severe angles

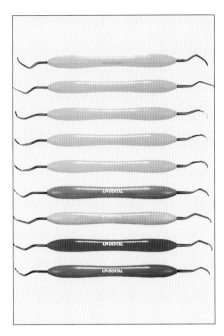

Fig 38 Assortment of universal curettes. *(top to bottom)* McCall 13S/14S, Mini McCall 13S/14S, LM 15/16, McCall 17/18, McCall 17S/18S, Goldman-Fox 3, Columbia 2R/2L, Columbia 4R/4L, and Columbia 13/14. (Courtesy of LM-Instruments.)

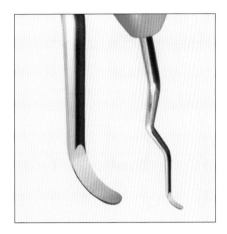

Fig 39 Blade *(left)* and shank *(right)* of a Gracey finishing curette. The working surface is inclined 20 degrees to the lower shank. There is only one cutting edge *(red line)* and a rounded tip.

are more suited for posterior teeth and deep pockets. The complete series of Gracey curettes is composed of nine double-ended instruments, two of which were recently added (Fig 41).

Although the Gracey 1/2 curette is a very commonly used anterior instrument in the Gracey set, the Gracey 5/6 curette is a more versatile anterior instrument with a longer lower shank that allows it to be used on premolars and molars with an opposite-arch or extraoral rest. The Gracey 7/8 curette is a buccal and lingual posterior instrument that is indispensable when used with a horizontal stroke in deep pockets and on line angles. The Gracey 11/12 curette for mesial surfaces and the Gracey 13/14 curette for distal surfaces are used for the posterior teeth.

Recent additions to the Gracey curette set are the Gracey 15/16 and 17/18 curettes. The Gracey

15/16 curette is a modification of the standard Gracey 11/12 curette and is designed for the mesial surfaces of posterior teeth. It consists of a Gracey 11/12 curette blade combined with a Gracey 13/14 curette shank. When an intraoral rest is used, it is often difficult or impossible to achieve optimal angulation with the Gracey 11/12 curette on the mesial surfaces of the posterior teeth, especially on the mandibular molars, because the upright instrument handle is obstructed by the opposite arch. The more acutely angled shank of the Gracey 15/16 curette allows better adaptation to posterior mesial surfaces when an intraoral fulcrum is used, and the modification has been well accepted by clinicians. If alternative fulcrums such as extraoral or opposite-arch rests are routinely used for the posterior mesial surfaces, the standard Gracey 11/12 curette still performs very well.

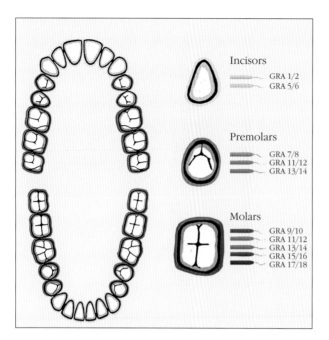

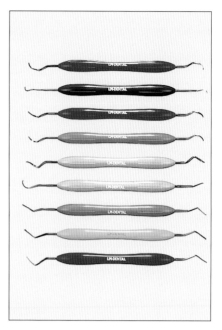

Fig 40 Guidance chart for the use of Gracey (GRA) curettes on different teeth and tooth surfaces.

Fig 41 Assortment of standard Gracey curettes. *(top to bottom)* Gracey 1/2, 3/4, 5/6, 7/8, 9/10, 11/12, 13/14, 15/16, and 17/18. (Courtesy of LM-Instruments.)

The new shank angulation of the Gracey 17/18 curette is a modification of the Gracey 13/14. The terminal shank is 3 mm longer with a more accentuated angulation to provide complete occlusal clearance and better access to all posterior distal surfaces. The horizontal handle position minimizes interference from the opposite arch and allows a more relaxed hand position when distal surfaces are scaled. The blade is also 1 mm shorter to allow better adaptation of the blade to the distal surfaces.

Gracey curettes are available with either a flexible finishing shank or a heavy rigid shank. The Gracey rigid curettes have a larger, stronger, less flexible shank and blade than the standard Gracey finishing curettes. The Gracey rigid curettes are designed for removal of moderate to heavy calculus. For supportive periodontal treatment, most clinicians prefer the enhanced tactile sensitivity provided by the thinner shanks and blades of the Gracey finishing curettes (Fig 42). New Gracey finishing curettes are usually still too large for use on well-maintained patients undergoing supportive periodontal treatment and therefore should be intentionally thinned by sharpening or used for initial scaling and root planing on patients with heavier calculus until they are reduced to the appropriate blade size.

The size of the curette blade, rather than its specific design, is the single most important factor in determining the success of subgingival instrumentation in both initial and supportive periodontal treatment. Blade size includes both the width and thickness of the blade. It is a critical factor in instrument selection because root debridement cannot be accomplished if the blade size is inappropriate for the type of tissue or area being treated. Probing depth, tissue consistency, amount of calculus, root morphology, furcation invasions, and accessibility of the area are all important conditions that influence the selection of curette blade size.

Following periodontal therapy, whether surgical or nonsurgical, the resolution of gingival inflammation generally results in firmer, tighter soft tissue. The large, heavy blades of standard new

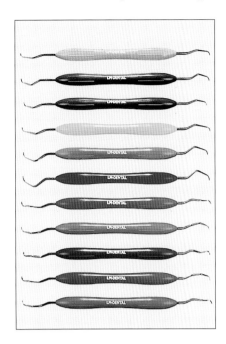

Fig 42 Assortment of Gracey finishing curettes. *(top to bottom)* Gracey 1/2, P3-P4, 3/4, 5/6, 7/8, 9/10, 11/12, 13/14, 15/16, 11/14 mesial-distal, and 12/13 mesial-distal. (Courtesy of LM-Instruments.)

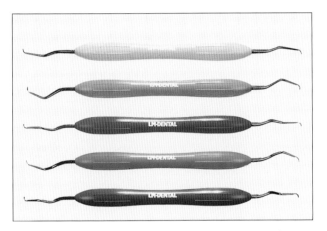

Fig 43 Assortment of Mini Gracey curettes. *(top to bottom)* Mini Gracey 1/2, 7/8, 11/12, 13/14, and 15/16. (Courtesy of LM-Instruments.)

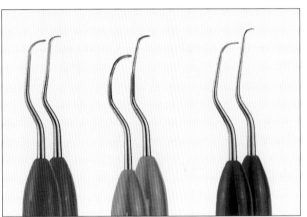

Fig 44 Comparison of standard *(left in each pair)* and Mini *(right in each pair)* Langer curettes. Mini Langer curettes 1/2 *(red)*, 3/4 *(green)*, and 5/6 *(blue)* have longer shanks and shorter working ends than the corresponding standard Langer curettes. (Courtesy of LM-Instruments.)

curettes are designed for removal of moderate to heavy calculus and should be used only when the tissue is loose and edematous. Their size may make it difficult to insert them to the base of the pocket when the gingiva is firm and nonretractable. Deep pockets with tight tissue and/or furcation involvement require the use of instruments with smaller, thinner, and more tactilely sensitive blades.

As a consequence, curettes with miniature blades and extended shanks have been designed. For example, the Mini-Five curettes (Hu-Friedy)

have shanks that are 3 mm longer and blades that are 50% thinner and shorter than those of standard Gracey curettes. Similar instruments are Mini Gracey curettes (Fig 43) and Mini Langer curettes (Fig 44) (LM-Instruments).

The shorter, thinner blade allows easier insertion and adaptation in deep, narrow pockets; furcations; developmental depressions; line angles; and deep, tight pockets on facial, lingual, or palatal surfaces. In areas where root morphology or tight tissue prevents full insertion of the stan-

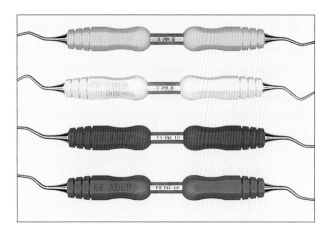

Fig 45 Mini Profil Gracey curettes. *(top to bottom)* Gracey 5 PM 6, 7 PM 8, 11 PM 12, and 13 PM 14. (Courtesy of Deppeler.)

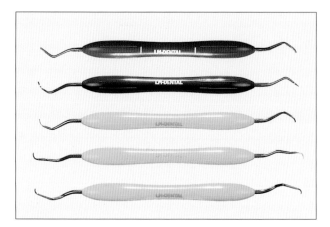

Fig 46 Special curettes. *(top to bottom)* Concavity diamond file SV 5-6, interproximal curette SV 1-3, interproximal curette SV 2-4, Syntette, and Mini Syntette. (Courtesy of LM-Instruments.)

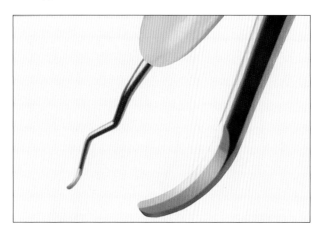

Fig 47 Shank *(left)* and blade *(right)* of a Syntette curette, a combination of universal and finishing curettes with two elliptic edges and a rounded tip. (Courtesy of LM-Instruments.)

dard Gracey or After-Five (Hu-Friedy) blade, the Mini-Five curettes or Mini Langer curettes can be used with vertical strokes, resulting in minimal tissue distention and no tissue trauma. In the past, the only solution in these areas of difficult access was to use the standard Gracey curettes with a short, toe-down, horizontal stroke.

The Mini Five curettes, along with other recently introduced mini-bladed instruments, have opened a new era in the history of root debridement by allowing superior access to areas that were previously extremely difficult or impossible to reach with standard hand instruments. However, these mini-bladed curettes with extended shanks should not be used routinely for all tooth surfaces in place of standard Gracey curettes. Rather they should be restricted to areas of difficult access. The new Mini Profil Gracey curettes (Deppeler), which

have an extrashort blade with a special curve and extrathick handles (cool grip), are another version of mini-bladed Gracey curettes (Fig 45).

In addition to the full assortments of universal curettes, Gracey curettes, and sickles, some specially designed hand instruments have been introduced during the last decade (Fig 46). The Concavity Diamond File SV 5-6 and the Furcation Diamond File SV 7-8 (LM-Instruments) are diamond-coated hand instruments for instrumentations in concavities and furcation areas. Standard and Mini Syntettes (LM-Instruments) are designed with two elliptic cutting edges and a rounded tip (Fig 47). The facial surface is formed as two facets with a 110-degree angulation (see Fig 37).

Syntette and Mini Syntette are both an ingenious combination of two special types of curette: the universal and the finishing curettes. Syntette

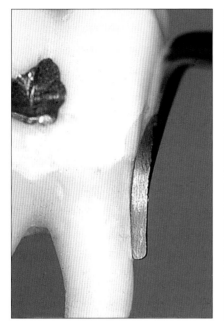

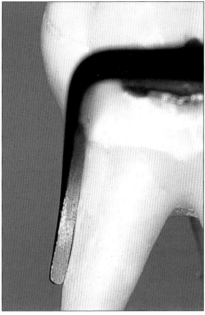

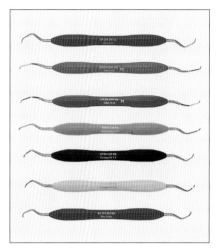

Fig 48a Interproximal curette SV 1-3 for the maxillary right and mandibular left quadrants. (Courtesy of Dr G. Svärdström.)

Fig 48b Interproximal curette SV 2-4 for the maxillary left and mandibular right quadrants. (Courtesy of Dr G. Svärdström.)

Fig 49 Limited set of hand instruments that should cover most root surfaces except for special irregularities and very deep, narrow pockets. (top to bottom) Gracey 9/10, Gracey 11/12, Gracey 13/14, Columbia 2R/2L, SV 1-3, SV 2-4, and Mini Sickle. (Courtesy of LM-Instruments.)

enables the clinician to work on both mesial and distal surfaces in the same interdental space, both vertically and horizontally, on both convex and concave surfaces. The working end can be adapted to the concavity of the root surface by varying the angle in the primary horizontal drawing movement. The instruments are particularly useful for debridement and root planing but less efficient for calculus removal.

The double-ended interproximal curettes SV 1-3 and SV 2-4 (see Fig 46) were specially designed by Svärdström for instrumentation of the approximal surfaces with horizontal strokes from the buccal side. These instruments have one cutting edge. One end is designed for treatment of the mesial surface and the other end for treatment of the distal surface of the same interdental space. The interproximal curette SV 1-3 is designed for

the maxillary right and mandibular left quadrants, 1 and 3 (Fig 48a), and SV 2-4 is designed for the maxillary left and mandibular right quadrants, 2 and 4 (Fig 48b).

In spite of these excellent possibilities for achieving accessibility to any difficult-to-reach area of subgingival root surfaces, many clinicians use a reduced set of four Gracey curettes supplemented by universal curettes and possibly a thin, straight Morse scaler for anterior teeth. Figure 49 shows a limited set of hand instruments that should cover most root surfaces. Figure 50 indicates where these different instruments should be used.

Fractured curette blades in deep pockets and furcations could be a complicated problem to solve. The initial step should be to locate the fractured blade by a combination of orthoradial and eccentric radiographs. Thereafter, the fractured

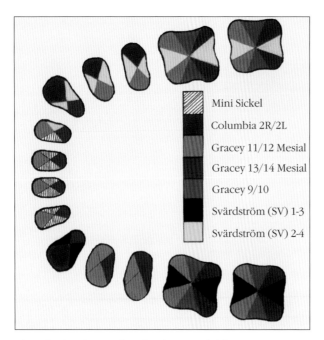

Fig 50 Guidance chart for the use of different instruments shown in Fig 49 on particular root surfaces. (Courtesy of Dr G. Svärdström.)

Mini Sickel

Columbia 2R/2L

Gracey 11/12 Mesial

Gracey 13/14 Mesial

Gracey 9/10

Svärdström (SV) 1-3

Svärdström (SV) 2-4

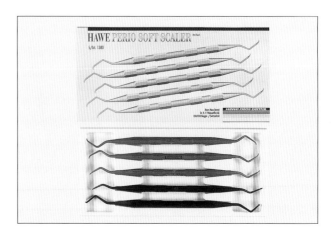

Fig 51 Plastic hand instruments for minimally invasive debridement of implants. (Courtesy of Hawe Neos.)

blade traditionally is removed by drawing the blade of a curette against the inner side of the soft tissue in a coronal direction while placing pressure with an index finger on the outer side of the tissue or by a mini-flap exposure. Another alternative is to use Schwarz Periotrievers (Daness Dental), a set of two double-ended, highly magnetized instruments designed for the retrieval of broken instrument tips from the periodontal pocket. These instruments are indispensable when the clinician has broken a curette tip in a furcation or deep pocket. The long, flat blade is for general use in deep pockets, and the contra-angled, blunt tip is for use in furcations. The tips are used in a probelike manner or swept horizontally in the pocket. The broken instrument tip will attach to the magnetized tip and can be gently drawn out of the pocket.

Several different companies are now manufacturing plastic instruments for use on titanium and other implant abutment materials. It is imperative that plastic rather than metal instruments be used for scaling to avoid scarring of and permanent damage to the implants. Implacare implant instruments (Hu-Friedy) have autoclavable stainless steel handles and plastic cone-socket tips. The paired implant maintenance replacement tips are available in three different designs: the Columbia 4R/4L curette, the 204S sickle scaler, and the H6/7 sickle scaler.

Implant-Prophy + instruments (Suter Dental) are available in the standard Gracey 5/6, 11/12, and 13/14 and Colombia 13/14 curette designs. They are made of a high-performance plastic that is very hard and can be resharpened with a specially designed sharpening stone that does not require lubrication. The instruments and the stone are all autoclavable.

Figure 51 shows Perio Soft Scaler plastic instruments (Hawe Neos) for instrumentation of implants.

Use of hand instruments

Patient position and ergonomic aspects. The patient's head must be correctly positioned from an ergonomic point of view. The patient should be in a supine position with the head bent back during

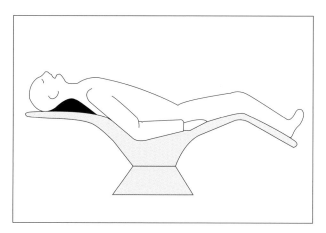

Fig 52a Position of the patient during instrumentation of the maxillary teeth.

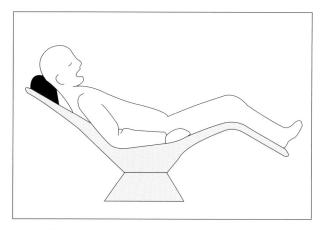

Fig 52b Position of the patient during instrumentation of the mandibular teeth.

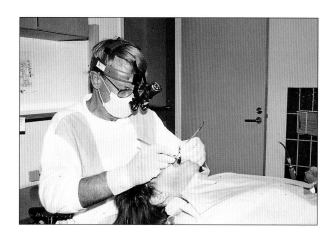

Fig 53 Use of a combination of a magnifying loupe (×3) and an additional zooming light to improve visibility during the clinical examination.

scaling of the maxillary teeth (Fig 52a). A small pillow placed under the shoulders will enable correct positioning of the head. When mandibular teeth are scaled, the patient should be sitting at an angle of approximately 30 to 45 degrees (Fig 52b). A small pillow can be placed behind the head to ensure correct positioning. Although the subgingival scaling procedure is performed more or less blindly, use of the combination of a magnification loupe (×3) and an additional zooming light (Orascoptic Research) improves detailed inspection of the operative field as well as clinical diagnoses (Fig 53).

Before subgingival instrumentation starts, detailed clinical and radiographic examinations have to be performed to assess root anatomy, probing depth, furcation involvement, local plaque-retentive factors such as calculus, rough root surfaces, and root resorptions, as well as the presence of subgingival plaque biofilms, purulent exudate, and bleeding on probing. Based on the comprehensive examinations, the clinician must decide whether all sites can be treated in only one session (one-stage treatment) or if the treatment has to be divided into two to four treatments performed in the same week. Most subgingival instrumentation should be performed under local anesthesia.

Effective hand instrumentation depends on four critical factors: *(1)* adequate access, *(2)* good adaptation, *(3)* effective angulation, and *(4)* thoroughness (complete root coverage). Failure to

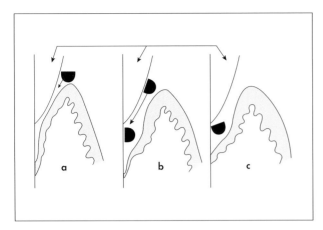

Fig 54 Insertion of the blade of the curette (a) to reach the base of the pocket (b) and subsequent adjustment to the correct angle against the root surface (c).

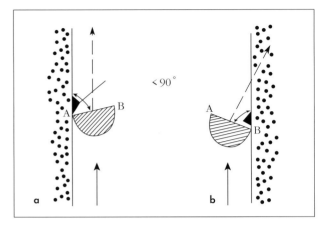

Fig 55 Angulation of the mesial edge (a) and the distal edge (b) of a universal curette to the approximal root surfaces of posterior teeth. (dashed arrows) Long axes of the handles of the instrument; (solid arrows) working direction; (A) mesial edge; (B) distal edge.

achieve any one or a combination of these factors results in subgingival instrumentation that is either unsuccessful or only partially successful.

The clinician should perform the steps of subgingival instrumentation in the following order:

1. Select the most suitable instrument.
2. Insert the blade to the base of the pocket using a light grasp.
3. Establish a working angulation.
4. Let the position of the handle and shank determine whether an intraoral or extraoral fulcrum is better and then establish the appropriate fulcrum and a firm grasp.
5. Position his or her own body according to the fulcrum.
6. Activate the stroke, and use the blade of the curette simultaneously as a probe for localization of calculus and as a blade for noninvasive removal of calculus and plaque biofilms.

For the curette to reach the bottom of the pocket, the facial surface of the blade must be inserted as parallel to the root surface as possible. Then the grasp is tightened to obtain a firm, secure grip, and the working part (blade) is opened by moving the shank away from the tooth until it assumes an angulation that is 70 degrees for Gracey curettes and more than 60 degrees and less than 90 degrees for universal curettes (Fig 54). Universal curettes

should be used at 80 to 85 degrees for scaling and at about 70 degrees for root planing and minimally invasive debridement (Fig 55).

Instruments for scaling and root planing must be used with a certain amount of pressure in very narrow spaces without damaging the surrounding tissue. Therefore, indispensable elements for optimum instrumentation are a correct grasp, a proper and stable finger rest, and effective strokes. To achieve a firm grip and a stable guide, a modified pen grasp must be used (Fig 56):

- The instrument is held in the thumb, the index finger, and the middle finger, which rests on the shank.
- The middle finger is extended, and the fingertip is placed on the side of the first part of the shank near the handle.
- The index finger is bent and slid backward on the handle.
- The thumb is bent and positioned on the opposite side of the handle, midway between the index and the middle fingers.

The triangular position of the fingers locks the curette as if it were in a vise, providing a firm guide, better control of the instrument, and greater tactile sensitivity. The finger rest must be as close as possible to the working area. The ring finger is used for this purpose, and the middle finger may

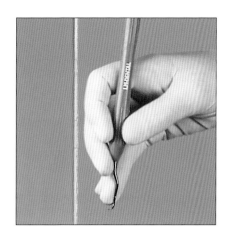

Fig 56 Modified pen grasp of the curette.

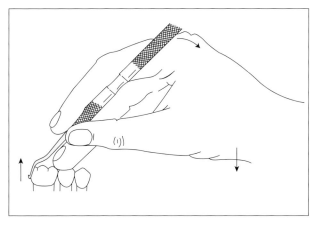

Fig 57a Tipping movement during the use of a curette. *(arrows)* Direction of movements.

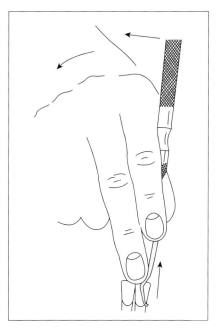

Fig 57b Turning movement during the use of a curette. *(arrows)* Direction of movements.

rest against it. A finger rest must be established in all cases, no matter what area is treated, what instrument is used, and whether a direct or an indirect view of the site to be treated is chosen.

In certain situations, to perform more effective instrumentation, the operator may be obliged to establish a finger rest that is not close to the working area. For example, an extraoral rest may be necessary, either on the chin so that the palm of the hand cups the mandible or on the reinforcing finger of the nonworking hand that pulls

back the cheek and at the same time pushes against the shank of the curette, thus increasing the pressure applied to the tooth surface during instrumentation. Whatever the choice, it is most important to establish and maintain a stable rest to permit a controlled and efficient instrumentation.

The two basic movements during instrumentation with curettes are tipping (Fig 57a) and turning (Fig 57b). Not only the wrist but also the arm has to be tipped during tipping movements.

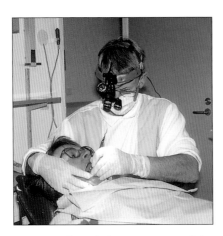

Fig 58 Clinical demonstration of the turning technique during instrumentation of mandibular teeth.

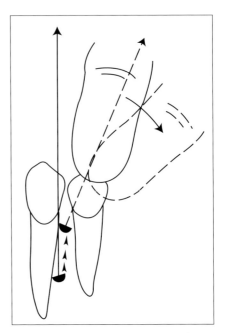

Fig 59 Finger rest of the middle finger for a well-controlled turning movement. *(arrows)* Direction of movements.

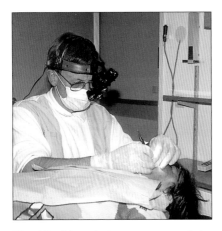

Fig 60 Clinical demonstration of the two-hand grip for well-controlled instrumentation of maxillary teeth.

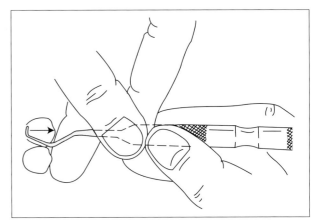

Fig 61 Two-hand grip for instrumentation of maxillary teeth. *(arrow)* Direction of movement.

> **Box 1**   Optimal operator positions for use of hand instruments
>
> The positions adopted by an operator during instrumentation are described in terms of the face of a clock.
>
> - **Right-handed operator:**
>   - At 8 o'clock, in front of the patient
>   - At 9 o'clock, beside the patient
>   - At 11, 12, or 1 o'clock, behind the patient
> - **Left-handed operator:**
>   - At 4 o'clock, in front of the patient
>   - At 3 o'clock, beside the patient
>   - At 1, 12, or 11 o'clock, behind the patient
> - **Ambidextrous operator[*]:**
>   - At 9 o'clock, beside the patient
>   - At 12 o'clock, behind the patient
>   - At 3 o'clock, beside the patient
>
> [*]The ambidextrous operator has many advantages because the ability to alternate the right hand with the left permits him or her to choose the most comfortable working position for each area to be treated, almost always with a direct view of the working area.

During turning movements, the middle finger or ring finger functions as a support to facilitate a well-controlled lever movement (Figs 58 and 59). In particular, during instrumentation of maxillary teeth, the two-hand grip is useful for well-controlled strokes (Figs 60 and 61).

During instrumentation with hand instruments, the operator must work in different positions in relation to the patient to be able to reach and treat the various areas of the mouth. Operators must choose the positions that they find most comfortable and that enable them to easily reach the areas to be treated and to work in most cases with a direct view. A direct view is especially useful during treatment of the lingual surfaces of incisors and the distal surfaces of molars.

The right-handed operator will use positions that are different from those used by an operator who is left-handed or ambidextrous. Box 1 describes the positions that are the most comfortable for reaching all areas of the oral cavity. If the suggested positions are used, the operator can avoid continuously moving the patient's head in attempts to obtain an adequate view of the area under treatment.

Instrumentation. The use of universal curettes, standard Gracey curettes, and special curettes (Syntette and interproximal curettes) on different tooth surfaces in maxillary and mandibular teeth is demonstrated by a right-handed operator in Figs 62 to 70.

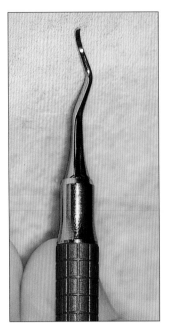

Fig 62a Goldman-Fox 3 universal curette (Hu-Friedy).

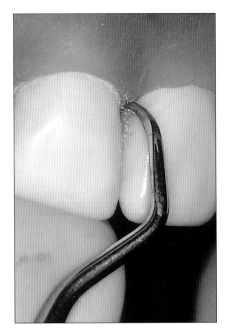

Fig 62b Use of Goldman-Fox 3 universal curette on the mesial surface of the maxillary left central incisor.

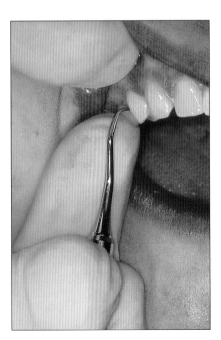

Fig 62c Use of Goldman-Fox 3 universal curette on the distal surface of the maxillary right canine.

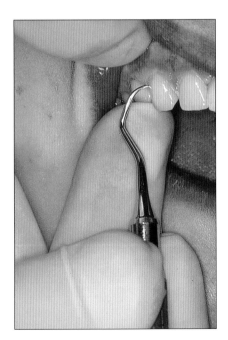

Fig 62d Use of Goldman-Fox 3 universal curette on the mesial surface of the maxillary right first premolar.

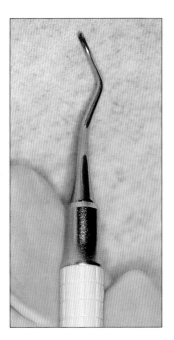

Fig 63a McCall 17/18 universal curette (Hu-Friedy), specially designed for molars.

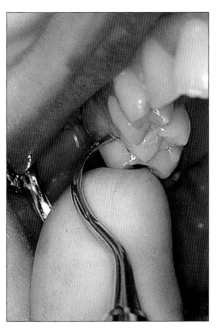

Fig 63b Use of McCall 17/18 universal curette on the mesial surface of the maxillary right first molar.

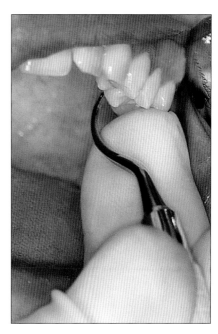

Fig 63c Use of McCall 17/18 universal curette on the mesial surface of the maxillary left first molar.

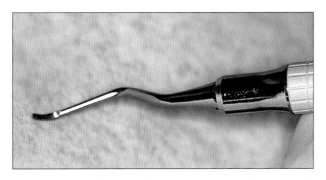

Fig 64a Columbia 2R/2L universal curette (Hu-Friedy), specially designed for anterior teeth.

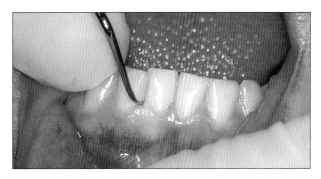

Fig 64b Use of Columbia 2R/2L universal curette on the mesial surface of the mandibular right lateral incisor.

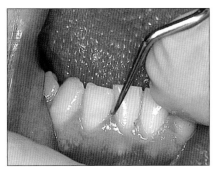

Fig 64c Use of Columbia 2R/2L universal curette on the distal surface of the mandibular right central incisor.

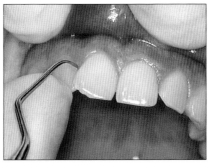

Fig 64d Use of Columbia 2R/2L universal curette on the mesial surface of the maxillary right lateral incisor.

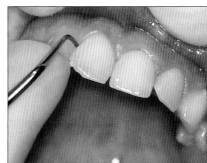

Fig 64e Use of Columbia 2R/2L universal curette on the distal surface of the maxillary right central incisor.

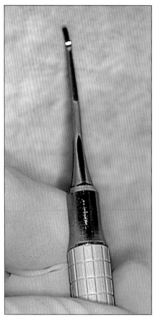

Fig 65a Gracey 1/2 curette (Hu-Friedy), slightly contra-angled for incisors and canines.

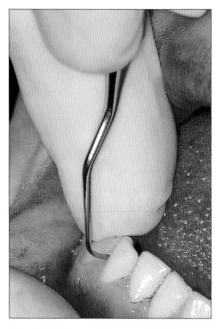

Fig 65b Use of Gracey 1/2 curette on the distal surface of the mandibular right lateral incisor.

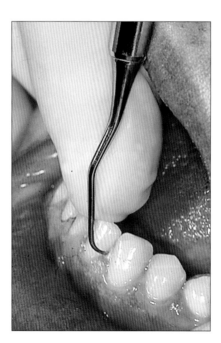

Fig 65c Use of Gracey 1/2 curette on the distal surface of the mandibular left lateral incisor.

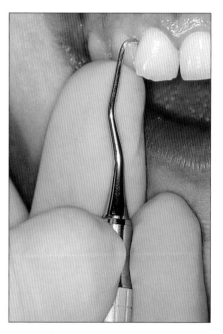

Fig 65d Use of Gracey 1/2 curette on the mesial surface of the maxillary right lateral incisor.

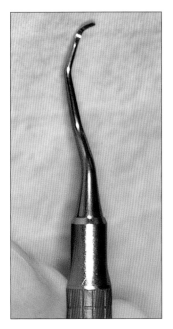

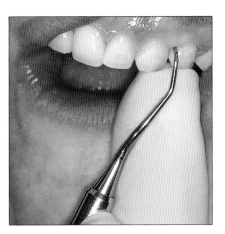

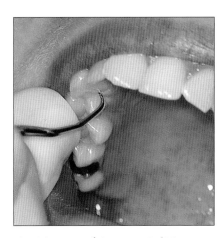

Fig 66a Gracey 11/12 curette (Hu-Friedy), angled to access the mesial surfaces of posterior teeth.

Fig 66b Use of Gracey 11/12 curette on the mesial surface of the maxillary left canine.

Fig 66c Use of Gracey 11/12 curette on the mesial surface of the maxillary right first premolar.

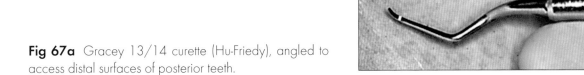

Fig 67a Gracey 13/14 curette (Hu-Friedy), angled to access distal surfaces of posterior teeth.

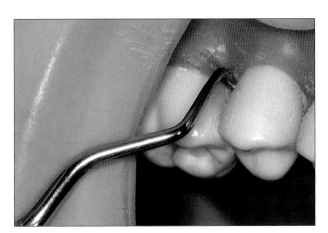

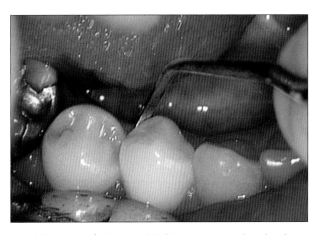

Fig 67b Use of Gracey 13/14 curette on the distal surface of the maxillary right second premolar in a model.

Fig 67c Use of Gracey 13/14 curette on the distal surface of the mandibular right first premolar.

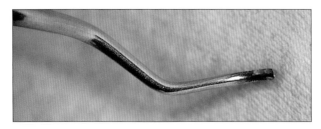

Fig 68a Syntette curette, specially designed with two off-set cutting edges (110 degrees) on one blade for debridement and root planing of all interdental surfaces, primarily in the posterior regions.

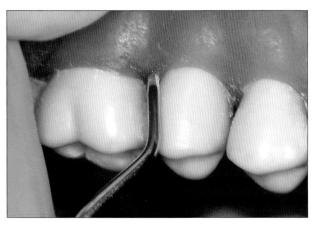

Fig 68b Use of Syntette curette on the distal surface of the maxillary right second premolar in a model.

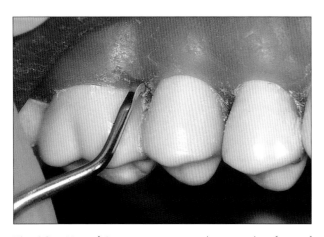

Fig 68c Use of Syntette curette on the mesial surface of the maxillary right first molar in a model.

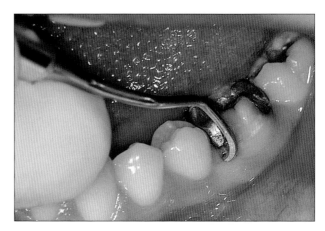

Fig 68d Use of Syntette curette on the mesial surface of the mandibular left first molar.

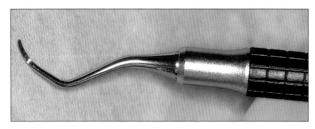

Fig 69a Interproximal curette SV 1-3, specially designed for horizontal instrumentation of approximal surfaces in the first and third quadrants.

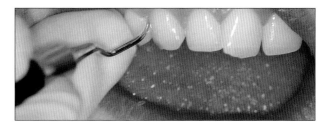

Fig 69b Use of interproximal curette SV 1-3 on the mesial surface of the maxillary right first premolar.

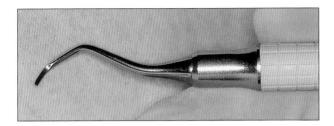

Fig 70a Interproximal curette SV 2-4, specially designed for horizontal instrumentation of approximal surfaces in the second and fourth quadrants.

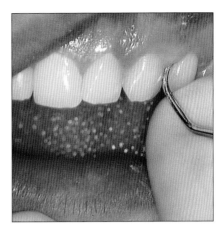

Fig 70b Use of interproximal curette SV 2-4 on the mesial surface of the maxillary left first premolar.

Sharpening. The efficacy of good instrumentation depends not only on the operator's skill but also on the quality of the instrument in use. Therefore, to perform effective scaling and root planing, all instruments must have sharp edges. This ensures that supragingival and subgingival treatment is efficient and precise and that calculus can be removed from the tooth surfaces with a limited number of strokes. Whenever calculus is located with a curette used as a probe in the coronal direction from the base of the pocket, it will be lifted away as efficiently and minimally invasively as possible if the curette has sharp edges. A curette with a blunt cutting edge must be pressed against the root surface with a greater force than is required when a sharp instrument is used.

Scaling with instruments that have blunt cutting edges often results in an incomplete removal of calculus but in the establishment of a smoothed root surface. Calculus that remains on such a smoothed root surface is difficult to detect with a periodontal probe. The cutting edge of the hand instrument, therefore, must be assessed repeatedly during scaling. This can be done by planing a plastic stick.

For efficient but minimally invasive root planing, the curette must have sharp edges and must have an angle against the root surface that is 10 to 20 degrees less than that employed during scaling.

Tal et al (1985) evaluated the wear of curette cutting edges during standardized root planing after 15 strokes and 45 strokes. Figures 71a and 71b show the blade of an unused curette. After 15 standardized root planing strokes, 77% of the tested curettes exhibited cutting edges with narrow wear bevels of 15 μm or less (Fig 72a). After 45 strokes, about 90% of all tested curettes exhibited cutting edges with wide wear bevels of more than 15 μm (Fig 72b).

Based on these results, hand instruments must be repeatedly sharpened during scaling and root planing procedures. However, for debridement (removal of subgingival biofilms) in maintenance patients, cutting edges that are even less sharp may work.

When curettes are sharp, they have acutely angled cutting edges with a 70-degree angulation. Sharpening an instrument adequately means restoring its cutting edges while conserving its original form and prolonging its durability. Figure 73 shows how the single cutting edges of the Gracey curettes must be sharpened and the angulation maintained. The two cutting edges of universal curettes should be sharpened as shown in Fig 74 to maintain a 70-degree angulation between the face of the blade and the lateral facets.

Sharpening of the hand instruments can be performed by hand with materials such as silicon carbide, India (artificial coarse-grained aluminum

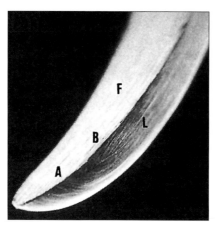

Fig 71a Previously unused sharp curette. The functional wire edges result from manufacturer sharpening. (A) Area investigated (1 mm from the tip); (B) area investigated (2 mm from the tip); (L) lateral surface; (F) facial surface (original magnification ×25). (From Tal et al, 1985. Reprinted with permission.)

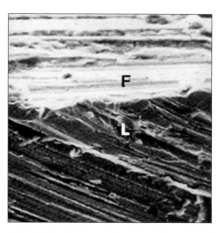

Fig 71b Increased magnification of the sharp curette. An exact meeting of the facial (F) and lateral (L) surfaces can be seen, as well as irregularities of the cutting edge (original magnification ×500). (From Tal et al, 1985. Reprinted with permission.)

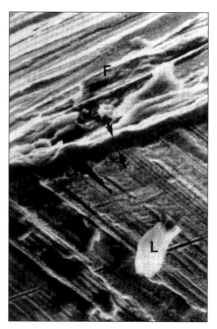

Fig 72a Mild deformation *(arrows)* of the cutting edge. (L) Lateral surface; (F) facial surface (original magnification ×500). (From Tal et al, 1985. Reprinted with permission.)

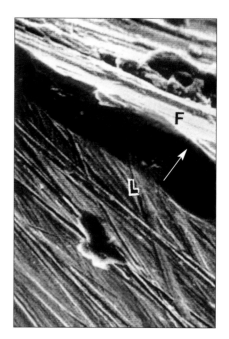

Fig 72b Severe deformation *(arrow)* of the cutting edge. (L) Lateral surface; (F) facial surface (original magnification ×500). (From Tal et al, 1985. Reprinted with permission.)

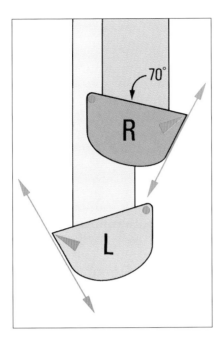

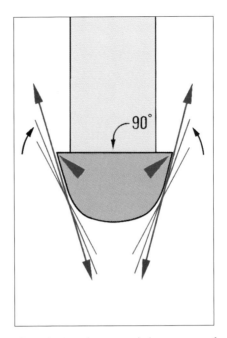

Fig 73 Angulation and sharpening of the single edges of Gracey curettes. (R) Right; (L) left.

Fig 74 Angulation and sharpening of the two edges of universal curettes.

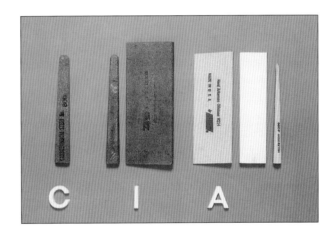

Fig 75 Sharpening stones for manual use. (C) Silicon carbide stone (Carborundum, Saint-Gobain); (I) India stones; (A) Arkansas stones.

oxide), and extrafine-grained Arkansas (aluminum oxide) sharpening stones (Fig 75). These stones are abrasive, granulous, and modeled into various shapes and sizes. The choice of shape of the stones depends on the design and condition of the instrument to be sharpened. For well-maintained instruments that are sharpened frequently during instrumentation, the light gray and extrafine Arkansas stones are used. However, if the instrument is extremely blunt, more abrasive sharpening stones such as the brown India or silicon carbide are required.

During sharpening, there must be a sufficient source of light in the working area and good stability of the stone and the instrument. Furthermore, the stone must be sterile if it is used during a treatment appointment because the instruments are then used immediately in the patient's oral cavity. Arkansas and India stones and the cylindric Arkansas stone should be the most frequently used sharpening stones. Sharpening stones may be used in two ways: either the stone is held firm while the working part of the instrument is stroked across it, or the stone is moved against the

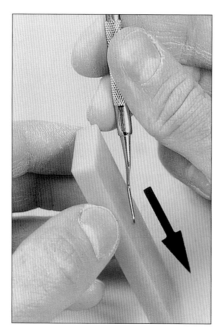

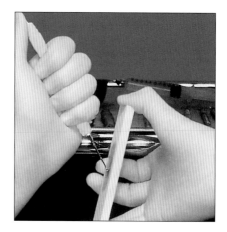

Fig 76 Sharpening of lateral surface of a universal curette against an Arkansas stone. There is about a 20-degree angle between the shank and the stone. *(arrow)* Direction of movement.

Fig 77 Sharpening of the lateral surface of a Gracey curette against an Arkansas stone. There is about a 40-degree angle between the shank and the stone.

working part of the instrument, which is held stationary. Most operators prefer to hold the stone firm and move the working part of the instrument (Figs 76 and 77).

The lateral surfaces of the working part of Gracey (see Fig 73) as well as universal curettes (see Fig 74) may be sharpened against the stone (see Figs 76 and 77). However, the edges of the universal curettes can also be sharpened by rotating the curved facial surface against a cylindric Arkansas stone. Whichever method is chosen, it is always necessary to understand the form and features of each instrument in order to sharpen it adequately.

To sharpen a Gracey curette, the operator must be very familiar with its shape and bear in mind the following features:

• The working part of a Gracey is curved.
• Each working part of the Gracey is offset at 70 degrees with respect to the last part of the shank.
• The blade has only one cutting edge, which is always the lower one.
• The cutting angle between the facial and lateral surfaces of the curette is 70 degrees; this means

that when the working part is applied to the stone, the angle between the facial surface and the surface of the stone must be 110 degrees.

Even more important as a guide for correct angulation during the sharpening procedure is the fact that the angle between the last part of the shank and the stone must be 40 degrees, about half of a right angle (see Fig 77). In addition, only a part of the lateral surface is in contact with the stone because the working part of the instrument is curved. Therefore, after it has been confirmed that the lateral surface has been correctly applied to the stone, it is necessary to move the entire length of the lateral surface, oscillating it with short movements from the extremity of the shank to the toe, and vice versa, as if it were a pendulum. If the lateral surface of the Gracey is kept continuously in contact with the stone and these short, slow, and regular strokes are performed, the cutting edge will be sharpened automatically and uniformly.

This method of frequent sharpening with low-abrasive Arkansas stones limits excessive wear of the instrument, which remains resistant because

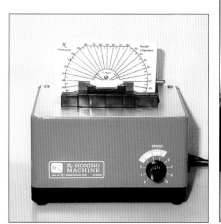

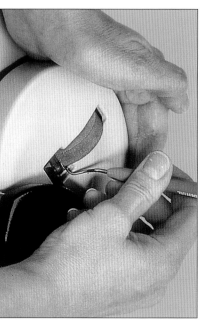

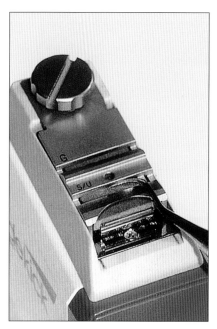

Fig 78 Rx Honing Machine.

Fig 79 LM Rondo Plus sharpening machine.

Fig 80 Sidekick grinding machine.

it narrows in width but is not reduced in thickness. In this way, it is possible to maintain the original design of Gracey curettes for many months. In addition, accessibility to the pocket is increased the more the width is reduced.

The same technique is also effective for sharpening Syntette curettes, but the procedure must be slightly modified because only the final part of the blade near the tip is curved, while the remaining part rests evenly on the stone. It is therefore necessary to perform two types of movements, maintaining an angle of 40 degrees between the final part of the shank and the surface of the stone:

1. The final part, near the tip, is sharpened with the same procedure described for Gracey curettes; the lateral surface is placed on the stone, and short oscillating movements are performed.
2. The rest of the working part is sharpened by placing the lateral surface on the stone and performing short, straight pulling strokes in one direction, thus making it possible to sharpen the entire extension of this part of the blade uniformly.

When the lateral surfaces of universal curettes are sharpened, the angle between the shank and the facial surface of the working part is 90 degrees (see Fig 74), and the angle of the cutting edge (the angle between the facial and lateral surfaces) is 70 degrees. Therefore, to maintain the correct angle of the cutting edges, the angle between the shank and the stone must be 20 degrees during the sharpening procedure (see Fig 76).

Mechanical devices for sharpening hand instruments are available on the market, which may be an alternative for operators not willing to learn the inexpensive and very efficient manual technique. However, for frequent sharpening during instrumentation, the manual use of sterile Arkansas stones is recommended from a hygienic point of view.

Figure 78 shows a mechanical sharpening machine (Rx Honing Machine, Rx Honing) in which the correct angle for the edge of the hand instrument can be chosen. The LM Rondo Plus sharpening machine (LM-Instruments) is equipped with a low-speed rotating sharpening stone (Fig 79). Recently, the Sidekick grinding machine (Hu-Friedy) was introduced (Fig 80). This machine is equipped with oscillating abrasive stones.

Table 2   Specifications of various ultrasonic scalers

Ultrasonic scaler	Energy system and frequency	Cooling system	Movement and amplitude of tip*				
			Longitudinal	Transverse	Circular	Elliptic	Three-dimensional
Amdent 830 (Amdent)	Piezoelectric 25,000 Hz	Internal	75–110 µm	–	–	–	–
Piezon Master 400 and 600 (EMS)	Piezoelectric 30,000 Hz	Internal	50–110 µm	–	–	–	–
Cavitron 3000 (Dentsply)	Magnetostrictive 30,000 Hz	Internal	120 µm	40 µm	–	+	–
Cavimed 200 (Dentsply)	Magnetostrictive 30,000 Hz	Internal	120 µm	40 µm	–	+	–
Hygienist (Lysta)	Piezoelectric 45,000 Hz	Internal	40 µm	–	–	–	–
Suprasson (Satelec)	Piezoelectric 29,000 Hz	Internal	75–110 µm	+	–	+	–
Odontoson 4 (Odonto-Wave)	Magnetostrictive 42,000 Hz	External	–	–	20 µm	–	+

*+/– signs indicate whether a specification applies to the scaler.

Ultrasonic scalers

Types

The first ultrasonic scaler, Cavitron (Dentsply), was introduced more than 50 years ago. Since then, development and improvement of more suitable machines have continued. The term *ultrasonic* is defined as "pertaining to mechanical radiant energy having a frequency beyond the upper limit of perception of the human ear, that is, beyond about 20,000 cycles per second (cps)." Whereas the ultrasonic scalers operate in the range of about 25,000 to 42,000 Hz (cps), frequencies as high as 2,000,000 Hz are used in medical and industrial units.

The development of ultrasonic energy in the dental unit is based on one of two concepts: The magnetostrictive effect and the piezoelectric effect. The amplitude of the tip of ranges from 10 to 120 µm. That means a total distance of 5 m/s by the tip of instruments with 25,000 Hz and 100 µm longitudinal amplitude. The movement can be longitudinal, circular, elliptic, and three-dimensional. Because of the heat generated, particularly with magnetostrictive instruments, the scalers must be cooled by external or internal water spray. Many of the ultrasonic scalers available and their specifications are presented in Table 2.

The effect of ultrasonic scalers on removal of calculus and plaque biofilm as well as iatrogenic removal of root cementum and roughness is strongly correlated to the power used, force of application, working time, angulation, shape and movement of the tip (longitudinal, lateral, circular, elliptic, or three-dimensional), cooling and irrigation system, and the operator's skill and technique. The iatrogenic effects of ultrasonic scalers and calculus removal compared to other scaling instruments were discussed earlier in this chapter (Jacobson et al, 1994; Jotikasthira et al, 1992; Kepic et al, 1990; Ladner et al, 1992; Lie and Leknes, 1985; Lie and Meyer, 1977; Ritz et al, 1991; Sherman et al, 1990).

Flemmig et al (1998a) assessed the depth and volume of defects resulting from in vitro root instrumentation with a piezoelectric ultrasonic scaler with a slim scaling tip. Combinations of the following working variables were analyzed: lateral forces of 0.5 N, 1.0 N, and 2.0 N; tip angulations of 0, 45, and 90 degrees; power settings of low, medium, and high; and instrumentation time of 10, 20, 40, and 80 seconds. Defects were quantified using a three-dimensional optical laser scanner.

Overall, lateral force had the greatest influence on defect volume, greater than either instrument power setting or tip angulation. Defect depth was most influenced by tip angulation, followed by lateral force and instrument power setting. At all power settings, the largest defects in volume and depth by far were found after a 45-degree tip angulation was combined with 2 N of lateral force. Flemmig et al (1998a) concluded that the efficacy of the assessed piezoelectric ultrasonic scaler may be adapted to various clinical needs by adjustment of the lateral force, tip angulation, and power setting. To prevent severe root damage, it is crucial that the scaler they assessed (Piezon Master 400, EMS) be used at a tip angulation of close to 0 degrees (for reviews on the iatrogenic and beneficial effects of ultrasonic scalers, see Adriaens and Adriaens, 2004 and Oda et al, 2004).

The early magnetostrictive ultrasonic scalers had very large, bulky tips, so their use was limited to the removal of supragingival calculus. It was not possible to use this type of instrument to perform adequate subgingival instrumentation. More modern ultrasonic instruments (eg, Piezon Master 400, 600, and Mini, EMS; US 30 Unicorn and Double, Amdent; Slimline, Dentsply; Odontoson M, Odonto-Wave) have thinner tips that make it easy to reach subgingival areas. Figures 81a to 81d show the piezoelectric Piezon Master 600 ultrasonic scaler, the extrathin tip for deep subgingival instrumentation, specially designed tips for approximal surfaces and furcation areas, and the plastic-coated tip, which is specially designed for minimally invasive debridement of implants.

Figures 82a and 82b show the new piezoelectric scaler US30 Double. It is equipped with a great assortment of thin tips that are fixed to disposable and autoclavable handles (Quick-a-tip), an advantage from a hygienic point of view.

In the piezoelectric scaler, the transducer is completely contained within the handpiece and is not connected to the working tip. The working tip is small and easily inserted into the handpiece. Alternating electric current applied to reactive crystals causes a dimensional change, which is then transmitted to the working tip as ultrasonic vibrations. These vibrations can dislodge tenacious calculus deposits from the tooth surface. The tip movement of the piezoelectric scaler is primarily linear (see Table 2). Some popular brands available on the market include Piezon Master, 27 to 30 kHz; ENAC, 30 kHz (Osada Electronics); Amdent, 25 kHz (Amdent); and Suprasson, 30 kHz (Satelec).

In the magnetostrictive scaler, either a stack of flat metal strips (Cavitron, 25 kHz) or a rod of ferromagnetic materials (Odontoson, 42 kHz) acts as the transducer. This magnetostrictive transducer comes attached to the working tip to constitute a handpiece insert. With passage of electric current, a coil within the handpiece insert reacts to the magnetic field by expanding and contracting in accordance with the alternating current. This rapid expansion and contraction result in vibrations that are transmitted to the working tip. The tip of the magnetostrictive scalers moves in an elliptic or circular manner (see Table 2).

Diamond-coated ultrasonic tips with three different grits have been designed for the magnetostrictive Cavitron machine in an attempt to increase the speed and efficiency of mechanical root preparation (Fig 83). They have been shown to be substantially faster for calculus removal in furcations in vitro (Steed et al, 1995) and in periodontal pockets in vivo (Yukna et al, 1997). However, a study by Lavespere et al (1996) showed that substantially greater root surface removal and greater residual root surface roughness occurred with diamond-coated ultrasonic inserts than with

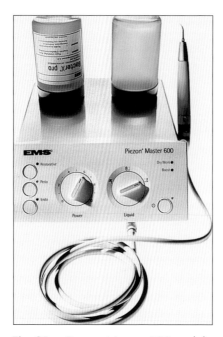

Fig 81a Piezon Master 600 mobile piezoelectric ultrasonic scaler with two reservoirs (350 mL each) for antimicrobial fluid coolant.

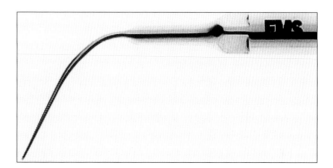

Fig 81b Extralong and extrathin PS tip.

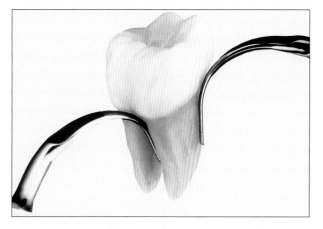

Fig 81c PC1 and PL2 tips for approximal surfaces and furcations.

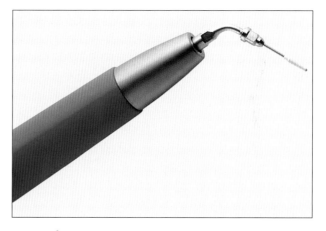

Fig 81d Plastic-coated PI tip for minimally invasive debridement of implants.

standard tips under standardized in vitro conditions. These results suggest that diamond-coated ultrasonic instruments should be used cautiously during subgingival instrumentation.

The magnetostrictive ultrasonic scalers produce a considerable amount of heat during instrumentation. About 50% of the electric energy is transformed to heat in the handle. Therefore, an efficient fluid cooling system is necessary. The benefit of this cooling system is that the cooling fluid can be used as a spray from a tiny hole near the tip of the instrument to simultaneously rinse away loosened calculus and microbial material from the pocket. Figure 84 shows how the cooling fluid is cavitated (also called *sonicated*) and widely spread around the tip of a magnetostrictive ultrasonic machine with elliptic movement. In contrast, the cooling fluid is cavitated and spread longitudinally around

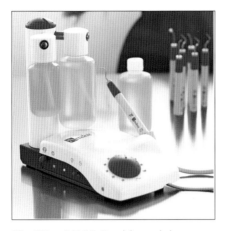

Fig 82a US30 Double mobile piezo-electric sonic scaler with autoclavable handles and two reservoirs for antimicrobial fluid coolant.

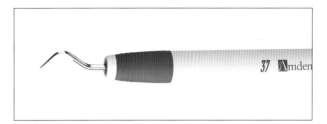

Fig 82b Autoclavable Quick-a-tip handle with the straight, long, and thin universal tip.

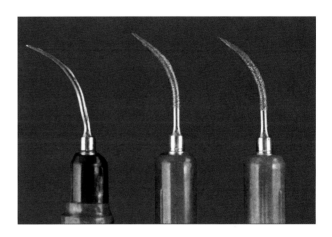

Fig 83 Tips for the Cavitron magnetostrictive ultrasonic machine. *(left to right)* Regular tip, fine-grit diamond-coated tip, and medium-grit diamond-coated tip.

the tip of a piezoelectric ultrasonic machine, offering better visibility during instrumentation compared with that provided by the magnetostrictive machines (Fig 85).

In addition, the piezoelectric ultrasonic machines produce less heat, need less application force and energy (see Table 2), and produce less root surface roughness than the magnetostrictive ultrasonic machines. For these reasons, piezoelectric ultrasonic machines have been more attractive than the magnetostrictive ultrasonic machines over the last decade.

To reduce the occurrence of bacteremia and improve the antimicrobial effect, it is beneficial to use a bactericidal cooling fluid, such as a 0.1% iodine solution. In a 12-year longitudinal study in more than 200 subjects with advanced periodon-

titis, Rosling et al (2001) showed that using 0.1% iodine solution as a cooling fluid together with a magnetostrictive ultrasonic machine in the maintenance program resulted in only a mean attachment loss of 0.3 mm per subject per 12 years, compared to loss of 0.9 mm when saline solution was used. Some piezoelectric ultrasonic scalers are equipped with one or two separate autoclavable reservoirs in which antimicrobial cooling fluids, such as 0.1% iodine solution, can be used (see Figs 81a and 82a).

The cavitation of the cooling fluid at the tip of ultrasonic scalers operating at high frequencies has a destructive effect on the plaque biofilm. The gram-negative periopathogens, including spirochetes, seem to be particularly sensitive to ultrasonication. Baehni et al (1992) showed that the

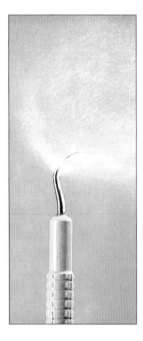

Fig 84 Widespread cavitated fluid coolant spray in a magnetostrictive ultrasonic scaler (Cavitron) during elliptic movement of the tip.

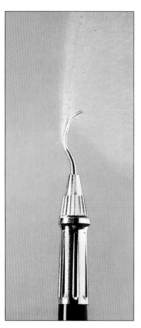

Fig 85 Longitudinal cavitated fluid coolant spray in a piezoelectric ultrasonic scaler during longitudinal movement of the tip.

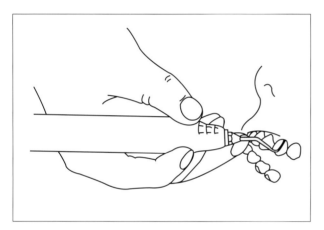

Fig 86a Fulcrum of the hand and finger during instrumentation with an ultrasonic scaler in the maxilla.

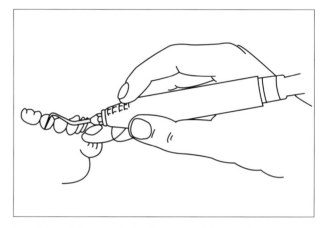

Fig 86b Fulcrum of the hand and finger during instrumentation with an ultrasonic scaler in the mandible.

use of a piezoelectric ultrasonic scaler caused a significantly initial reduction in spirochetes and other motile rods in diseased periodontal pockets. This reduction was related to the duration of instrumentation: 10 or 30 seconds.

Use of ultrasonic scalers

The application force of the tip along the tooth surface must not exceed 50 g, and a force of 20 g should be enough for removing calculus. Greater application force will result in excessive loss of root cementum.

Similar to the use of hand instruments, the use of ultrasonic scalers requires a fulcrum for the hand or fingers (Figs 86a and 86b). However, during instrumentation with ultrasonic scalers, an extraoral fulcrum can also be used.

To prevent iatrogenic development of roughness, the tip has to be continuously moved in contact with the root surface. The power (the length of the movement of the tip) used should be as lim-

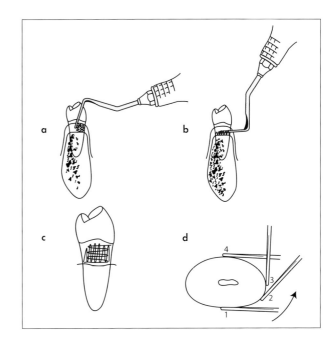

Fig 87 *(a)* Brushlike overlapping back-and-forth movements with the ultrasonic tip in a vertical position and parallel to the root surface. *(b and c)* Horizontal overlapping instrumentation with the tip until the entire surface has been covered. *(d)* During horizontal instrumentation, only the side of the tip, and not the lateral endpoint, must touch the tooth surface to prevent hammering action and iatrogenic effects. Different correct horizontal positions of the tip (1–4) are shown.

ited as possible to reduce iatrogenic loss of tooth substance. For debridement in maintenance patients, the minimum power should be used; in untreated patients with heavy amounts of calculus, more power, but not increased application force, may be necessary.

Excessive supply of cooling fluid will reduce the visibility and increase the difficulty of evaluating the surfaces; this problem is most common when magnetostrictive ultrasonic scalers are used.

As the movement of the tip is linear with piezoelectric ultrasonic scalers, and mainly linear with magnetostrictive ultrasonic scalers, the side of the tip will work against the root surface. Thus, a hammering movement and iatrogenic loss of tooth substance are prevented. However, contact with bonded veneers and cemented restorations should be avoided during instrumentation.

The length of the tip movement is greatest at the distal end and is almost 0 at the middle. Therefore, only the most distal 1 to 3 mm of the tip will be used to maximum effectiveness. The most frequent position of the tip is vertical and parallel to the root surface (Fig 87). The tip should start at the base of the pocket and move in a coronal direction with systematic overlapping back-and-forth brushlike movements to cover the entire root surface. Thereafter, the tip is used horizontally on the same

surface until the entire surface is instrumented. The completeness of deposit removal is assessed with an appropriate evaluation instrument.

Ultrasonic scalers should not be used on patients with cardiac pacemakers without consultation with their cardiologist, and they should be used with caution on patients with infectious diseases such as AIDS, tuberculosis, and hepatitis because of aerosol production in the treatment room. A 30-fold increase of airborne microorganisms is produced by ultrasonic scalers. Ultrasonic scalers produce bacteremias similar to hand scaling, so precautions are indicated for patients at risk for bacterial endocarditis.

The tip has to be discarded before 2 mm of the length is lost to wear, normally after 6 months if the instrument is used frequently.

Vector system (modified ultrasonic scaler)

A modified ultrasonic system (Vector ultrasonic system, Dürr), generating vibrations at a frequency of 25 kHz, has been introduced (Fig 88). The Vector scaler is fitted with six piezoceramic disks as an ultrasonic machine instead of the four disks fitted to conventional piezoelectric ultrasonic scalers, so more energy is available. The horizontal vibration of the device is converted by a resonating ring in vertical vibration, resulting in a par-

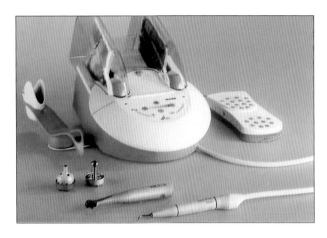

Fig 88 Complete Vector modified ultrasonic unit.

allel movement of the working tip to the root surface. Furthermore, the energy from the instrument is transmitted to the root surface and the periodontal tissues by a suspension of hydroxyapatite particles and water, comparable to ultrasonic cleaning baths. The suspension is not sprayed in an aerosol by the instrument but held hydrodynamically on the instrument by the linear ultrasonic movement. The particle suspension works like toothpaste, removing deposits and plaque biofilms from even the most difficult areas. Thus the cleaning and polishing effect on the root surfaces is increased. However, root planing will not be achieved.

A newly developed handset transmits the increased ultrasonic output directly to the special Vector scaler instrument. Because the fluid is conducted inside the instrument, the aerosol formation that normally occurs during the use of traditional ultrasonic scalers is almost completely avoided in the same way as with the periodontal hand instruments. This also enables the simultaneous use of polishing particles. The increase of ultrasonic output achieved by the additional piezoceramic disks enables the most stubborn of deposits to be removed rapidly as well.

The autoclavable (134°C) Vector handpiece is usefully shaped. Dismantled, it can be optimally cleaned. The same applies to the scaler handset, which is also equipped with a rotating joint. The base station contains the fluids that can be added by pressing a button during treatment. The functions can be called up at the base station or by the foot-operated switch in a very user-friendly way: Vector fluid can be turned on or off with preselected intensity and kickdown. The flexible hand-

set rest can be attached to the base station on the left or right to suit individual preferences.

The assortment of tips is made in stainless steel and carbon fiber–reinforced plastic. The metal tips should only be used for removal of calculus in untreated patients (Fig 89). The carbon fiber–reinforced plastic tips in combination with the Vector fluid polish are recommended for minimally invasive debridement in maintenance patients with scaled and root planed natural teeth and in implant patients (Fig 90).

Preliminary clinical results have shown that the use of the Vector ultrasonic instrument caused less pain during the treatment of periodontal lesions than did cleaning with hand instruments or a conventional ultrasonic system (Braun et al, 2003). Furthermore, results from another study, evaluating the healing of human intrabony defects following nonsurgical periodontal treatment with the Vector instrument clinically and histologically, revealed a significant gain of clinical attachment after 6 months. The histologic evaluation revealed that healing is predominantly characterized by formation of a long junctional epithelium along the instrumented root surface (Sculean et al, 2003).

In a 6-month randomized controlled clinical study, Sculean et al (2004a) showed similar improvements in probing depth and clinical attachment when they compared instrumentation with a hand instrument and the Vector ultrasonic scaler. In another 6-month clinical study, Kocher et al (2005) found no difference in clinical effects and pain during instrumentation with the Vector instrument, piezoelectric ultrasonic scaler, and a Slimline Cavitron magnetoelectric ultrasonic scaler.

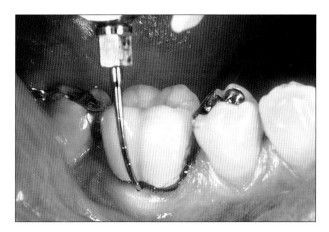

Fig 89 Curved stainless steel Vector tip in situ during scaling.

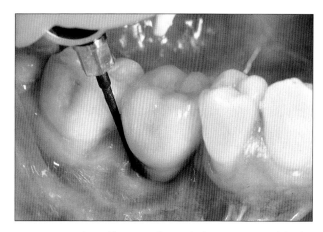

Fig 90 Carbon fiber-reinforced plastic tip, suitable for minimally invasive debridement of natural teeth as well as implants.

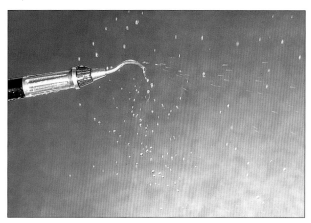

Fig 91 Because the tips of sonic scalers have much lower frequency than the tips of ultrasonic scalers, the fluid coolant will not be cavitated. Therefore, the cleaning and flushing effect in the pocket is very limited.

In vitro, the loss of tooth substance with the Vector stainless steel tip and polishing fluid seems to be similar to that obtained with conventional ultrasonic scalers (Braun et al, 2005). However, data on the long-term clinical and iatrogenic effects of frequent instrumentation with this instrument are still lacking.

Sonic scalers

Sonic instruments utilize mechanical rather than electric vibrations of the working tip. The sonic scaler tip vibrates by compressed air from the dental unit with frequencies ranging from 2,000 to 6,000 Hz. Titan sonic scaler, 6.5 kHz (Star Dental); SonicFlex, 6.0 kHz; Quixonic sonic scaler, 6.0 kHz (Dentsply); and Emie560, 6.0 kHz (Micron) are examples of this type of instrument. The handpiece is composed of a hollow rod, a rotor, and several rubber O rings. Compressed air is forced through the hollow rod in the handpiece. The rotor is a 6-mm-wide thin metal ring that encircles the hollow rod above a series of the scientifically angled holes. The air escapes through the 10 holes and causes the rotor to vibrate, which in turn triggers vibration of the entire rod.

The working motion of the sonic scaler is generally elliptic but irregular. The length of the tip movement is about 0.2 mm. The application force is normally 20 to 100 g. At forces greater than 100 g, the tip will stop. Although a coolant is not necessary, its use enhances the effect through acoustic streaming. However, because sonic scalers have a lower frequency than ultrasonic scalers, no cavitation of the cooling fluid occurs (Fig 91). The irrigation and flushing effect is also minimal compared to that of ultrasonic scalers. Sonic scalers have been widely used because their price is less than that of ultrasonic scalers and because they can be directly connected to the regular air pressure outlet on dental units. They are compact and easy to sterilize. Their effect on calculus removal is at least as good as that of ultrasonic scalers, but their iatrogenic effects on the root surfaces are worse (for a recent review, see Walmsley et al, 2008).

PER-IO-TOR system

Design

A clean and smooth root cementum is of great importance for good healing of diseased periodontal pockets and for successful minimally invasive debridement if subgingival plaque biofilms reform, as discussed earlier in this chapter. However, the thickness of the cementum in the coronal third of the root is originally only 0.03 to 0.10 mm. Therefore, only a total of 10 to 20 strokes with a sharp curette (Coldiron et al, 1990; Fig 92) and 5 to 10 rotations with a 15-μm-grit diamond bur (Ritz et al, 1991) may result in the complete removal of the root cementum. This can lead to an infection of the pulp (see Fig 19; Adriaens et al, 1988a, 1988b; Hirsch et al, 1989). Additionally, microflora and their toxins in infected root canals may go the other way (ie, into the periodontal pocket), which will disturb the healing of periodontitis (Ehnevid et al, 1995) and may reduce the success of regenerative therapy. Supragingivally removed root cementum and exposed, bacterially invaded dentinal tubules may increase the risk for development of root caries.

Significantly more plaque will reaccumulate subgingivally on root surfaces with deep grooves created by invasive instrumentation with rotating diamond burs than on root surfaces that have been instrumented less invasively with a hand curette (Leknes et al, 1994). Even supragingivally, plaque reaccumulation is significantly correlated to surface roughness (Quirynen et al, 1990).

Heavy scaling and root planing should only have to be performed initially in patients with untreated periodontitis. Repeated invasive scaling and root planing must be regarded as a treatment failure. Badersten et al (1984b) showed that the long-term effect of one initial scaling, root planing, and debridement on periodontal attachment and probing depth in patients with advanced periodontal disease was at least as successful as three initial repeated instrumentations with 1-month intervals, particularly in the deepest pockets, when excellent gingival plaque control was established by self-care and needs-related intervals of PMTC (Fig 93). Thus it may be concluded that the need for scaling and root planing should be very limited in practices in which a majority of patients are in the maintenance phase of treatment. In maintenance patients, minimally invasive subgingival debridement (removal of re-formed subgingival biofilms) in a few sites is the most invasive treatment that should be necessary when gingival plaque control by self-care and PMTC have been failing and scaling has been restricted to supragingival calculus lingually in mandibular anterior teeth and buccal surfaces of maxillary molars in patients who form salivary calculus rapidly. For example, about 90% of the adult patients in Sweden should be regarded as maintenance patients, and a majority receive needs-related supportive care by dental hygienists.

PER-IO-TOR instruments (see Fig 21) have been designed to solve some of the problems related to instrumentation with hand instruments, sonic and ultrasonic scalers, and rotating diamond burs. The basic concept is illustrated in Fig 94. The instruments are mechanically driven with reciprocating strokes of 1.0 to 1.5 mm long. The instrument is designed so that when the working side faces the root surface, the plaque biofilm and calculus can be scraped off and the rough root cementum planed during reciprocal vertical movements along the root. However, further removal of root cementum is prevented as soon as the root cementum is cleaned and planed because of the special design.

The working parts are the essentially right-angled cutting edges, formed between the opposed side walls of a recessed groove and the smooth aligned areas of the working side of the instrument. When the plaque biofilm and calculus have been removed and the root cementum is planed, the surface parts will contact and rest against the flat faces of the root cementum surface and will form load-relieving surfaces that absorb the pressure of the tool and restrain the cutting edges. During continued use of the instrument, these parts of the instrument will slide along the

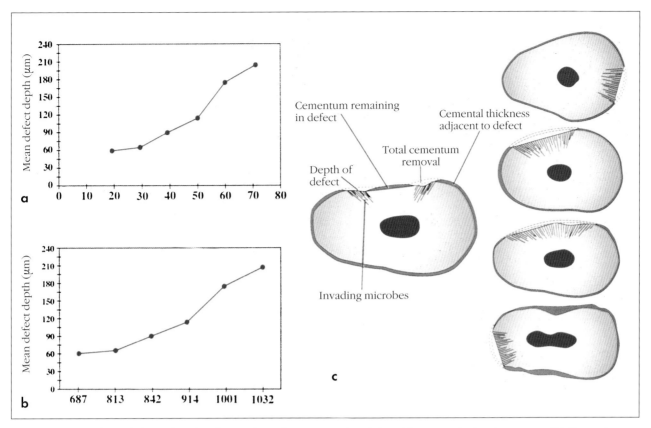

Fig 92 Root surface defect related to the number of curette strokes (a) and force applied to the curette (b). Typical types of root defects formed by the curette during root planing (c). (Modified from Coldiron et al, 1990.)

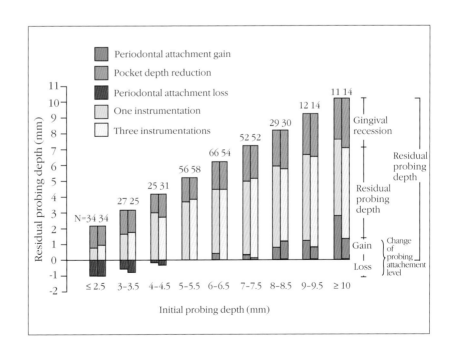

Fig 93 Mean amounts of gingival recession, residual probing depth, and change in probing attachment level at 24 months in relation to initial probing depth. (Modified from Badersten et al, 1984b. Reprinted with permission.)

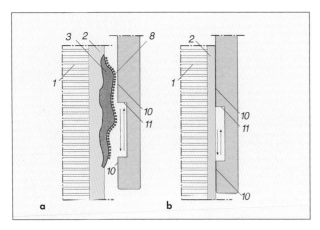

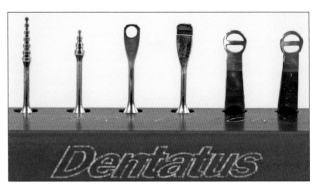

Fig 94 Basic minimally invasive principle of the PER-IO-TOR instruments. *(a)* Before treatment. *(b)* Final outcome as a consequence of the design. (1) Root dentin with dentinal tubules; (2) rough unplaned root cementum *(yellow)*; (3) subgingival calculus *(gray)*; (8) plaque biofilm *(red)*; (10 and 11) principal design of the PER-IO-TOR instruments with essentially right-angled cutting edges formed between (10) the opposed side walls of a recessed groove and (11) the smooth aligned surface of the working side.

Fig 95 Shape of the six reciprocating PER-IO-TOR instruments. *(left to right)* PER-IO-TOR 1, 2, 3, 4, 5, and 6, made of surgical stainless steel.

tooth surface, and the cutting edges will not perform any further scraping action, thus preventing removal of any significant degree of root cementum and exposure of the dentin; this result is in contrast to the action of more invasive instruments, such as hand instruments and ultrasonic scalers, which remove mineralized tooth substance, cementum, and root dentin continuously when they are used (see Fig 21).

PER-IO-TOR instruments have the following specific characteristics (Fig 95):

• They are specially designed reciprocating instruments that will optimize cleaning and planing of the rough root cementum and prevent further removal of root cementum once the surface is clean and smooth. Therefore, there are grooves with right-angled cutting wedges between smooth plane surfaces.

• The special size, shape, and assortment of instruments allow access to any area of diseased and rough root surfaces.

• Mechanically driven instruments with 1.0- to 1.5-mm reciprocating strokes are easy to use and do not cause ergonomic problems (Axelsson, 1993).

In vitro and in vivo studies have confirmed that the PER-IO-TOR instruments are less invasive and result in smoother root surfaces than, for example, sonic scalers, ultrasonic scalers, and hand instruments. In an in vitro study, Jotikasthira et al (1992) showed that the spatula-shaped PER-IO-TOR 4 instrument resulted in a smoother root surface and less loss of tooth substance than sonic scalers, in particular, as well as ultrasonic scalers (Fig 96). In another in vitro study, Mengel et al (1994) showed that 2 to 3 minutes' nonstop use of the PER-IO-TOR

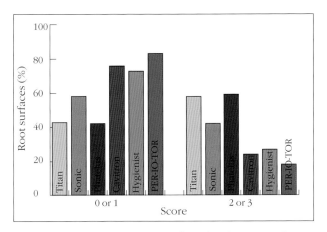

Fig 96 Roughness and loss of tooth substance after instrumentation. (0 or 1) Smooth or slightly roughened cementum surface; (2 or 3) definitely corrugated or completely removed cementum. (Modified from Jotikasthira et al, 1992. Reprinted with permission.)

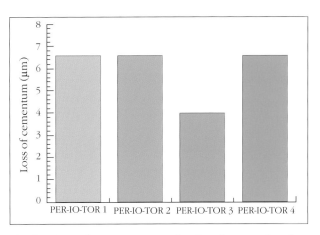

Fig 97 Loss of root cementum after 2 to 3 minutes' scaling and root planing with different PER-IO-TOR instruments. (Modified from Mengel et al, 1994. Reprinted with permission.)

instruments resulted in only a 4- to 6-μm loss of root cementum (Fig 97). That quantity represents approximately the amount that has to be removed to plane the rough outer surface of root cementum during root planing and debridement. In vivo studies (Kocher et al, 2001b; Rühling et al, 2005) have shown that subgingival instrumentation with PER-IO-TOR instruments resulted in smoother root surfaces than sonic scalers and ultrasonic scalers and less loss of tooth substance than hand curettes, sonic scalers, and regular ultrasonic scalers and performed similarly to polytetrafluoroethylene-coated ultrasonic tips (see Figs 22 to 25).

Use of PER-IO-TOR instruments

PER-IO-TOR precision surgical stainless steel instruments are designed for use in either the old EVA contra-angle handpiece (Dentatus) or the new Profin contra-angle handpiece (Dentatus), which represents an improvement over the EVA contra-angle handpiece. In the latter, the instruments are self-steering because they can freely rotate 360 degrees during the reciprocating movement and automatically follow the shape of the tooth surfaces. Profin is similar to EVA, but in addition, the instruments can be locked in six secured angles or positions during the reciprocating movement (Fig 98). Both the handpieces will

result in 1.0- to 1.5-mm reciprocating strokes of the instruments.

The speed of the instrument should be adjusted to suit the comfort of both the patient and the operator. However, the recommended speed should be between 10,000 and 15,000 rpm, equaling 20,000 to 30,0000 single strokes per minute. The new handpiece is equipped with water spray, and some versions also have a fiber-optic light. However, the creation of excessive heat is not a problem with the use of a low-speed reciprocating instrument in the wet subgingival environment, unlike with the use of rotating instruments and ultrasonic scalers.

Initially, the operator should practice the use of the different PER-IO-TOR instruments with a water spray on wet teeth without old, heavy amounts of calculus, directly after extraction and disinfection but without dehydration of the root surface, that is, under conditions that resemble the in vivo clinical setting: the root surface contaminated by saliva, exudates, blood, and so on.

The speed must not be too low because vibration could cause patient discomfort. Higher pressure is necessary than for the other tips and instruments of the Profin Directional and EVA systems. In contrast to sonic scalers and particularly ultrasonic scalers, PER-IO-TOR instruments provide superior tactile feedback during use.

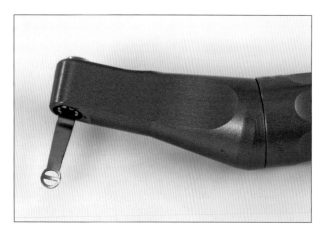

Fig 98 Profin contra-angle handpiece with a PER-IO-TOR 5 insert.

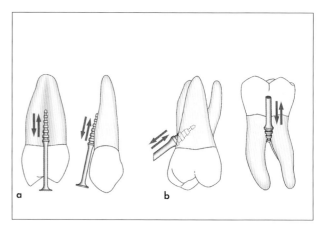

Fig 99 Application of PER-IO-TOR 1 *(a)* and PER-IO-TOR 2 *(b)*. *(arrows)* Direction of movement.

Gross scaling with hand or ultrasonic instruments could be the first step in scaling for new patients with heavy deposits of calculus. Then the final detailed scaling, root planing, and debridement procedures can be carried out with PER-IO-TOR instruments. In maintenance patients (90% of the Swedish population), initial gross scaling should not be necessary if initial treatment and the needs-related maintenance program have been effective. The demanding, time-consuming conventional subgingival scaling and root planing procedure should be necessary only once, as discussed earlier in the chapter (Badersten et al, 1984b). Only a few at-risk surfaces with recurrent periodontal disease may need an additional, minimally invasive subgingival scaling and root planing; for the most part, only debridement of reformed subgingival biofilms with the PER-IO-TOR instruments is necessary.

PER-IO-TOR 1 and 2 are circular, tapered instruments with circumferential ridges and are specially designed for access to root grooves and furcation areas (Fig 99). PER-IO-TOR 1 is thinner than PER-IO-TOR 2. The instrument is specially designed to allow access to and treatment of root surfaces with root grooves in narrow bone pockets and furcation areas. For example, the instrument provides good access for treatment of the mesial root surfaces of the maxillary first premolars and the distal root surfaces of the maxillary second molars, which are normally difficult to reach for subgingival scaling and root planing.

Figure 100 shows the spatula-shaped PER-IO-TOR 3 and 4. PER-IO-TOR 3 is an extrathin eyelet spatula-shaped instrument to be used horizontally or diagonally on flat or slightly convex approximal surfaces in very narrow interproximal spaces where the thicker spatula-shaped PER-IO-TOR 4 has no access, for example, at the mandibular incisors. PER-IO-TOR 4 is a spatula-shaped instrument with a groove on the working side. It is thicker but more efficient than PER-IO-TOR 3. Therefore, this instrument is the first choice for every accessible flat or convex approximal surface. It can be used horizontally as well as diagonally. Even vertical instrumentation can be carried out on root surfaces if the crown of the tooth does not block the correct direction parallel to the root surface.

When using the PER-IO-TOR 4, it is very important to ensure that the working side with the notch is pressed against the root surface before treatment is started.

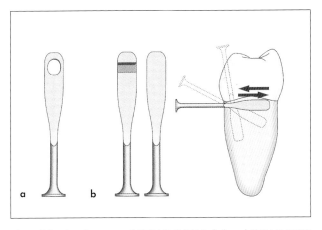

Fig 100 Application of PER-IO-TOR 3 *(a)* and PER-IO-TOR 4 *(b)*. *(arrows)* Direction of movement.

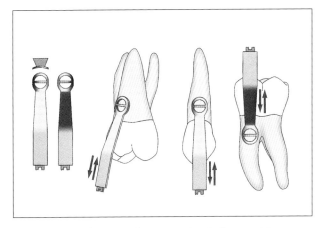

Fig 101 Application of PER-IO-TOR 5. *(arrows)* Direction of movement.

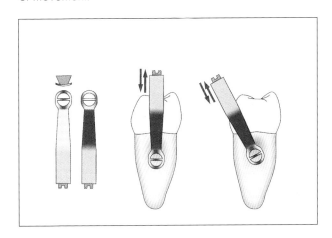

Fig 102 Application of PER-IO-TOR 6. *(arrows)* Direction of movement.

PER-IO-TOR 5 (Fig 101) has a concave working surface for vertical use on convex buccal and lingual surfaces as well as on the line angles. PER-IO-TOR 6 (Fig 102) has a convex working surface for vertical or diagonal use on concave approximal surfaces.

The use of the different PER-IO-TOR instruments will be demonstrated on extracted teeth with apical-marginal communication and heavy amounts of calculus from patients with advanced untreated periodontitis. However, for the sake of efficiency, the first step in vivo should be to use a sharp curette as a probe in a coronal direction from the base of the pocket. Whenever calculus is located, it should simultaneously be lifted away without invasive removal of root cementum. An alternative for initial treatment could be a piezo-electric ultrasonic scaler with an extralong and extrathin tip, as discussed earlier. This is a logical

course because PER-IO-TOR instruments are minimally invasive and should only be used for the final minimally invasive scaling, root planing, and debridement. However, although PER-IO-TOR instruments are much less efficient in removal of calculus than are hand instruments and ultrasonic scalers, PER-IO-TOR can be used successfully to remove large deposits (Figs 103a and 103b).

Figure 104a shows an extracted untreatable maxillary molar with a gross amount of calculus up to the apical region and in the furcation area. However, most often, scaling, root planing, and debridement are performed on the coronal third of the root. Again, initial scaling normally should start with the use of a sharp curette, which also offers excellent facility for locating calculus and other surface roughness. However, in this case, PER-IO-TOR 2 was used from the beginning in the furcation area between the mesiobuccal and palatal

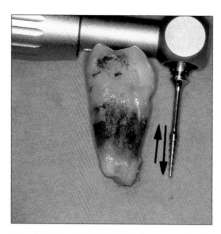

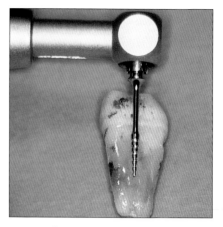

Fig 103a PER-IO-TOR 1, particularly designed for vertical use in root grooves and narrow furcation areas. *(arrows)* Direction of movement.

Fig 103b Use of PER-IO-TOR 1 on the approximal surface of an extracted premolar with a shallow root groove and extensive calculus.

roots (Fig 104b), resulting in a surface that was not only clean but also extremely smooth, similar to glass (Fig 104c), which could not have been achieved after instrumentation with fine-grit diamond burs, curettes, sonic, or ultrasonic scalers. PER-IO-TOR 4 was used for instrumentation of the remaining part of the mesial surface (Fig 104d).

PER-IO-TOR 5 and 6 are specially designed for convex and concave root surfaces, respectively (Figs 105 and 106). Figures 107a and 107b show the use of PER-IO-TOR 5 on the mesiobuccal convex part of a mandibular left third molar and the result. In another patient with advanced untreated periodontitis, an untreatable right mandibular molar was extracted. It exhibited gross calculus, particularly on the distal root, even around the apex (Fig 108a). With the permission of the patient, immediately after extraction of the tooth, PER-IO-TOR 5 was tested strictly on the most prominent convex buccal part of the distal root (Fig 108b). Initially, the most proximal part of the instrument was used as a shovel for gross scaling. Thereafter, the inner concave surface with its smooth surfaces and 90-degree protected edges was used for the final scaling and root planing. Figure 108c shows the result after 20 seconds' instrumentation.

Clinical use of the PER-IO-TOR instruments is exemplified with some cases. Figures 109 and 110 show PER-IO-TOR 2 in function on the buccal surfaces of two maxillary first molars with grade I furcation involvement. If the furcation area is very narrow and deep, for example, on the distal surface of the maxillary second molars or the mesial surface of the maxillary first premolars, PER-IO-TOR 1 is substituted for PER-IO-TOR 2.

PER-IO-TOR 1 and 2 should be used to recontour the furcation areas in a manner similar to that used with rotating diamond tips; initially, the bottom of the furcation area is reached tactilely before the instrument is used. The instrument is then gradually used coronally as well as mesially and distally, strictly following the shape of the furcation area during the instrumentation procedure. In contrast to the use of the diamond tip, with PER-IO-TOR the furcation area is only cleaned and planed and not recontoured.

When PER-IO-TOR 4 is used, the working side with the groove initially has to be positioned properly, firmly against the root surface (see Fig 100b). Figure 111 shows the instrument in function diagonally on the distal surface of a maxillary central incisor. In very narrow interproximal spaces such as mandibular incisors, PER-IO-TOR 4 may be replaced with the eyelet PER-IO-TOR 3. On the flat or slightly convex approximal surfaces of the molars, PER-IO-TOR 4 is especially efficient in a horizontal or slightly diagonal direction (Figs 112 and 113).

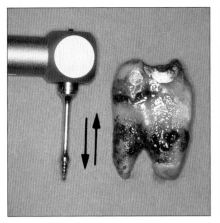

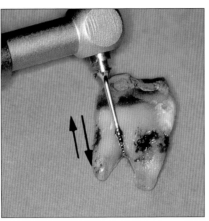

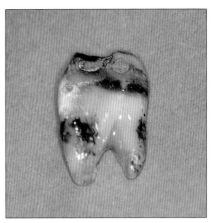

Fig 104a Extracted maxillary molar with heavy amounts of calculus on the apical two thirds of the roots. *(arrows)* Direction of movement.

Fig 104b Use of PER-IO-TOR 2 in the furcation area. *(arrows)* Direction of movement.

Fig 104c Extremely smooth and shiny root surface in the furcation area after instrumentation.

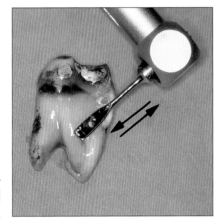

Fig 104d Use of spatula-shaped PER-IO-TOR 4 on the remaining approximal surface. *(arrows)* Direction of movement.

Figure 114a shows a large accumulation of calculus located on the apical third of the distal root of the mandibular left second premolar in combination with a narrow three-wall intrabony pocket. Even this extensive accumulation was removed by PER-IO-TOR 4, as shown in Fig 114b, 4 months after treatment, which also reveals initial repair of the intrabony pocket. However, the process was more time consuming than using, for example, a Mini Langer Gracey 5/6 curette (extralong shank and short blade) for the initial gross scaling and then following with PER-IO-TOR 4 for the final scaling and root planing.

PER-IO-TOR instruments can be used for open debridement, scaling, and root planing, in which the root surfaces are exposed for improved access by open flap surgery (Figs 115 and 116).

Figure 117 shows the three rotary versions of the PER-IO-TOR instruments (7R, 8R, and 9R). The straight and conical PER-IO-TOR 7R should be used for scaling, root planing, and debridement vertically along the root surfaces and especially in root grooves. The convex and pointed PER-IO-TOR 8R is designed for the same purpose on root concavities. PER-IO-TOR 9R is a concave and pointed tip specially designed for scaling, root planing, and debridement in furcation areas (Fig 118).

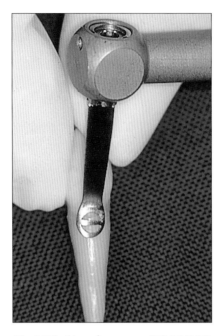

Fig 105 Use of concave PER-IO-TOR 5 on the convex buccal root surface of a premolar.

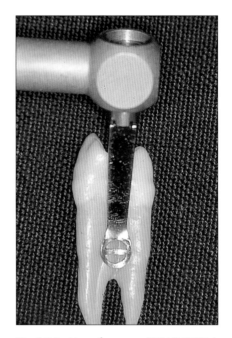

Fig 106 Use of convex PER-IO-TOR 6 on the concave approximal surface of a premolar.

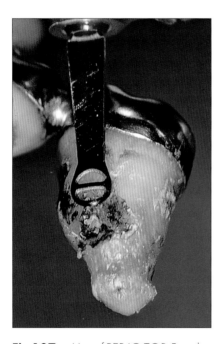

Fig 107a Use of PER-IO-TOR 5 on the mesiobuccal convex part of a mandibular third molar with a heavy amount of calculus.

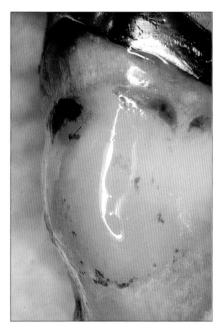

Fig 107b Result on the instrumented part of the root.

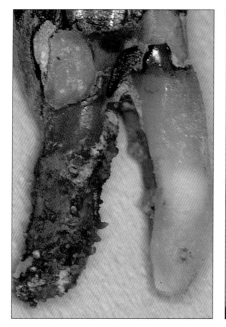

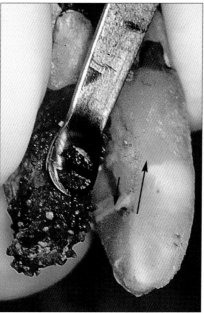

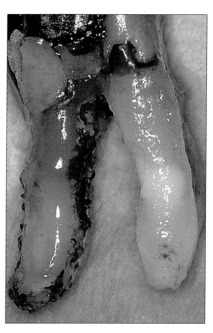

Fig 108a Mandibular second molar exhibiting a tremendous amount of calculus around the distal root.

Fig 108b Use of PER-IO-TOR 5 only on the most prominent part of the convex buccal surface. *(arrows)* Direction of movement.

Fig 108c Extremely smooth and shiny instrumented part of the root.

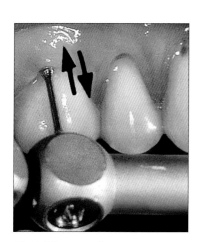

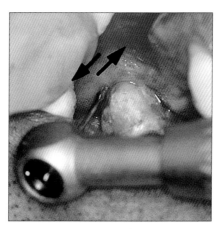

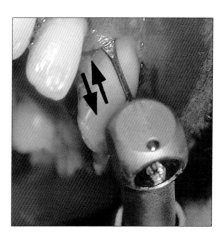

Fig 109 Use of PER-IO-TOR 2 in the furcation area of a maxillary first molar with degree I involvement. The instrument is used at about a 20-degree angulation. *(arrows)* Direction of movement.

Fig 110 Use of PER-IO-TOR 2 in the furcation area of a maxillary first molar with degree I to II furcation involvement. The instrument is used at about a 45-degree angulation. *(arrows)* Direction of movement.

Fig 111 Use of PER-IO-TOR 4 diagonally on the distal surface of a maxillary central incisor. *(arrows)* Direction of movement.

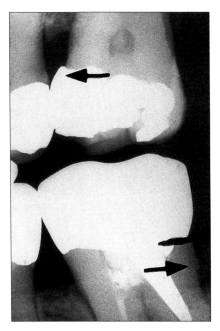 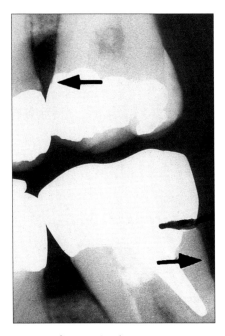

Fig 112a Radiograph showing subgingival calculus on the distal root surface of a mandibular second molar *(bottom arrow)* and restoration overhang *(top arrow)* on the mesial surface of the maxillary second molar.

Fig 112b Result after instrumentation with PER-IO-TOR 4 on the distal surface of the mandibular second molar *(bottom arrow)* and recontouring of the restoration on the maxillary molar *(top arrow)* with Lamineer diamond and tungsten-coated reciprocating double knife–shaped tips.

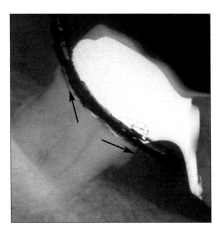 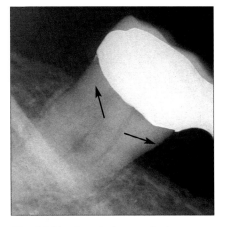

Fig 113a Radiograph showing subgingival calculus *(arrows)* on the mesial and distal root surfaces of a mandibular second molar.

Fig 113b Result *(arrows)* after instrumentation with PER-IO-TOR 4.

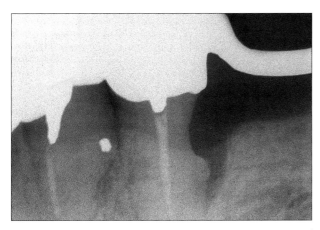

Fig 114a Radiograph showing a large accumulation of calculus on the apical third of the distal root surface of a mandibular second premolar and an intrabony pocket.

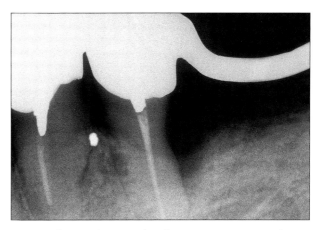

Fig 114b Result 4 months after instrumentation with PER-IO-TOR 4. Some repair of the intrabony pocket has already been achieved.

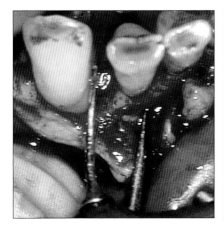

Fig 115 Use of PER-IO-TOR 4 on the mesial surface of a mandibular right canine during regenerative treatment of an intrabony pocket.

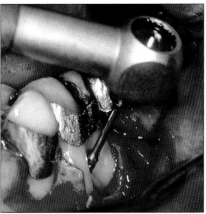

Fig 116 Use of PER-IO-TOR 2 to treat advanced furcation involvement on the buccal surface of a mandibular left first molar during regenerative therapy.

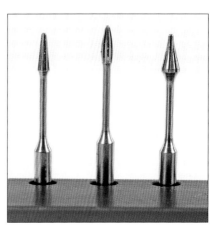

Fig 117 Shape of the rotary PER-IO-TOR instruments. *(left to right)* PER-IO-TOR 7R, 8R, and 9R.

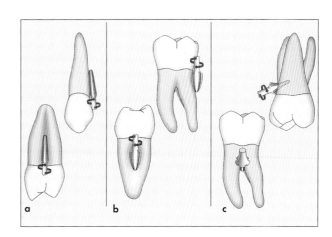

Fig 118 Application of PER-IO-TOR 7R *(a)*, PER-IO-TOR 8R *(b)*, and PER-IO-TOR 9R *(c)*.

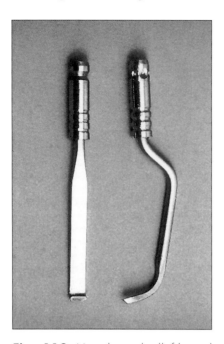

Fig 119 Hoe-shaped *(left)* and curette-shaped *(right)* Perioplaners. (From Hänggi et al, 1991. Reprinted with permission.)

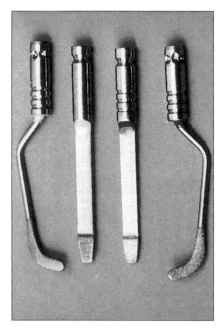

Fig 120 Diamond-coated (40- and 15-µm) Periopolishers. (From Hänggi et al, 1991. Reprinted with permission.)

Perioplaners and Periopolishers

A certain contra-angle (Mikrona) has been designed for scaling and root planing with reciprocating instruments. The amplitude of the instruments is 0.4 mm. The contra-angle can be adapted to regular electric-powered engines.

The contra-angle can be used with Perioplaners (Mikrona) and Periopolishers (Mikrona). There are two different Perioplaner instruments, one shaped like a universal curette and one shaped like a hoe (Fig 119). The curette-shaped instrument is used for the approximal surfaces and has to be secured in one of eight available positions. The hoe-shaped scaler is used for buccal and lingual surfaces and can be used with a freely rotating insert.

Four Periopolisher instruments are available (Fig 120). Two flat, golf club–shaped diamond-coated instruments (40 or 15 µm) are designed for the approximal surfaces and should be se-cured in one of eight different positions. Two diamond-coated (40 or 15 µm) instruments with flat tips are designed for buccal and lingual surfaces.

Hänggi et al (1991) evaluated the loss of root substance in vitro by using Perioplaners, Periopolishers, and Perio-Set rotating diamond-coated burs (Intensiv), which are specially designed for scaling. Table 3 shows the mean loss of root substance per 1 and 12 strokes related to type of instrument and force of application (100 to 500 psi).

The in vitro data indicated that the Perioplaner instruments (500 psi) and Periopolisher instruments (40 µm + 200 psi), used at a speed of 20,000 strokes per minute (engine greater than 10,000 rpm), will result in complete removal of coronal root cementum (30 to 100 µm) in less than 1 second (1 second = 330 strokes). This would result in exposure of dentinal tubules (see Fig 19). The invasive effect of these instruments on the root surface would probably be diminished in vivo in a wet periodontal pocket.

Table 3   Loss of root substance after scaling with various instruments*

Instrument	No. of measurements	Force of application (psi)	Mean loss of root substance per 12 strokes (μm)	Mean loss of root substance per stroke (μm)
Perioplaner				
Curette-shaped	20	250	51.5	4.3
	20	500	92.3	7.7
Hoe-shaped	20	250	53.7	4.5
	20	500	98.8	8.2
Periopolisher				
Golf club–shaped (15 μm)	20	100	27.1	2.3
	20	200	37.0	3.1
Golf club–shaped (40 μm)	20	100	44.8	3.7
Perio-Set				
Diamond-coated burs (15 μm)	20	100	42.1	3.5
	20	200	59.6	4.9

*Data from Hänggi et al (1991).

Rotating instruments

In vitro studies have shown that rotating diamond burs are more efficient in removal of calculus than other scaling instruments but are also by far the most damaging in terms of removing root cementum and producing iatrogenic root surface roughness (Leknes et al, 1994; Lie and Meyer, 1977; Ritz et al, 1991; see Fig 13). Even with extra fine (15-μm) grit diamond burs (Perio-Set 415), 120 μm of the root substance was lost after 15 seconds with an application force of 100 p (Ritz et al, 1991). The thickness of the root cementum in the coronal third of the root is only 30 to 100 μm. Therefore, such invasive instruments should be used only when the aim is to recontour the root, for example, to recontour root grooves and grade I furcation involvement.

Laser instruments

LASER is an acronym for *light amplification by stimulated emission of radiation*. The process of lasing occurs when an excited atom is stimulated to emit a photon before the process occurs spontaneously. Spontaneous emission of a photon by one atom stimulates the release of a subsequent photon and so on. This stimulated emission generates a very coherent (synchronous waves), monochromatic (a single wavelength), and collimated form (parallel rays) of light that is found nowhere else in nature. Lasers can concentrate light energy and exert a strong effect, targeting tissue at an energy level that is much lower than that of natural light. The photon emitted has a specific wavelength that depends on the state of the electron's energy when the photon is released. Two identical atoms with electrons in identical states will release photons with identical wavelengths.

The characteristics of a laser depend on its wavelength. Wavelength affects both the clinical applications and the design of the laser. The wavelength of lasers is measured in nanometers. The wavelength of lasers used in medicine and dentistry generally range from 193 to 10,600 nm, representing a broad spectrum from the ultraviolet to the far infrared range. The lasers most commonly used in dentistry, carbon dioxide (CO_2), neodymium:yttrium-aluminum-garnet (Nd:YAG), and erbium:yttrium-aluminum-garnet (Er:YAG), have wavelengths of 10,600 nm (far infrared), 1,064 nm (near infrared), and 2,940 nm (infrared), respectively.

CO_2 and Nd:YAG lasers are the lasers most commonly used for surgical procedures performed on oral soft tissues, and they were the first to have handpieces adapted for intraoral use. However, these two lasers are not suitable for treatment of mineralized tissues such as the tooth because of severe side effects. Among other things, the extreme heat generated may kill the pulp and damage the root surface.

The primary emphasis of utilizing lasers only on soft tissues was changed in 1997 with US Food and Drug Administration safety clearance for the use of the Er:YAG laser on hard tissues such as enamel, cementum, and bone. The Er:YAG laser has a wavelength (2,940 nm) that is ideal for absorption by hydroxyapatite and water, making it more efficient in ablating enamel and dentin than any previously introduced laser. This wavelength corresponds to the absorption coefficient of water, causing water to evaporate into steam in the tissues being irradiated and resulting in a microexplosion of the hard tissue. This process of ablation generates very little heat in the underlying tissues and minimal elevation of the pulpal temperature. The laser energy produced at the 2,940-nm wavelength is absorbed by water 15,000 times more than is the Nd:YAG laser wavelength of 1,064 nm. Therefore, tissue destruction caused by the ER:YAG laser is probably not related to thermal effects, as with other types of lasers, but to the microexplosions associated with the water evaporation within the cementum and other dental hard tissues.

The Er:YAG laser utilizes a fiber-optic delivery system with an accompanying helium-neon laser as an aiming beam because the wavelength is invisible. It is essential to use a water spray to wet the surface during laser radiation to achieve maximum efficiency of tissue removal with minimal heat generation. The surface is left with an acid-etched appearance microscopically. This fact, in combination with the absence of tactile feedback, means that root planing cannot be achieved with laser apparatuses.

The Er:YAG laser has demonstrated the best application of laser use directly on hard tissue, leaving the least thermal damage and creating a surface that suggests biocompatibility for soft tissue attachment. Studies have demonstrated the ability of the Er:YAG laser to remove lipopolysaccharides from root surfaces, facilitate removal of the smear layer after root planing, remove calculus and cementum, and leave a surface similar to an acid-etched appearance with a scalelike texture (Gutknecht et al, 2001). The effects on the root surface from this laser show an absence of the melting, charring, and carbonization that are observed with the use of Nd:YAG or CO_2 lasers. However, any additional benefits of applying the Er:YAG laser to root surfaces compared to root planing alone have not been substantiated. Damage to the cementum surface occurs from laser irradiation despite water coolant, and no study has shown attachment of human gingival fibroblasts to a root surface previously treated by the Er:YAG laser.

Frentzen et al (2002) reported that, although Er:YAG laser scaling achieved complete debridement clinically, laser scaling at a panel setting of 160 mJ/pulse (output energy 100 or 200 mJ/pulse and calculated energy density 18.8 or 14.5 J/cm² per pulse in the use of 1.1- and 0.5-mm chisel tips, respectively) and 10 Hz with water spray resulted in greater loss of cementum and dentin in vitro compared to mechanical scaling. They believed that this loss should be taken into account in the clinical situation. The crater depth of the treated root surface was approximately 40 and 80 µm with the use of the 1.65- and 1.10-mm tips, respectively.

Figures 121 to 123 from their study show histologic cross sections of root surfaces instrumented with a curette, an ultrasonic scaler, or an Er:YAG laser with a 1.10-mm tip (Key II, KaVo). In

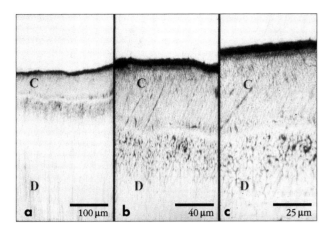

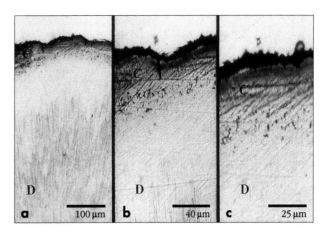

Fig 121 Micrographs of a root surface scaled with hand instruments. The cementum (C) surface is evenly covered by a smear layer. (D) Dentin (original magnifications ×100 *[a]*; ×250 *[b]*; ×400 *[c]*). (From Frentzen et al, 2002. Reprinted with permission.)

Fig 122 Micrographs of a root surface instrumented with an ultrasonic device. The cementum (C) surface is smooth and covered by a smear layer; however, this layer is less condensed than it is following hand instrumentation. (D) Dentin (original magnifications ×100 *[a]*; ×250 *[b]*; ×400 *[c]*). (From Frentzen et al, 2002. Reprinted with permission.)

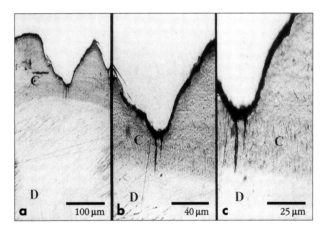

Fig 123 Micrographs of a laser-scaled root surface (1.10-mm tip). There are no signs of carbonization or denaturation, but deep grooves are visible. (D) Dentin (original magnifications ×100 *[a]*; ×250 *[b]*; ×400 *[c]*). (From Frentzen et al, 2002. Reprinted with permission.)

this study, relatively high energy was used. However, although the efficiency of laser scaling can be easily improved by using a higher output power, the power output should be selected carefully, balancing effectiveness and the avoidance of unnecessary tissue removal. Improvement of the effectiveness of laser scaling should rely on other variables, such as pulse repetition rate and pulse duration, rather than only on an increase of energy output.

Thus, the Er:YAG laser does not accomplish selective ablation of dental calculus in vitro because the tissue underlying dental calculus is also removed during laser scaling. For safe and effective clinical use, a combination of a higher pulse repetition rate and lower energy outputs is recommended to increase the efficiency of calculus ablation and simultaneously decrease the loss of cementum. Under such conditions of irradiation, the efficiency is improved without increasing the uncomfortable vibration stress experienced by patients. At the same time, selective calculus removal using the Er:YAG laser may be more feasible.

The angulation of the application tip to the root surface also has a strong influence on the amount of root substance removed during Er:YAG laser irradiation. Thus the angulation of the application tip is another important factor for decreasing root substance removal.

Supragingival laser scaling of the enamel surface using the Er:YAG laser is contraindicated because it is difficult to achieve complete calculus removal without affecting the underlying enamel. However, in subgingival scaling, the removal of not only calculus but also contaminated cementum may be clinically acceptable to some extent. Further in vitro and in vivo studies are required to determine a suitable combination of laser irradiation settings, such as energy output and pulse rate, in conjunction with the irradiation method, tip angulation, and type of contact tip used that will avoid excessive removal of sound root substance during Er:YAG laser subgingival scaling.

Schwarz et al (2001) reported clinical data of nonsurgical periodontal treatment, comparing Er:YAG laser irradiation with conventional scaling and root planing in a randomized, controlled clinical study using a split-mouth design in 20 patients. Periodontal pockets of 110 teeth with subgingival calculus with moderate to advanced periodontal destruction were treated under local anesthesia with either the Er:YAG laser or scaling and root planing using hand instruments. Er:YAG laser treatment was performed using chisel-type contact tips (1.10×0.50 mm or 1.65×0.50 mm) at the panel setting of 160 mJ/pulse (energy output of 100 and 120 mJ/pulse and energy density of 18.8 and 14.5 J/cm^2 per pulse for 1.10- and 1.65-mm tips, respectively) and 10 Hz with water coolant. The laser treatment was performed in a coronal to apical direction in parallel paths, with the fiber tip inclined 15 to 20 degrees to the root surface. The laser treatment required less time than the scaling and root planing treatment.

At a 6-month posttreatment evaluation, pockets subjected to the laser treatment showed results similar to those subjected to scaling and root planing in terms of reduction of bleeding on probing, probing depth, and clinical attachment level. In particular, the laser group presented a significantly greater reduction of bleeding on probing and improvement of clinical attachment level

than did the scaling and root planing group. Furthermore, the difference in treatment outcomes between laser and hand instrumentation was much more significant in deeper pockets. This can probably be explained by the combined antibacterial effect, reduction of endotoxins, and greater accessibility of laser instrumentation than hand instruments in deep pockets. Schwarz et al (2003) also reported that the clinical attachment gain obtained following nonsurgical Er:YAG laser periodontal treatment was maintained over a 2-year period.

Sculean et al (2004b) compared the effectiveness of an Er:YAG laser to that of an ultrasonic scaler for nonsurgical periodontal treatment. Twenty patients with moderate to advanced periodontal destruction were randomly treated in a split-mouth design. The periodontal sites were treated with a single episode of subgingival debridement using either an ultrasonic instrument or an Er:YAG laser device (energy output of 120 mJ/pulse; energy density of 14.5 J/cm^2 per pulse; 10 Hz) combined with a calculus detection system with fluorescence induced by 655-nm indium-gallium-arsenide-phosphide diode laser radiation (DIAGNOdent pen, KaVo). Six months following treatment, there was a statistically significant improvement in the mean values of bleeding on probing, probing depth, and clinical attachment level in both groups. However, no statistically or clinically significant differences were observed between the treatment modalities.

The effects of the Er:YAG laser as well as the long-term effect of repeated laser treatment must be demonstrated in further randomized controlled trials and a subsequent meta-analysis. With respect to healing after Er:YAG laser scaling, no histologic studies have been reported. Further studies are necessary to clarify the histologic attachment of periodontal tissues to the irradiated root surface in vivo.

The Er:YAG laser also has some shortcomings when used for subgingival scaling. For clinical application in periodontal pockets where the operator cannot visualize the irradiated target, special tips should be designed to facilitate insertion into the periodontal pocket and detection of the presence of dental calculus on the surface because no tactile feedback is achieved. For example, the laser

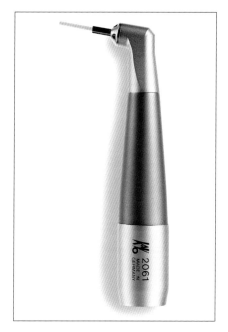

Fig 124a KaVo Key Laser handpiece 2061 for periodontal treatment, which is equipped with a water spray system and fiber tips rotatable through 360 degrees.

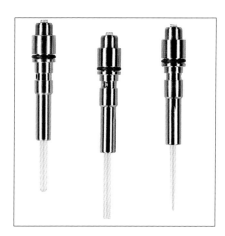

Fig 124b Exchangeable optical prisms for the KaVo Key Laser handpiece 2061 in various sizes for subgingival instrumentation, surgery, and treatment of peri-implantitis.

apparatus for caries detection (DIAGNOdent) has recently been supplemented with a wireless instrument for subgingival calculus detection (DIAGNOdent pen). Also, because Er:YAG laser irradiation causes splashing of water and blood from pockets as a result of explosive ablation, adequate high-speed evacuation by means of not only intraoral suction but also an extraoral evacuation apparatus is required to prevent contamination by blood and water splatter.

Use of the Er:YAG laser for treatment of peri-implantitis may also be a promising field; however, further studies are required to assess application of lasers in implant maintenance therapy.

With the KaVo Key Laser handpiece 2061 (KaVo), the laser energy emerges from an optical prism (Figs 124a and 124b). It is specially developed for treatment in the periodontal pocket. The optical prism is rotatable through 360 degrees and is thus adaptable to the position of the tooth.

Cooling is provided by an integrated water spray system that additionally flushes out the dis-

placed concrement particles. All KaVo laser handpieces are sterilizable and can be easily attached to the coupling of the flexible laser tube.

However, the use of laser apparatuses also has some disadvantages. Laser light interacts with target tissues not only in the contact irradiation mode but also in the noncontact irradiation mode. Therefore, inadvertent irradiation of the patient's eyes, throat, and delicate oral tissues outside the target site may occur during treatment and must be prevented. Particular care must be taken to avoid accidental irradiation of the eyes. The most important precaution in laser surgery is the use of glasses for eye protection. During laser treatment, protective eyewear, specifically blocking the wavelength of the laser in use, must always be worn by the patient, operator, and assistant. The laser beam may be reflected off shiny metal surfaces of dental instruments, such as retractors or mouth mirrors, which can cause accidental irradiation to adjacent tissues.

Use of wet gauze packs occasionally may be useful for protection of the oral tissues surrounding the surgical site from accidental beam impact. In addition, adequate high-speed evacuation is necessary to capture the laser plume, which is a biohazard. Contact with tooth enamel during periodontal treatment should be avoided during CO_2 and Er:YAG laser emission because they easily cause melting or ablation.

There also exists a risk of excessive tissue destruction by direct ablation and thermal side effects on periodontal tissues during irradiation in periodontal pockets. Improper use of lasers could cause further destruction of the intact attachment apparatus at the bottom of pockets as well as excessive ablation of the root surface and gingival walls. A root surface with major thermal damage could render the tissue incompatible for normal cell attachment and healing. Thermal injury to the pulpal tissue and underlying bone tissue would also be concerns with some lasers, especially those exhibiting deep penetration (CO_2 laser and Nd:YAG laser). Therefore, thermal injury must be prevented by the use of proper irradiation conditions and techniques.

Regarding the laser apparatus, development of new laser systems and improvement of currently available laser systems, such as miniaturization of device sizes and advances in performance, are required. Also, new contact probes must be developed because accessibility of contact probes in periodontal pockets is limited by complex root morphology and furcated roots.

The cost of the laser apparatus is still somewhat prohibitory, and this has prevented the spread of laser treatment among general practitioners. However, the price is expected to decrease with developments in laser technology and with increasing demand (for detailed reviews on the use of lasers for periodontal therapy, see Aoki et al, 2004; Schwarz et al, 2008; and the position paper by the Research, Science, and Therapy Committee of the American Academy of Periodontology, 2002).

Air-powered cleaning devices

Air-powered abrasive devices have the unique ability to remove plaque and stain from areas difficult to reach with other instruments, such as narrow interproximal embrasure surfaces, grooves, and crevices. These instruments have been used during the past decade to facilitate the removal of supragingival plaque and stains (eg, Prophy-Jet, Dentsply; Air-Flow, EMS; Prophyflex II, KaVo).

They operate by directing a fine slurry of pressurized air, water, and abrasive particles (sodium bicarbonate) against the tooth surface. The suggested working tip pressure is 55 psi.

The head of the Air-Flow device is the nozzle (Fig 125). It consists of two ducts: an outer ring duct for the water supply and an inner duct for a mixture of air and sodium bicarbonate. At the tip of this concentric nozzle construction, these streams meet in a fine spray, whose precision is appropriate for well-directed treatment.

The ideal distance between the Air-Flow nozzle and the tooth is 3 to 5 mm. The ideal angle between the Air-Flow nozzle and the tooth surface is 30 to 60 degrees toward the incisal edge. This enlarges the surface to be cleaned. The jet that strikes the tooth glances off at the angle of reflection and is captured by a suction tube. The nozzle must be directed at the tooth and used with circular movements. Staining is a cosmetic problem, particularly in smokers and patients who have been rinsing with chlorhexidine. Even severe staining can be efficiently removed with an air polisher (Figs 126a and 126b). Because of the abrasiveness of the powder (sodium bicarbonate), air polishing has been recommended for use only on tooth enamel. Its use on root surfaces and resin composite restorations should be avoided.

Atkinson et al (1984) showed in vitro that 30 seconds' nonstop use of a Prophy-Jet stream directed at a fixed point resulted in a craterlike defect up to $636\,\mu m$ in depth. In contrast, 30 seconds of constant movement over the root surface resulted in a $25\text{-}\mu m$ loss of root substance. Galloway and Pashley (1987) evaluated the amount of root cementum and dentin removed related to exposure time. They found considerable loss of tooth substance after 5 seconds. The loss was strictly related to exposure times from 5 to 60 seconds.

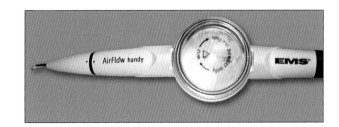

Fig 125 Air-Flow air abrasion handpiece.

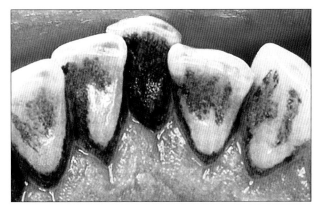

Fig 126a Staining on the lingual surfaces of the mandibular incisors in a heavy smoker before air abrasion.

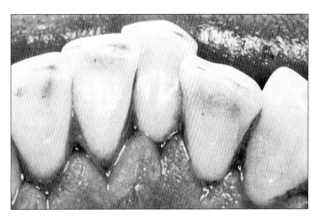

Fig 126b Result after air abrasion.

Horning et al (1987) found that during open flap surgery, 80 μm of root cementum was abraded away after 40 seconds of exposure to the air-powder spray. Petersilka et al (2003a) evaluated defect depth and defect volume after instrumentation with Prophy-Jet using conventional sodium bicarbonate powder for 5, 10, and 20 seconds; a combination of low, medium, and high powder and water settings; distances of 2, 4, and 6 mm; and angulations of 45 and 90 degrees. The results showed that exposure time had the greatest influence on the volume and depth of the resulting defects. Variations in distance affected depth but not volume. The worst (most invasive) combination led to a maximal defect depth of 475 μm within 20 seconds. Again, it must be observed that the thickness of the root cementum on the coronal third of the root ranges from only 30 to 100 μm.

However, a low-abrasive air polishing powder (Cleanpro Prophy Powder, EMS) has been introduced for use in the Air-Flow handpiece. It consists of small, water-soluble, minimally abrasive glycine particles. On approximal surfaces, the use of this low-abrasive powder in the Air-Flow handpiece removed significantly more subgingival plaque biofilms down to a 5-mm probing depth than did curettes in a split-mouth study in maintenance patients (Petersilka et al, 2003c). Similar results were also achieved on buccal and lingual sites within 3 to 5 mm subgingivally (Petersilka et al, 2003b). However, the abrasive loss of tooth substance on root surfaces with long-term use still has to be evaluated, as does the development of root dentin sensitivity and root caries.

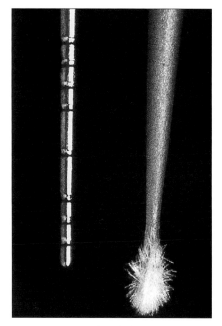 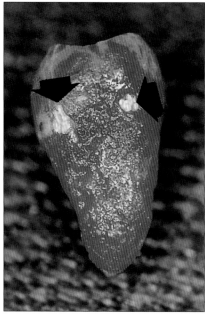 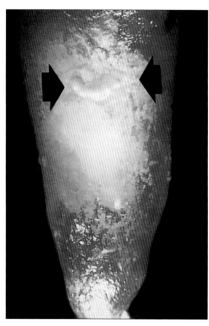

Fig 127 Microbrush *(right)* compared with Williams periodontal probe *(left).* (From Carey and Daly, 2001. Reprinted with permission.)

Fig 128 Dense erythrosin staining on an untreated periodontally involved root surface. *(arrows)* Bur notches. (From Carey and Daly, 2001. Reprinted with permission.)

Fig 129 Debrided root surface showing little erythrosin stain. *(arrows)* Bur notches. (From Carey and Daly, 2001. Reprinted with permission.)

Subgingival Microbrush

Researchers in Australia wondered if a disposable, flexible Microbrush (Microbrush) would provide access and effectively remove subgingival plaque biofilms (Carey and Daly, 2001). To test this hypothesis, they selected 30 periodontally involved teeth scheduled for extraction in 26 adults. There were 14 posterior teeth and 16 anterior teeth. They selected a Microbrush similar in size to a periodontal probe (Fig 127). These brushes come in various sizes and are used in dentistry to apply liquids such as varnishes, etchants, resins, and disclosing solutions.

Prior to extraction, the area was anesthetized, and one proximal surface was cleaned with the Microbrush for 2 minutes. The subgingival surface was rubbed vigorously with the Microbrush. The brush was frequently dipped in saline solution to remove blood and debris. The other proximal surface was untouched and served as the control. The teeth were then carefully extracted, immersed in

2% erythrosin disclosing solution for 10 minutes, rinsed for 5 minutes in running water, and left to air dry.

These root surfaces were examined and photographed under a stereomicroscope. The 30 undebrided proximal surfaces were stained on 100% of the surface. The disclosing solution revealed a thick layer of plaque biofilm (Fig 128). The Microbrush-treated teeth showed an average staining of 16% of the surface, and the staining was thin and discontinuous (Fig 129). Plaque removal with the Microbrush showed no differences between anterior or posterior teeth or between mesial and distal surfaces.

SEM evaluations were also performed. Control surfaces showed thick, organized collections of bacteria. Microbrush-treated surfaces showed variable amounts of debris with no regular structure. The Microbrush was able to remove plaque from the surface of calculus deposits but did not reach areas below the edge of the deposits or in crevices on the deposits. The next step will be a clinical study to determine tissue response to Microbrush debridement.

This study is a new approach to subgingival removal of plaque biofilms using a flexible, disposable, plastic Microbrush. This approach may become a useful adjunct to conventional instrumentation for both initial and maintenance therapy. In addition, a well-motivated and well-trained maintenance patient could use this method together with a bactericidal solution such as 0.1% iodine or triclosan-containing fluoride toothpaste in selected risk pockets as a supplement to debridement and PMTC by dentists and dental hygienists.

CONCLUSIONS

For successful treatment of periodontitis, both supragingival plaque and the subgingival microflora have to be removed and controlled. Subgingival instrumentation can be performed nonsurgically (closed and blindly) or in combination with flap surgery (open and visibly).

The goals of subgingival instrumentation are:

- Removal of attached plaque biofilms and the nonattached microflora and its products from the gingival sulcus and periodontally diseased pockets
- Removal of plaque-retentive factors, particularly calculus
- Minimally invasive root planing without exposure of the root dentin
- Establishment of optimal gingival plaque control by self-care and needs-related intervals of PMTC to prevent subgingival recolonization by microflora

Several studies have shown that complete removal of plaque biofilms and calculus seldom is achieved during nonsurgical instrumentation. Studies have also shown that instrumentation during open flap surgery may fail to remove all biofilms.

However, in spite of the fact that more plaque biofilms remain in deep pockets after nonsurgical therapy than after open flap debridement, the total reduction of the subgingival microflora mostly results in improved periodontal health if excellent gingival plaque control is established through self-care and needs-related intervals of PMTC. The exception may be teeth with grade II and III furcation involvement. The generally good long-term clinical results, even after nonsurgical therapy, are attributable to a combination of effective host response to residual microorganisms and efficient maintenance care.

Hand instruments

Hand instruments are the most frequently used instruments for debridement, scaling, and root planing. During the last few decades, double-ended curettes have dominated the market. The double-ended curette consists of a handle, two shanks, and two curved blades. There are two main groups of curettes: universal and Gracey curettes. In addition, there are some specially designed curettes, such as Syntette curettes and Svärdström approximal curettes.

Advantages of hand instruments

- They provide superior tactile sensitivity from the sharp blade on the root surface compared to all other instruments, which is important for locating calculus and root planing.
- There is a large assortment of instruments for accessibility to difficult-to-reach areas, including deep pockets.
- Mini-bladed curettes provide good adaptation to root morphology.
- Hand instruments do not generate heat and therefore do not require water spray or high-speed evacuation, resulting in better visibility.
- They do not produce an aerosol contaminated by microorganisms from the patient and dental unit water lines.
- Curettes can be used in combination with irrigation with bactericidal solutions (0.1% iodine), and the pocket can be filled with this solution to reduce bacteremia.
- The cost is low, and the instrument may last for 6 months with normal use.

Disadvantages of hand instruments

- Proper blade angulation is required.
- Sharpening of the blade is required.
- Heavy lateral pressure is necessary to achieve calculus removal.
- Hand instruments are more tiring for the clinician.
- Use of hand instruments has greater potential to cause carpal tunnel syndrome or other repetitive motion injuries in the operator.

Ultrasonic scalers

The development of ultrasonic energy in the dental unit is based on one of two concepts: the magnetostrictive effect or the piezoelectric effect. The amplitude of the tip ranges from 10 to 120 µm. That means a total distance of 5 m/s by the tip instruments with 25,000 Hz and 100-µm longitudinal amplitude. The movement can be longitudinal, circular, elliptic, or three-dimensional. The movement of the tip is longitudinal in piezoelectric ultrasonic scalers, while it is elliptic in magnetostrictive scalers. Because of the heat generated, particularly with magnetostrictive instruments, the scalers must be cooled with external or internal water spray.

Advantages of ultrasonic scalers

- Cavitation effectively removes and disrupts plaque biofilms.
- The new assortment of thin and straight as well as curved tips have improved accessibility to deep pockets, root grooves, and grade II and III furcation involvement.
- Pocket irrigation can simultaneously be performed when bactericidal cooling fluid is used.
- Tips do not need sharpening.
- Use of ultrasonic scalers does not require a firm finger rest.
- Their use requires less time than do hand instruments.
- They are used with a light touch.
- Ultrasonic scalers are particularly efficient for gross scaling.

Disadvantages of ultrasonic scalers

- They provide very limited tactile sensitivity of root surfaces and thus are not suitable for root planing.
- High power and strong application force, for example, during gross scaling, will result in advanced loss of root substance.
- Use of an incorrect angulation will result in deep iatrogenic defects.
- They produce a contaminated aerosol, allowing the spread of bacteria as well as viruses from infected patients.
- Water evacuation is required.
- Not all handpieces can be autoclaved.
- Use of ultrasonic scalers may represent a risk in patients with pacemakers.
- Equipment and tips are expensive compared to hand instruments.

Vector system

The Vector scaler is fitted with six piezoceramic disks as an ultrasonic machine instead of the four disks fitted to conventional piezoelectric ultrasonic scalers, making more energy available. The horizontal vibration of the device is converted by a resonating ring into vertical vibration, resulting in a parallel movement of the working tip to the root surface. Furthermore, the energy from the instrument is transmitted to the root surface and the periodontal tissues by a suspension of hydroxyapatite particles and water, comparable to ultrasonic cleaning baths. The particle suspension works like toothpaste, removing deposits and plaque biofilms from even the most difficult areas. Thus, the cleaning and polishing effects on the root surfaces are increased, but root planing will not be achieved.

Advantages of Vector system

- Compared to regular ultrasonic scalers and hand instruments, the subgingival cleaning and polishing effects should be better because of the special piezoelectric ultrasonic technique in combination with the polishing suspension of hydroxyapatite.

- The carbon fiber–reinforced plastic tip is particularly useful for minimally invasive debridement of natural teeth and implants.

Disadvantages of Vector system

- As with ultrasonic scalers, the tactile sensitivity of the instrument on the root surface is very limited, and thus root planing cannot be achieved.
- The effect of long-term use on loss of root substance is unknown.
- The price of the Vector unit is relatively high.

Sonic scalers

Advantages of sonic scalers

- They are efficient for gross scaling.
- Sonic scalers are about half the price of ultrasonic scalers.
- They are easy to connect to the regular air pressure outlet on dental units.

Disadvantages of sonic scalers

- Sonic scalers have more severe iatrogenic effects than do ultrasonic scalers.
- Sonic scalers cannot be used for root planing and minimally invasive debridement.
- The price of a handpiece is considerably higher than that of a curette.

PER-IO-TOR instruments

PER-IO-TOR instruments have been designed to supplement hand instruments, sonic and ultrasonic scalers, rotating diamond burs, and laser instruments. The instrument, inserted in the periodontal pocket against the subgingival plaque biofilm and calculus on the rough root cementum, is designed so that, when the working side faces the root surface, the plaque biofilm and calculus can be scraped off and the rough root cementum planed. When the plaque biofilm and calculus have been removed and the root cementum is planed, the surface parts will contact and rest against the flat faces of the root cementum surface to form load-relieving surfaces that bear the pressure of the tool and restrain the cutting edges. As these parts of the instrument slide along the tooth surface, the cutting edges will not perform any further scraping action, thus preventing removal of any significant degree of root cementum and exposure of the dentin.

Advantages of PER-IO-TOR instruments

- They are specially designed reciprocating instruments that will optimize cleaning and planing of the rough root cementum and prevent further removal of root cementum once the surface is clean and smooth. Therefore, there are grooves with right-angled cutting wedges between smooth plane surfaces.
- Because of this design, the PER-IO-TOR instruments are minimally invasive and especially suitable for debridement and root planing, as well as final scaling.
- The special size, shape, and assortment of instruments, allow access to any area of the diseased and rough root surfaces.
- They are mechanically driven instruments with 1.0- to 1.5-mm reciprocating strokes or rotary strokes, are easy to use, and do not cause ergonomic problems.
- They provide superior tactile sensitivity compared to ultrasonic scalers, sonic scalers, laser instruments, air polishers, and rotating diamond burs.
- The PER-IO-TOR instruments are made in surgical stainless steel and will last for years. If necessary, they can easily be sharpened.
- The price of the PER-IO-TOR instruments and handpiece (Profin) is reasonable.

Disadvantages of PER-IO-TOR instruments

- PER-IO-TOR instruments are not suitable for initial gross scaling in patients with untreated periodontal disease because they are minimally invasive.
- Final scaling may be more time-consuming than it is with the use of the other scaling instruments.

- In teeth with grade II or III furcation involvement, rotating PER-IO-TOR 8R and 9R and ultrasonic scalers with thin, specially designed tips will offer better accessibility than reciprocating PER-IO-TOR instruments.

Perioplaners and Periopolishers

This system is based on a special contra-angle handpiece and different reciprocating tools. One universal curette-shaped instrument with a wedge and one hoe-shaped instrument with an edge are designed for root planing (Perioplaners). Two flat, golf club–shaped diamond-coated instruments (Periopolishers) are designed for instrumentation of the approximal surfaces and two flat diamond-coated instruments are designed for the buccal and lingual surfaces.

Advantages of Perioplaners and Periopolishers

- Use of mechanical reciprocating instruments should result in less ergonomic problems than hand instruments.
- Because both of these instruments are very aggressive, they can be used for gross scaling in untreated patients.

Disadvantages of Perioplaners and Periopolishers

- Studies have shown that both Perioplaners and Periopolishers remove as much root substance per second as rotating diamond-coated burs (about 4 to 8 μm per stroke). Therefore, these instruments are too invasive to be used for debridement and root planing.
- The limited assortment of instruments may provide less accessibility than the great assortment of hand instruments, ultrasonic scalers with extrathin tips, and PER-IO-TOR instruments.

Rotating instruments

Rotating diamond-coated burs provide efficient removal of calculus but can remove damaging levels of root cementum. Use of these invasive instruments should be limited to recontouring of the root.

Advantages of rotating instruments

- They are very efficient for rapid, gross scaling and recontouring of root grooves and grade I or II furcation involvement. However, because of their invasiveness, they should be used supragingivally or during flap surgery when visibility is good, and then only with great caution.
- Their cost is low, and they can be used in the regular handpiece.

Disadvantages of rotating instruments

- Rotating instruments are too invasive to be used for final scaling, debridement, and root planing.
- The instrumentation will result in iatrogenic plaque-retentive horizontal grooves on the root surfaces.

Laser instruments

The process of lasing occurs when an excited atom is stimulated to emit a photon before the process occurs spontaneously. The characteristics of a laser depend on its wavelength. The wavelength affects both the clinical applications and the design of the laser. The lasers most commonly used in dentistry are CO_2, Nd:YAG, and Er:YAG lasers. For nonsurgical scaling, only the Er:YAG laser should be used.

Advantages of laser instruments

- The antimicrobial effect of laser instruments in very deep diseased pockets seems to be greater than that provided by other scaling instruments.
- Laser instruments efficiently remove endotoxins and smear layers from the root surfaces, which may improve healing after instrumentation.
- Studies have shown lasers to have effects on clinical variables and to achieve calculus removal that is similar to those of hand instruments and ultrasonic scalers.

Disadvantages of laser instruments

- The surface is left with an acid-etched appearance microscopically. This fact, in combination with the absence of tactile feedback during use, means that root planing cannot be achieved with laser apparatuses.
- With relatively high energy output, very severe loss of root substance, including craterlike defects (40 to 80 µm deep), can occur. Therefore, the power output must be selected carefully; it is safer to improve the efficacy by modifying pulse repetition and duration than by increasing power.
- Supragingival scaling on enamel surfaces is contraindicated because of the risk for severe ablation of the enamel surface.
- Eye protection with special glasses is necessary for the operator, patient, and assistant.
- The patient's throat and oral tissues outside the target site have to be protected.
- Adequate high-speed evacuation to capture the laser plume is necessary.
- Reflection of the laser beam from shiny metal surfaces has to be avoided.
- The periodontal attachment at the bottom of the pockets may be destroyed.
- Excessive ablation of the root surface and thermal injury of the pulp may occur if laser instruments are misused.
- Laser apparatuses are very expensive.

Air-powered cleaning devices

Air-powered abrasive devices have the unique ability to remove plaque and stains from areas that are difficult to reach with other instruments, such as narrow interproximal embrasure surfaces, grooves, and crevices. They operate by directing a fine slurry of pressurized air, water, and abrasive particles (sodium bicarbonate) against the tooth surface.

Advantages of air-powered cleaning devices

- They provide fast and efficient removal of plaque and staining supragingivally on tooth enamel.
- Low-abrasive powder can be useful for debridement in shallow pockets (5 mm or less).

Disadvantages of air-powered cleaning devices

- Because of the severe abrasiveness of regular powder, they should not be used on root surfaces and resin composite restorations.
- They have a relatively high cost.

Subgingival Microbrushes

Microbrushes, normally used in dentistry to apply liquids such as varnishes and etchants, have been used experimentally to remove subgingival plaque.

Advantages of subgingival Microbrushes

- They can be used for subgingival removal of nonmineralized biofilm from at-risk surfaces in shallow pockets (of 5 mm or less) by a well-motivated and well-instructed patient in combination with an antimicrobial toothpaste.
- Microbrushes are very inexpensive.

Disadvantages of subgingival Microbrushes

- Accessibility in very deep pockets and furcation involvements is limited.
- Semimineralized plaque biofilms cannot be removed.

(For reviews on scaling, root planing, and debridement with different instruments, see Adriaens and Adriaens, 2004; Aoki et al, 2004; Drisko and Lewis, 1996; Oda et al, 2004; Pattison, 1996; and Umeda et al, 2004.)

CHAPTER 2

INITIAL INTENSIVE THERAPY FOR HEALING OF INFECTIOUS INFLAMED PERIODONTAL TISSUES

The optimal goals of periodontal therapy are:

- Elimination of etiologic factors (periopathogenic microflora) and plaque-retentive factors
- Healing of infectious inflamed periodontal tissues
- Repair and regeneration of lost periodontal tissues
- Maintenance of healthy periodontal tissues by needs-related supportive care (secondary prevention) after successful therapy

Years of research and clinical experience have revealed the methods and materials that provide the best chances for predictable healing of sites affected by periodontal disease. A protocol that emphasizes an initial phase of intensive therapy will promote rapid healing of infectious inflamed tissues, thereby reducing the Plaque Formation Rate Index (PFRI). This initial phase is followed by supplemental needs-related therapy to heal any sites with refractory disease or to address aggressive forms of periodontitis (see chapter 3).

ETIOLOGY OF PERIODONTAL DISEASES

Gingivitis and periodontitis are unquestionably caused by microorganisms; that is, both are infectious diseases. These microorganisms colonize the gingival region of the tooth surfaces, supragingivally as well as subgingivally, forming dentogingival plaque, a so-called biofilm. In diseased pockets, microorganisms also grow subgingivally, without attaching to the tooth surfaces, and may invade the periodontal tissues (Frank and Voegel, 1978; Listgarten, 1976; Saglie et al, 1982a, 1982b).

Löe and coworkers (1965) showed that, if dental plaque was allowed to accumulate undisturbed, students with healthy gingiva developed clinical signs of gingivitis within 2 or 3 weeks; on resumption of oral hygiene, the inflammation subsided within a week.

The thickness of the plaque biofilm gradually increased to a maximum after about 10 days. In addition, the assortment of bacteria increased, particularly gram-negative rods and spirochetes. In a 6-week study, Lang and coworkers (1973) showed that no clinical signs of gingival inflammation appeared if plaque was thoroughly removed at least every second day; with less frequent plaque removal, only every third or fourth day, gingivitis developed. Listgarten (1976) found that the thickness of de novo accumulated plaque increased dramatically from the second day to the third and fourth days. Similarly, Bosman and Powell (1977) induced experimental gingivitis in a group of students. If plaque removal was carried out only every third or fifth day, gingival inflammation persisted; however, healing occurred within 7 to 10 days in two groups of students who cleaned their teeth at least every second day.

These studies provided evidence that prevention of gingivitis should be based on plaque control: Thorough mechanical cleaning of all tooth surfaces every second day is more effective than daily cosmetic brushing of the buccal and lingual surfaces that are not at risk.

Experimental animal studies have shown that untreated, plaque-induced gingivitis can eventually progress to periodontitis (Lindhe et al, 1975; Saxe et al, 1967). In humans, although gingivitis is very common, chronic periodontitis develops in a minority of individuals and sites, and aggressive periodontitis develops in fewer than 10%. At the First European Workshop on Periodontology (Lang and Karring, 1994), the consensus was that periodontitis is always preceded by gingivitis. Prevention of gingivitis should also, therefore, prevent periodontitis (for details on the classification and pathogenesis of gingivitis and periodontal diseases, see chapter 5 in volume 3 of this series [Axelsson, 2002]).

Etiologic hypotheses

Three different hypotheses about the etiology of periodontal diseases have been proposed: the nonspecific plaque hypothesis, the ecological plaque hypothesis, and the specific plaque hypothesis.

Nonspecific plaque hypothesis

Since the aforementioned studies of experimental gingivitis and periodontitis were conducted, the nonspecific plaque hypothesis has been the most frequently and successfully tested hypothesis for the prevention and control of gingivitis and periodontitis. It asserts that many of the microorganisms in the heterogenous mixture in the plaque (biofilm) could play a role in the development of gingivitis and periodontal diseases and that these diseases are a result of the overall interaction of the microflora with the host (Theilade, 1986). It also explains why, in longitudinal clinical studies, frequent use of self-care methods for mechanical removal or disruption of the biofilm, supplemented by needs-related professional mechanical tooth-cleaning (PMTC) and subgingival debridement, has been so successful in the prevention and control of gingivitis and periodontitis (Axelsson and Lindhe, 1977, 1981a, 1981b; Axelsson et al, 1991, 2004; Badersten et al, 1981, 1984a, 1984b, 1985a,

1985b, 1985c, 1985d, 1987a, 1987b; Lövdal et al, 1961; Söderholm, 1979; Suomi et al, 1971).

Ecological plaque hypothesis

The ecological plaque hypothesis proposes that a change in a key environmental factor (or factors) will trigger a shift in the balance of the resident plaque microflora and that this change might predispose a site to disease (Marsh, 1994). The occurrence of potentially pathogenic species as minor members of the resident plaque microflora would be consistent with this proposal. Under the conditions that prevail in health, these organisms would be only weakly competitive and might be suppressed by intermicrobial antagonism, so that they would constitute only a small, clinically insignificant percentage of the plaque microflora. Microbial specificity in disease would be attributed to the fact that only certain species are competitive under the altered environmental conditions.

It is a basic tenet of microbial ecology that a major change to an ecosystem produces a corresponding disturbance in the stability of the resident microbial community. With respect to the etiology of periodontal diseases, this may be exemplified by the following sequences: Undisturbed gingival plaque gradually results in gingivitis, manifested by edema of the gingival margin (pseudopocket formation) and secretion of gingival crevicular fluid. The resultant improved nutritional conditions and lowered redox potential in the gingival sulcus favor subgingival growth of gram-negative anaerobic microorganisms, including the most important periopathogens (Fig 130).

The ecological plaque hypothesis explains why surgical elimination of pockets, supported by excellent control of gingival plaque in the subsequent maintenance program, is a successful method for treatment of periodontal diseases (Axelsson and Lindhe, 1981b; Lindhe and Nyman, 1984; Nyman et al, 1975; Rosling et al, 1976a, 1976b; Westfelt et al, 1983b). On the other hand, periodontal surgery without well-maintained gingival plaque control will accelerate the progression of lost periodontal tissues (Nyman et al, 1977).

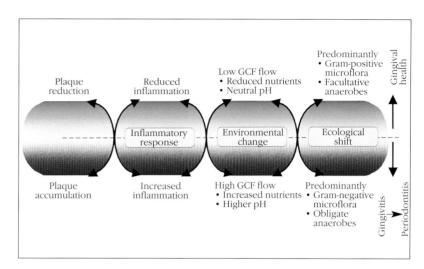

Fig 130 Ecological plaque hypothesis and the prevention of periodontal disease. (Modified from Marsh, 1994.)

Specific plaque hypothesis

The specific plaque hypothesis proposes that, of the diverse collection of microorganisms that constitute the resident plaque microflora, only a very limited number are actively involved in disease. This hypothesis, however, fails to explain satisfactorily those occasions when disease is diagnosed in the apparent absence of putative pathogens or when pathogens are present at sites with no evidence of disease.

There is a consensus that *Porphyromonas gingivalis (Pg)*, *Aggregatibacter actinomycetemcomitans (Aa)*, and *Tannerella forsythia (Tf)*, formerly known as *Bacteroides forsythus*, in particular, as well as *Prevotella intermedia (Pi)* and *Treponema denticola (Td)*, should be considered true periopathogens, strongly correlated to the etiology of periodontal diseases (American Academy of Periodontology, 1996). Both *Pg* and *Aa* are regarded as exogenic, transmissible periopathogens, and *Tf*, *Pi*, and *Td* are considered to be opportunistic bacteria.

Several studies have shown a relationship between *Aa* and aggressive "early-onset" periodontitis. A prospective study (Machtei et al, 1997) showed that periodontal pockets containing *Tf* exhibited seven times higher risk for further loss of periodontal attachment than did *Tf*-negative

sites. It has also been shown that *Aa* and *Pg* in particular may invade the periodontal soft tissues (Madianos et al, 1996; Sandros et al, 1994; Sreenivasan et al, 1993), which may partly explain why diseased periodontal pockets sometimes fail to heal when treated by nonsurgical subgingival debridement alone but may respond to mechanical removal of the subgingival biofilm in combination with administration of antibiotics.

Socransky et al (1998) have shown that bacterial species exist in complexes in subgingival plaque biofilms. The data were derived from 13,261 subgingival plaque samples taken from the mesial aspect of each tooth in 185 adult subjects. Each sample was individually analyzed for the presence of 40 subgingival species using checkerboard DNA-DNA hybridization. Associations were sought among species using cluster analysis and community ordination techniques. Five major complexes were consistently observed (Fig 131).

The first group (the red complex) consists of *Tf*, *Pg*, and *Td*, which are closely related to the etiology of periodontal diseases. The second group (the orange complex) consists of a closely related core group, including members of the *Fusobacterium nucleatum* and *Fusobacterium periodonticum* subspecies, *Pi*, *Prevotella nigrescens*, and *Peptostreptococcus micros*. Species associated

87

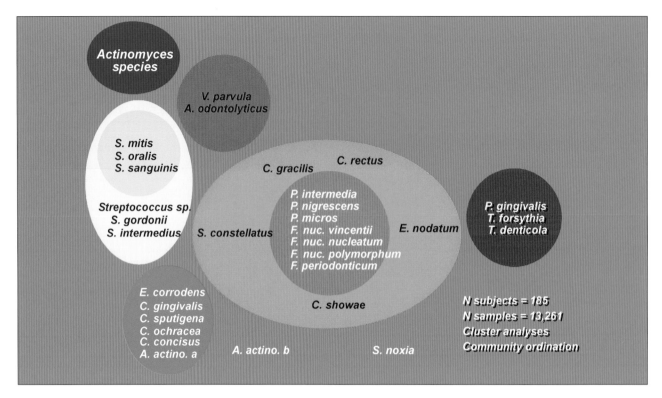

Fig 131 Associations among subgingival species, derived from checkerboard DNA-DNA hybridization analysis of subgingival plaque samples. (From Socransky et al, 1998. Reprinted with permission.)

with this group included *Eubacterium nodatum*, *Campylobacter gracilis*, *Campylobacter rectus*, *Campylobacter showae*, and *Streptococcus constellatus*. The third group (the yellow complex) consists of *Streptococcus sanguis*, *Streptococcus oralis*, *Streptococcus mitis*, *Streptococcus gordonii*, and *Streptococcus intermedius*. The fourth group (the green complex) comprises *Capnocytophaga gingivalis*, *Capnocytophaga sputigena*, *Capnocytophaga ochracea*, *Campylobacter concisus*, *Eikenella corrodens*, and *Aa* serotype a. The fifth group (the blue and purple complexes) consists of *Veillonella parvula*, *Actinomyces odontolyticus*, and other *Actinomyces* species. *Aa* serotype b, *Selenomonas noxia*, and *Actinomyces naeslundii* genospecies 2 (*Actinomyces viscosus*) were outliers with little relation to each other and the five major complexes.

The first (red) complex related strikingly to clinical measures of periodontal disease, particularly probing depth and bleeding on probing (Socransky et al, 1998). Figure 132, from a study by Ximénez-Fyvie et al (2000) of 22 periodontally healthy subjects and 23 subjects with periodonti-

tis, shows the amount and distribution of microbial complexes supragingivally and subgingivally.

According to the specific plaque hypothesis as well as the ecological plaque hypothesis, there should also be differences in the subgingival microflora of healthy pockets, shallow pockets, and deep diseased pockets. In a study by Socransky et al (1991), the subgingival profiles of deep diseased periodontal sites were compared with healthy sites in the same individuals. Statistically significant differences were found in the mean subgingival counts of many species, particularly for species in the red and orange complexes, between the healthy and diseased sites in subjects with advanced periodontitis. Moreover, there were marked differences, for virtually all species examined, between periodontally healthy sites in a group of periodontally healthy subjects and periodontally healthy sites in subjects with chronic periodontitis. The differences were most marked for species in the orange and red complexes. Thus, healthy sites in periodontitis-susceptible subjects may be at far greater risk for future de-

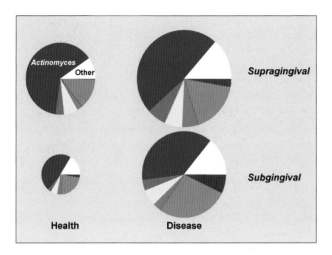

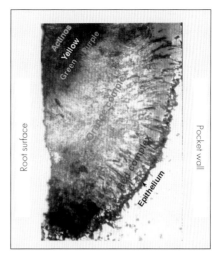

Fig 132 Mean percentage DNA probe counts of microbial groups in supragingival and subgingival plaque samples from periodontally healthy subjects and subjects with periodontitis. The species are classified into seven microbial groups based on the description of Socransky et al (1998). The areas of the pies have been adjusted to reflect the mean total counts at each of the sample locations. The percentages of red, orange, and blue (*Actinomyces*) species in healthy and diseased subjects are significantly different ($P <$ .001), and the green complex species differ ($P <$ .05) after the data are adjusted for seven comparisons. (From Ximenez-Fyvie et al, 2000. Reprinted with permission.)

Fig 133 Histologic section of human subgingival dental plaque. The tooth surface is to the left and the epithelial lining of the periodontal pocket is to the right. Bacterial plaque attached to the tooth surface is evident toward the upper left of the section, while a second zone of organisms can be observed lining the periodontal pocket wall. The suspected location of species in the different complexes has been indicated (toluidine blue–methylene blue stain; original magnification ×400). (Courtesy of Dr M. Listgarten. From Socransky and Haffajee, 2005. Reprinted with permission.)

velopment of periodontitis than healthy sites in periodontally healthy subjects.

Species that make up the different complexes also appear to be distributed differently at different regions of the periodontal pocket or sulcus and in the plaque biofilm (Fig 133). The red complex seems to be located in the most apical surface of the biofilm and in direct contact with the pocket wall (Socransky and Haffajee, 2005).

In addition to local factors, there are also important modifying factors unique to each host that may markedly affect the subgingival biofilm composition. For example, Socransky et al (2000) found that there was a significantly elevated amount of the red complex species (*Pg, Tf,* and *Td*) and seven members of the orange complex in sites with probing depths greater than 6 mm among subjects who tested positive for polymorphism of the proinflammatory cytokines interleukin 1α and interleukin 1β, compared to the amount found in subjects who tested negative.

It has also been shown that subjects who are obese (body mass index greater than 35) exhibit a significantly higher percentage of sites with plaque and bleeding on probing, as well as significantly greater mean probing depth and mean attachment level, than do subjects who are not obese. Obesity is also associated with increased counts and proportions of certain periopathogens, including *Tf* (Socransky and Haffajee, 2005).

On the other hand, most studies have shown no significant differences in the prevalence of periopathogens in smokers and nonsmokers, in spite of several studies showing that smokers exhibit significantly more loss of periodontal support than do nonsmokers (Preber et al, 1992; Stoltenberg et al, 1993).

The geographic location may also influence the composition of the subgingival microflora. Haffajee et al (2004) examined the composition of the subgingival microflora in subjects with chronic periodontitis from four different countries: Brazil, Chile, Sweden, and the United States. The data indicated marked differences among the four populations in the proportions of 39 test species, particularly red complex species, among the four subject groups. No significant difference was detected among the four groups in the proportions of *Tf*, although this was the dominant red complex species in Swedish subjects. On the other hand, Swedish subjects exhibited significantly lower levels of *Pg* and *Td* than did the other three populations. There were no significant differences among groups in terms of clinical features, although the racial and ethnic backgrounds of the subjects differed, and the percentage of current smokers ranged from 2% in the Brazilians to 62% in the Swedish subjects.

Differences in the subgingival microbiota of subjects with comparable levels of disease in different geographic locations could affect therapeutic outcomes. It is likely that subjects with different microbial profiles will respond differently to a given periodontal therapy. In addition, these microbial differences among subjects may partly explain the differences in disease severity in different regions of the world (Van Winkelhoff et al, 2005; for review, see Rylev and Kilian, 2008).

Microbiologic testing

For the past few decades, anaerobic culture has been regarded as the gold standard for evaluation of the subgingival periopathogenic microflora. The advantages are that unexpected species may be detected and antibiotic sensitivity or resistance can be evaluated. The main disadvantages are that not all the subgingival microflora are cultivable and, in order to be cultured, the sampled bacterial species must be viable.

The most recent and promising techniques for detection of periopathogens are the nucleic acid probe assays, which use a piece of DNA or RNA—a whole genomic probe, a cloned probe, or a synthetic oligonucleotide probe—to hybridize to complementary nucleic acid sequences in the target microorganisms.

The advantage of these techniques is that the microbial cells in the samples need not be viable. However, to date, the techniques do not allow an-

tibiotic sensitivity testing, and the range of species identified is limited by the number of DNA probes currently available. With the new so-called checkerboard DNA-DNA hybridization technology, up to 40 different species in up to 28 teeth per subject have been evaluated. Chairside DNA probe tests are now available.

From a cost-effectiveness aspect, there is general agreement that microbiologic tests for periodontal pathogens are indicated only for those patients in certain categories: patients exhibiting aggressive or refractory periodontitis; patients about to undergo extensive prosthetic, implant, or regenerative therapy; and patients susceptible to cardiovascular diseases.

Role of herpesviruses

During the last decade, an increased interest has been focused on the role of viruses as an etiopathogenic factor in cooperation with periopathogenic microbiota, particularly in subjects with sites exhibiting aggressive periodontitis. Although specific infectious agents are of key importance in the development of periodontitis, it is unlikely that a single agent or even a small group of pathogens is the sole cause or modulator of this heterogenous disease. Since the mid-1990s, herpesviruses have emerged as putative pathogens in various types of periodontal disease (Contreras and Slots, 2000). In particular, human cytomegalovirus and Epstein-Barr virus seem to play important roles in the etiopathogenesis of severe types of periodontitis.

Genomes of the two herpesviruses occur at high frequency in progressive periodontitis in adults, localized and generalized aggressive (juvenile) periodontitis, human immunodeficiency virus–associated periodontitis, acute necrotizing ulcerative gingivitis, periodontal abscesses, and some rare types of advanced periodontitis associated with medical disorders (Slots, 2002; Saygun et al, 2004b). Human cytomegalovirus infects periodontal monocytes, macrophages, and T lymphocytes, and Epstein-Barr virus infects periodontal B lymphocytes. Herpesvirus-infected inflammatory cells release tissue-destroying cytokines and may have diminished ability to defend against bacterial challenge. Herpesvirus-associated periodontal sites also tend to harbor elevated levels of periopathogenic bacteria (Slots, 2002; Saygun et al, 2004a).

Prolonged periods of latency interspersed with periods of active herpesvirus infection may in part be responsible for the burstlike episodes of periodontitis disease progression. Tissue tropism of herpesvirus infections may also explain the localized pattern of tissue destruction in most types of periodontitis. Frequent reactivation of periodontal herpesviruses may account for the rapid periodontal breakdown in some patients who exhibit little dental plaque. The absence of a herpesvirus infection or of viral reactivation may explain why some individuals carry periopathogenic bacteria while still maintaining periodontal health.

Among the many arguments supporting the involvement of herpesviruses in human periodontal disease are the following observations:

- Herpesvirus-positive periodontitis lesions harbor increased levels of periopathogenic bacteria.
- There exists an apparent association between active infection with human cytomegalovirus and progressive periodontitis.
- An association between herpesviruses and acute necrotizing ulcerative gingivitis has been demonstrated.
- Periodontal inflammatory cells contain nucleic acid sequences of herpesviruses.
- Infection of periodontal inflammatory cells with herpesvirus has the potential to profoundly alter the host defense.
- Herpesviruses have the potential to increase the expression of tissue-damaging cytokines and chemokines in periodontal inflammatory and connective tissue cells.

(For a detailed review on the role of herpesviruses as an etiopathogenic factor for periodontal diseases, see Slots, 2005.)

In conclusion, analysis of clinical and laboratory data indicates that the etiology of periodontal diseases is not satisfactorily explained by the nonspecific plaque hypothesis, the ecological plaque hypothesis, or the specific plaque hypothesis alone but rather is explained by a combination of all three hypotheses as well as viral in-volvement. All of these factors must be taken into account if efficient causative periodontal therapy is to be achieved (for details on the etiology of periodontal diseases, see volume 3 of this series [Axelsson, 2002] and Socransky and Haffajee, 2005).

METHODS AND MATERIALS FOR INITIAL INTENSIVE THERAPY

Among the presently available methods to prevent periodontal diseases, dental plaque control is regarded as the first choice because it is directed toward the elimination of the etiologic factors of gingivitis and periodontitis, namely, the pathogenic microflora that colonizes the tooth surfaces. Studies in human have shown that high-quality plaque control can prevent and control gingivitis and periodontitis in children as well as adults (for review, see Axelsson, 1994, 1998, 2004).

Plaque control can be achieved through mechanical or chemical methods of self-care or professionally by dentists or dental hygienists. Plaque control programs based on needs-related combinations of these methods are, to date, the most successful means for prevention and control of gingivitis and periodontitis.

For successful healing of infectious inflamed tissues, the following methods and materials for initial intensive therapy may be integrated, based on the individual's needs:

- Mechanical plaque control by self-care
- PMTC
- Chemical plaque control (self-care and professional)
- Minimally invasive scaling, root planing, and debridement
- Early extraction of untreatable teeth and elimination of plaque-retentive factors

Mechanical plaque control by self-care

The effectiveness of self-care mechanical plaque control depends on the patient's motivation, knowledge, and manual dexterity; the quality of oral hygiene instructions; and the type of oral hygiene aids used. Many oral hygiene aids are available; the clinician should assess the individual needs of the patient and recommend appropriate aids.

Procedures

Toothbrushing is the most widely used mechanical means of personal plaque control throughout the world. Enthusiastic use of the toothbrush is not, however, synonymous with a high standard of oral hygiene. The toothbrush has very limited access to the wide approximal surfaces of the molars and premolars. Clinical, visual verification of plaque removal by toothbrushing does not mean that the bacteria have been removed completely from the tooth surfaces.

Different methods have been recommended to systematize the toothbrushing procedure. In recent decades, the Bass method (Bass, 1954) has been the most frequently recommended. Proper use of the Bass method twice daily can prevent the formation of supragingival plaque on buccal and lingual surfaces accessible to the toothbrush; furthermore, dental plaque can be removed at least 1 mm subgingivally (Waerhaug, 1981b; for review on the effectiveness of manual toothbrushes, see van der Weijden and Hioe, 2005).

However, studies comparing the plaque-removing effect of different toothbrushing methods have shown that, with all methods, the effect on the approximal tooth surfaces is very limited, particularly in the molar and premolar regions (Gjermo and Flötra, 1970). Therefore, toothbrushing must be supplemented with special interproximal toothcleaning aids, such as dental floss or tape, toothpicks, and interdental brushes. Electric toothbrushes also have been shown to be very effective plaque control aids, particularly in patients with low dexterity, persons with disabilities, and young children (for review, see van der Weijden et al, 1998).

On the approximal surfaces of molars and premolars, use of flat, fluoridated dental tape combined with a fluoride toothpaste is recommended for children and young adults. By applying the so-called rubbing technique, either holding the tape by hand or in a special holder, the patient can remove plaque 2 mm subgingivally on the approximal surfaces of the molars (Waerhaug, 1981a).

It has also been shown in vivo that a pointed, triangular toothpick inserted interproximally can maintain a plaque-free region 2 to 3 mm subgingivally (Mörch and Waerhaug, 1956). The resilience of the gingival papilla allows plaque removal apical to the subgingival margins of restorations, which are surfaces at risk for recurrent caries (Figs 134a and 134b). Subgingival removal of interproximal dental plaque is likely to be more decisive than supragingival plaque control for prevention of periodontitis. Therefore, a fluoridated, pointed, triangular toothpick is a particularly suitable oral hygiene aid for approximal toothcleaning in adults with accessible interdental spaces (Fig 135). The best time to apply the cleaning power of toothpaste as a fluoride vehicle is just as the gingival papilla is depressed.

For individuals with advanced periodontal disease, with wide interdental spaces and particularly with exposed root surfaces, interdental brushes are recommended. Unfortunately, most interdental brushes are circular in cross section. Their effectiveness would probably be enhanced if the brush shape were triangular instead of circular (Figs 136a and 136b). Other special supplementary oral hygiene aids include interdental toothbrushes for tipped or rotated teeth, lighted mouth mirrors for self-diagnosis, Super Floss (Oral-B) for cleaning around fixed partial denture pontics, and tongue scrapers. Special self-care aids for those with physical disabilities are also available (Fig 137).

A fundamental principle of any preventive effort is that the maximum positive effect is achieved where the risk for disease is greatest. The patient has the greatest chance of being able to see positive results in his or her hygiene efforts if the person concentrates initially on key-risk teeth and key-risk surfaces. For example, in a toothbrushing population, the maximum effect may be seen at the approximal surfaces of the molars and premolars. However, interdental cleaning is practically nonexistent and not an established habit in most countries. Thus, in toothbrushing populations, needs-related toothcleaning is currently not practiced. The adult patient today tends to disrupt dental plaque principally from those tooth sur-

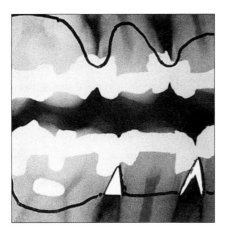

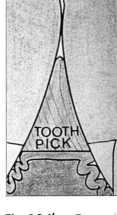

Fig 134a Bitewing radiograph of a 50-year-old Scandinavian. The location of the gingival margin and papillae is marked. Placement of two pointed (wedge-shaped and triangular) toothpicks is illustrated.

Fig 134b Triangular pointed toothpick inserted interdentally. Delivery of fluoride from toothpaste is also enhanced by depression of the gingival papilla. (Illustration by J. Waerhaug, courtesy of the University of Oslo.)

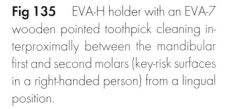

Fig 135 EVA-H holder with an EVA-7 wooden pointed toothpick cleaning interproximally between the mandibular first and second molars (key-risk surfaces in a right-handed person) from a lingual position.

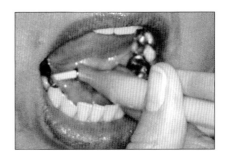

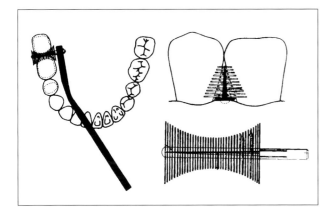

Fig 136a Tailor-made interdental brush as it should look.

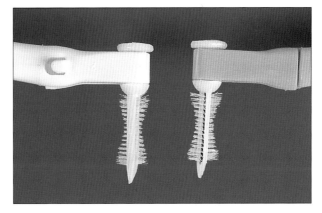

Fig 136b Tailor-made interdental brush shown in long section from the back *(left)* and front *(right)*. The flat, smooth back side presses down on the buccal and lingual papillae in the posterior teeth, thereby facilitating 2- to 3-mm subgingival removal of plaque biofilms. The different lengths of the bristles optimize the accessibility and cleaning effect of the line angles. The pointed triangular tip facilitates entry into interproximal spaces.

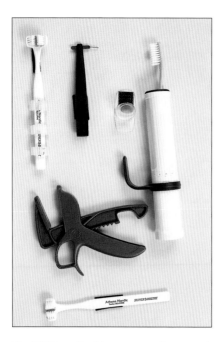

Fig 137 Oral hygiene aids specially designed for elderly or physically disabled persons with poor manual dexterity.

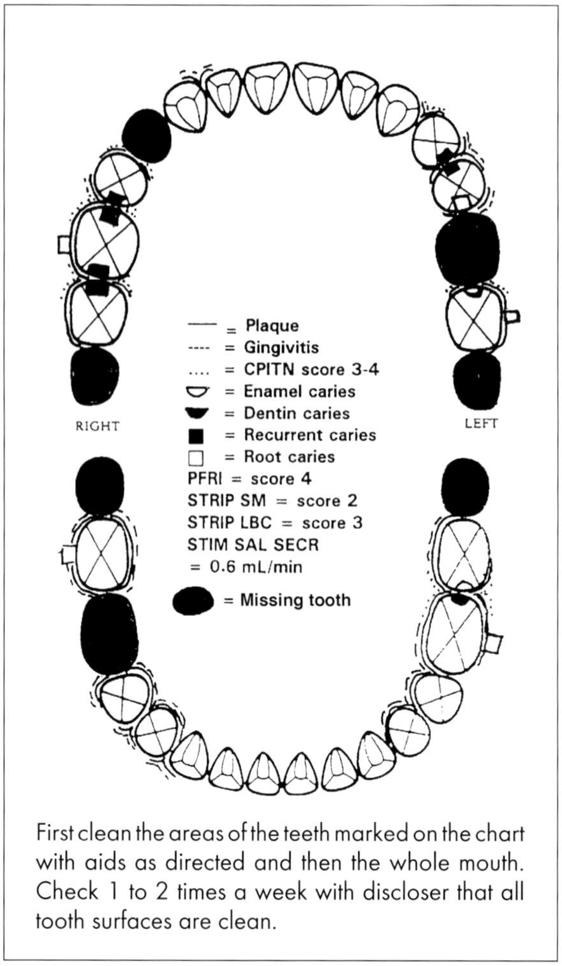

— = Plaque
---- = Gingivitis
.... = CPITN score 3-4
▽ = Enamel caries
▼ = Dentin caries
■ = Recurrent caries
□ = Root caries
PFRI = score 4
STRIP SM = score 2
STRIP LBC = score 3
STIM SAL SECR
= 0.6 mL/min

⬤ = Missing tooth

RIGHT   LEFT

First clean the areas of the teeth marked on the chart with aids as directed and then the whole mouth. Check 1 to 2 times a week with discloser that all tooth surfaces are clean.

Fig 138 Sample toothcleaning chart. (CPITN) Community Periodontal Index of Treatment Needs; (SM) *Streptococcus mutans*; (LBC) *Lactobacillus* count; (STIM SAL SECR) salivary secretion rate.

faces that are least susceptible to disease (ie, facial and lingual surfaces).

Patient motivation

The first condition for successful establishment of needs-related toothcleaning habits is a well-motivated, well-informed, and well-instructed patient. *Motivation* is defined as readiness to act or the driving force behind a person's actions. Greater responsibility has been described as the motivating factor of longest duration. People's actions are also governed by the needs they feel they have. Therefore, training the patient in self-diagnosis is of great importance.

In this context, risk profiles (Axelsson, 1998, 2002; Lang and Tonetti, 2003; see also chapter 5) and a toothcleaning chart (Axelsson, 1998, 2004) are useful tools (Fig 138). On the basis of the joint (patient-professional) observations of disease factors outlined on the risk profile and the toothcleaning chart, the PFRI (Axelsson, 1991), and the location of plaque in the patient's mouth, the patient should be encouraged to make suggestions about the choice of oral hygiene aids and, above all, the order of priorities for cleaning.

Thereafter, it is extremely important that the sharing of responsibilities be discussed. The primary responsibility of the patient is daily care of his or her teeth. The necessary oral hygiene methods should be specified. When the sharing of responsibilities is complete, a "contract" could be drawn up and signed by the parties involved. An agreement that an individual has put his or her name to is more emotionally binding than a hasty verbal affirmative.

However, even with such an agreement, there is a high risk that these habits will not become firmly established. When new oral hygiene habits are established, they should be linked firmly to preestablished habits. The new habit should always be carried out immediately prior to the established habit because the risk that the older habit will not be performed is minimal.

This principle of behavioral science is called the *linking method* and has been described in a dental context (Weinstein and Getz, 1978). If the patient has irregular oral hygiene habits, an interview should reveal already established habits that, in terms of frequency and point in time during the day, happen to coincide well with the proposed oral hygiene routine. According to the linking method, oral hygiene should be scheduled immediately prior to the patient's daily routine. For example, needs-related toothcleaning in patients with well-established daily toothbrushing habits should start with interproximal cleaning in the molar and premolar regions immediately before use of the toothbrush (for details on plaque formation and self-care methods of mechanical plaque control, see chapters 1 and 2 in volume 4 [Axelsson, 2004]).

Professional mechanical plaque control

PMTC is the selective removal of plaque—not only supragingivally but also 1 to 3 mm subgingivally—from *all* tooth surfaces, using mechanically driven instruments and fluoride prophylaxis paste. It is performed by specially trained personnel, such as a dental hygienist or dentist. In essence, the term *professional gingival plaque removal (control)* may more accurately describe this procedure.

The buccal, lingual, and occlusal surfaces of teeth are generally at low risk or no risk for the development of destructive periodontal diseases. Hence, prophylaxis or polishing with a rotating rubber cup and prophylaxis paste that is primarily aimed at these surfaces should not be regarded as

PMTC. If calculus and deep subgingival plaque biofilms are also removed, the procedure is usually referred to as *scaling* or *debridement* (see chapter 1).

Procedures

Axelsson and Lindhe (1974, 1978, 1981a) described the use of PMTC in children and adults and recommended using the following materials for these procedures:

- Plaque-disclosing pellets or tablets
- Profin contra-angle handpiece (a modification of the EVA prophylaxis contra-angle handpiece, Dentatus) and reciprocating triangular pointed tips
- Prophylaxis contra-angle handpiece and rotating rubber cup
- Fluoride-containing prophylaxis paste (medium abrasive)
- Syringe for injecting the prophylaxis paste interproximally

Because PMTC must be directed to the tooth surfaces normally neglected by the patient, disclosure of the accumulated dental plaque is the first step in this technique. Significant plaque growth is often found in the mandibular lingual embrasures of the molars and premolars (Fig 139). Plaque is almost always present in the interproximal spaces if continuous plaque is visible in the line angles, and this can be verified by probing.

A disposable syringe facilitates the application of fluoride prophylaxis paste to the interproximal spaces. Approximal application should always be started from the lingual aspect of the mandibular teeth. This is a rational means of applying the fluoride prophylaxis paste to all approximal surfaces. When paste is already applied to the surfaces requiring maximum attention, mechanical cleaning can be carried out very quickly (Fig 140).

A specially designed prophylaxis contra-angle handpiece (Profin) with reciprocating V-shaped flexible tips or triangular pointed tips is used for interproximal PMTC. The tips are self-steering and reciprocating with 1.0- to 1.5-mm strokes (Fig 141). When entering the interproxi-

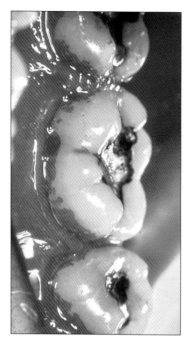

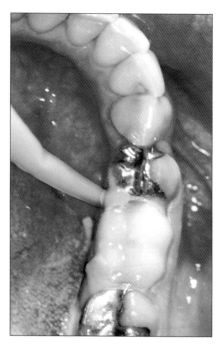

Fig 139 Typical pattern of disclosed plaque on the lingual and approximal surfaces of the posterior mandibular teeth in a patient with poor oral hygiene.

Fig 140 Syringed application of fluoride prophylaxis paste.

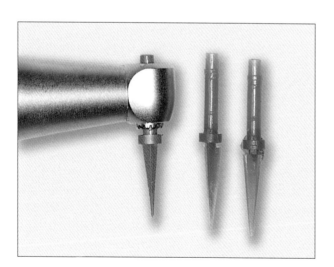

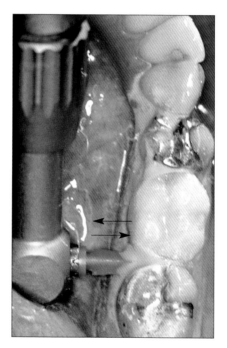

Fig 141 Profin Prophy contra-angle handpiece and V-shaped, pointed, flexible plastic tips.

Fig 142 Needs-related PMTC always commences from the lingual surfaces of the mandibular molars. *(arrows)* Direction of movement.

mal space, the tip will have a 10-degree coronal angle until the papilla is pressed down. The resilience of the papilla will result in an expected cleaning effect 2 to 3 mm subgingivally. A suitable speed for the contra-angle handpiece is approximately 7,000 rpm (15,000 strokes per minute or 250 strokes per second). The direction of the tip should continually be adjusted vertically and horizontally to reach the entire approximal surface. At the same time, fluoride prophylaxis paste is applied to all instrumented surfaces.

PMTC should always commence from the lingual surface of the mandibular molars (Fig 142). When the approximal surfaces have been carefully instrumented from the more easily accessible lingual side, they are then instrumented from the buccal side; this is followed by cleaning of the maxillary interproximal surfaces, lingual embrasures, and buccal surfaces. A regular prophylaxis contra-angle handpiece and rotating rubber cup, combined with application of the same prophylaxis paste, are recommended for PMTC on lingual and buccal surfaces. Hand instruments, such as curettes, may also be used to remove partly mineralized plaque in the gingival sulcus as well as more deeply located subgingival plaque biofilms (see chapter 1).

The frequency of PMTC should be based on individual needs to maximize its cost effectiveness.

Preventive effects

Experimentally, it has been shown that after a single PMTC, the volume of gingival exudate decreases continuously during the first 24 to 28 hours and does not regain the preexperimental level until 1 week later (Gwinnett et al, 1975). Three sessions of PMTC, at 2-day intervals, will normally induce healing of inflamed gingivae within 1 week. Indirectly, this results in a reduction in plaque formation rate. Studies have shown that the reaccumulation rate of gingival plaque is directly correlated to the degree of gingival inflammation (Axelsson, 1987; Ramberg et al, 1995) and the quantity of gingival exudate (Saxton, 1975). Therefore, frequent initial PMTC, followed up at needs-related intervals in the maintenance program, enhances the patient's own oral hygiene efforts by removal of

mature, partially mineralized plaque and reduces the rate of formation of new plaque.

The fluoride ions in prophylaxis paste gain access to the cleaned approximal surfaces, even subgingivally, increasing the potential for remineralization of enamel caries and root caries on these key-risk surfaces. This reduces the risk for future plaque-retentive factors such as secondary caries, restoration overhangs, and unfinished subgingival margins.

PMTC may also be expected to have a strong patient-motivating effect if it is carried out in a needs-related fashion, similar to the oral hygiene procedures proposed earlier. The patient experiences PMTC as a positive treatment form and attempts to maintain the feeling of cleanliness with his or her own efforts (Glavind, 1977).

In contrast, so-called prophylaxis or polishing with only a rotating rubber cup and prophylaxis paste on the nonrisk buccal and lingual surfaces cleaned daily by the patient by toothbrushing is a waste of time and will only discourage the patient.

After PMTC, re-formation of perceptible complex plaque in the dentogingival region is normally retarded for several days, compared to about 1 to 2 days after oral hygiene measures carried out by the patient. PMTC should completely remove supragingival plaque from all tooth surfaces and plaque to at least 1 to 3 mm subgingivally; ie, it provides gingival plaque control.

Frequent PMTC also influences the composition of the subgingival microflora and reduces the number of periopathogens (Dahlén et al, 1992; Hellström et al, 1996; Katsanoulas et al, 1992; McNabb et al, 1992; Ximénez-Fyvie et al, 2000). After subgingival root surface instrumentation, frequent PMTC can prevent recolonization by subgingival microflora (Magnusson et al, 1984; Mousquès et al, 1980). Ximénez-Fyvie et al (2000) showed that frequent PMTC during a 3-month period after a single subgingival debridement resulted in a subgingival microbial profile comparable to that observed in periodontal health. This profile was still maintained at the final examinations 9 months after completion of therapy.

PMTC has favorable effects on periodontitis, particularly in patients with moderately deep pockets (4 to 6 mm). A number of studies have shown that frequent PMTC sessions with no prior subgingival scaling can lead to a reduction in the probing depth, in addition to a gradual decrease in the number of subgingival microflora (Dahlén et al, 1992; Hellström et al, 1996). These favorable results may be attributed to the repeated 2- to 3-mm subgingival plaque removal approximally accomplished by the PMTC. In contrast, self-care methods of supragingival plaque control conceivably have little effect on the subgingival microflora of deep periodontal pockets.

After initial subgingival instrumentation (scaling, root planing, and debridement), even more significant results should be achieved. In a selected group of patients with advanced periodontitis, Badersten et al (1984b) compared the effect of one session of subgingival scaling and root planing with three sessions, at 1-month intervals, in a 24-month split-mouth study. After the initial instrumentation of single-rooted teeth, the patients were recalled for repeated oral hygiene education and PMTC at intervals based on individual need. The initial probing depths varied from 2.5 to 11.0 mm.

The results were evaluated by recording plaque scores, bleeding on probing, probing depths, and probing attachment levels. During the final 15 months of the 24-month experimental period, no further changes of the recorded variables were noted. No differences in results were observed between the effects of single and repeated instrumentation. Thus, it appears that deep periodontal pockets in incisors, canines, and premolars may be successfully treated by a single initial session of meticulous subgingival instrumentation together with adequate gingival plaque control. The results also suggest that subgingival recolonization by microorganisms during the healing phase, which causes recurrence of disease, may not be a major clinical problem if high-quality gingival plaque control is established.

In a more recent study, Wennström et al (2005) showed that a single full-mouth ultrasonic debridement resulted in similar positive results on probing depth and attachment gain as quadrant scaling and root planing in patients with chronic periodontitis—and was much less time consuming.

Thus, after a single session of meticulous scaling, root planing, and debridement, avoiding aggressive removal of the root cementum, the health of the periodontal tissues can be maintained by excellent gingival plaque control, which includes self-care supplemented by PMTC at needs-related intervals. The need for repeated subgingival scaling should be regarded as an unfavorable response to treatment (for details on PMTC, see Axelsson, 2004; for a systematic review of studies based on professional mechanical plaque removal, see Needleman et al, 2005).

Chemical plaque control

Chemical plaque control can be achieved through self-care or professionally. By far the most efficient plaque control programs are those combining mechanical and chemical methods: self-care supplemented by needs-related PMTC and professional chemical plaque control (PCPC). For example, in mechanical plaque control achieved through self-care, the toothpaste used usually contains not only an abrasive agent but also antiplaque or antimicrobial agents such as sodium lauryl sulfate, stannous fluoride, triclosan plus zinc citrate, triclosan plus copolymers, triclosan plus pyrophosphate, or chlorhexidine gluconate (CHX).

Antiplaque and antimicrobial preparations (excluding antibiotics) suitable for self-care are available in a variety of vehicles, including toothpastes, mouthrinses, irrigants, gels, and chewing gums. For PCPC, several types of antiplaque and antimicrobial preparations are available, including pocket irrigants, gels, slow-release agents (varnishes), and controlled slow-release agents (PerioChip, Dexcel).

Chemical plaque control should always be regarded as a needs-related supplement to, and not as a substitute for, mechanical plaque control. Therefore, the choice of agent and frequency of use for self-care and professional care should be related to the individual patient's oral health status and predicted risk for oral disease.

Self-care procedures

The agents are applied with high frequency: one to three times per day, regularly or intermittently. Accessibility and efficacy are good supragingivally but very limited subgingivally and interproximally in the molar and premolar regions, particularly for mouthrinsing. The method is compliance dependent and relatively costly for regular daily use unless the agent is incorporated in toothpaste.

Professional procedures

The frequency should be based on needs, and PCPC generally is more frequent during the initial intensive period to heal inflamed periodontal tissues as soon as possible and thereby reduce the PFRI. The accessibility is high because the agent is professionally applied. The duration of effect can be extended by using slow-release agents, such as CHX-thymol varnish (Cervitec, Ivoclar Vivident) and gels, and controlled slow-release agents, such as PerioChip (CHX).

Goals

Chemical plaque control may be used for a variety of purposes:

- To prevent plaque formation
- To reduce the PFRI
- To control plaque formation
- To reduce, disrupt, or remove existing plaque
- To alter the composition of the plaque microflora
- To exert bactericidal or bacteriostatic effects on microflora implicated in caries and periodontal diseases
- To alter the surface energy of the tooth and thereby reduce plaque adherence
- To inhibit the release of virulence factors from plaque bacteria

Although many antimicrobial agents would appear to be suitable for plaque control, few have demonstrated clinical efficacy because of inherent problems in the mode of action of agents in the mouth and difficulties in incorporation in dental products. Although many of these agents exhibit broad-spectrum antimicrobial activity in the laboratory, they may display valuable selective properties on plaque.

However, long-term use of dental products containing antimicrobial agents must not (1) disrupt the natural balance of the oral microflora, (2) lead to colonization by exogenous organisms, or (3) lead to the development of microbial resistance. Several products that satisfy these criteria are now available and are clinically effective in helping to control plaque and gingivitis. As new agents and combinations of agents with improved antiplaque and antimicrobial properties are developed, the challenge will be to increase efficacy while preserving microbial homeostasis in the mouth.

Accessibility is critical for the effect of chemical plaque control agents and varies greatly for different delivery systems. For efficacy, the agent has to reach the site of action and be maintained at the site long enough to have a sustained effect. A study illustrating this point was conducted by Bouwsma et al (1992). Once-daily use of a wooden triangular interdental cleaner was more effective in reducing interdental bleeding than twice-daily rinsing with CHX, undoubtedly because the CHX rinse did not reach the interproximal sites, whereas the mechanical interdental cleaner did.

Classification of plaque control agents

Chemical plaque control agents can be classified in the following groups:

- Cationic agents
- Anionic agents
- Nonionic agents
- Other agents
- Combination agents

Cationic agents are generally more potent antimicrobials than anionic or nonionic agents because they bind readily to the negatively charged bacterial surface. Cationic agents can interact with both gram-positive and gram-negative bacteria and, by virtue of their antimicrobial properties, reduce the number of viable bacteria on the tooth surfaces or reduce the pathogenicity of established dental plaque. The following groups of cationic agents have been tested or used as chemical plaque control agents:

- Bisbiguanide detergents: CHX and alexidine
- Quaternary ammonium compounds: cetylpyridinium chloride, benzethonium chloride, and domiphen bromide
- Heavy metal salts: copper, tin, and zinc
- Pyrimidines: hexetidine
- Herbal extracts: sanguinarine

Of these, CHX is by far the most efficient and frequently used agent, followed by heavy metal salt compounds, such as stannous fluoride and zinc citrate. CHX is still the most efficient chemical antiplaque agent and is regarded as the gold standard; it has served as a positive control in most recent studies on chemical plaque control. A disadvantage is brown staining of the teeth and the tongue after some weeks' use, particularly from mouthrinses. Therefore, CHX is not generally acceptable for long-term daily use. On the other hand, CHX is frequently and successfully used intermittently for 2 to 3 weeks in self-care mouthrinses, gels, varnishes, and controlled slow-release devices by professionals.

CHX is only bacteriostatic and not bactericidal. It is not suitable for subgingival irrigation because of the rapid turnover of gingival crevicular fluid in diseased pockets. Therefore, bactericidal 0.5% iodine solution is recommended as an irrigant during subgingival debridement.

The anionic sodium lauryl sulfate is the most frequently used detergent in toothpastes; it is also used in mouthrinses.

Cationic agents are inactivated by anionic agents. Therefore, use of CHX mouthrinse is not recommended immediately after use of toothpastes that contain anions such as sodium lauryl sulfate and monofluorophosphate.

The most successful and frequently used nonionic plaque control agents, triclosan and Listerine (McNeil), both belong to the category of noncharged phenolic compounds:

- Phenol
- Thymol
- Listerine (thymol, eucalyptol, menthol, and methyl salicylate)
- Triclosan
- 2-Phenylphenol
- Hexylresorcinol

Listerine (named after Lister, the father of the antiseptics) was tested for efficacy against oral bacteria as early as 1884 by the legendary W. D. Miller. Listerine mouthrinse has been used for more than 100 years by millions of consumers, particularly in the United States. Its effect on plaque and gingivitis, although well documented, is less potent than that of CHX (Axelsson and Lindhe, 1987). Triclosan, currently incorporated in commercial toothpastes and mouthrinses, is now the most important chemical plaque control agent in oral hygiene products for self-care. However, its well-documented effect on plaque and gingivitis is also less potent than that provided by CHX (Ramberg et al, 1996). Like other phenolic compounds, both Listerine and triclosan have an anti-inflammatory effect.

The substantivity of triclosan is limited. To increase its substantivity, triclosan has to be combined with other compounds. The most successful combinations to date are with copolymer (Colgate, Colgate-Palmolive) and with zinc citrate (Pepsodent, Church & Dwight). Both combinations are used in fluoride toothpastes. The former is also used in fluoride mouthrinses. Significant reduction of gingivitis and probing depths with daily use of toothpaste containing triclosan and copolymer was shown in a 3-year randomized controlled study (Rosling et al, 1997).

Because the plaque biofilm is a complex aggregation of various bacterial species, it is therefore unlikely that one single agent can be effective against the complete flora. Combining two or more agents with complementary inhibiting modes of action may enhance the efficacy and reduce the adverse effects of chemical plaque control agents, offering promising prospects for new and more effective chemical plaque control agents. Examples of combined agents are heavy metal ions (eg, Zn^{2+}) plus CHX or sodium lauryl sulfate; triclosan plus copolymer or zinc citrate; and stannous fluoride plus amine fluoride.

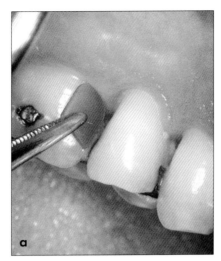 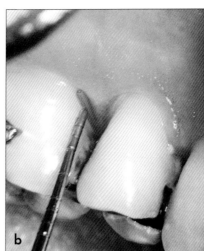

Figs 143a and 143b Placement of the PerioChip in the periodontal pocket using suitable forceps.

Optimizing effectiveness

For chemical plaque control agents to achieve their optimal effect, existing well-organized supragingival and subgingival biofilms must be mechanically eliminated or ruptured because of the limited penetrability and accessibility of these agents and their delivery systems (for example, mouthrinses, irrigants, and gels).

For better compliance and cost effectiveness, the strategy for chemical plaque control by self-care should be to optimize the use of safe, efficient toothpastes. For professional use, the strategy should be to optimize safe, efficient, slow-release and controlled slow-release agents and devices.

PerioChip is a biodegradable chip for sustained and direct delivery of CHX to the periodontal pocket. It is a 4.00 × 5.00 × 0.35-mm orange-brown rectangular chip, rounded on one end. The device weighs 7.40 mg and contains 2.50 mg of CHX in a gelatin matrix. The chip is biodegradable and indicated for use in periodontal pockets that are 5.00 mm or deeper.

The chip, which is very user friendly, is inserted in the pocket with suitable forceps. By grasping the flat end of the chip, the clinician can place the round end into the periodontal pocket (Figs 143a and 143b). It is recommended that the area to be treated be dry because a wet chip may become soft and more difficult to insert. The entire procedure takes less than 1 minute.

No retention system is required. The patient should refrain from mechanical interdental cleaning for 10 days to avoid dislodging the chip. The chip biodegrades in 7 to 10 days and does not require an additional appointment for removal.

Two multicenter studies with a randomized, controlled split-mouth design have shown that a combination of scaling and root planing and placement of a PerioChip results in a significantly greater reduction in probing depth in pockets deeper than 5 mm and a significantly greater gain in clinical periodontal attachment than do scaling and root planing alone (Jeffcoat et al, 1998; for details on methods and materials for chemical plaque control, see volume 4 [Axelsson, 2004]).

Minimally invasive scaling, root planing, and debridement

For details on methods and materials for minimally invasive scaling, root planing, and debridement, see chapter 1.

Role of initial intensive treatment

Traditionally, the initial treatment of new, untreated patients consisted of four to six consecutive sessions of comprehensive scaling, root planing, and debridement at 1- to 2-week intervals. Such quadrant or sextant therapy might result in a reinfection of previously disinfected areas by bacteria from an untreated region. Within 1 week, a mature biofilm can be formed.

In addition, not all the subgingival microflora and subgingival biofilms are eliminated by nonsurgical mechanical instrumentation alone. Socransky et al (1991) found about 10^8 colony-forming units per pocket in untreated patients with severe periodontitis, and the numbers increased with increasing probing depths. The microflora in such patients is characterized by a large proportion of periopathogens and a small proportion of beneficial species (Socransky and Haffajee, 2002). Immediately after subgingival instrumentation, about 10^5 colony-forming units per deep pocket remain (Goodson et al, 1991b; Maiden et al, 1991). Moreover, directly after subgingival scaling, root planing, and debridement, 5% to 80% of roots still exhibit residual plaque biofilms and calculus over an area up to 30% (Petersilka et al, 2002), particularly in furcations, narrow osseous defects, and deep pockets and when performed by clinicians with reduced experience and skill.

Seven days after subgingival instrumentation, the total number of subgingival species has increased almost to the baseline values in deep pockets. However, the flora has changed to a small proportion of periopathogens and a large proportion of beneficial species (Harper and Robinson, 1987; for a review, see Umeda et al, 2004).

If the protective root cementum has been removed by invasive scaling and root planing, the recolonizing bacteria will not only cover the exposed root dentin but also invade the dentinal tubules. These bacteria are inaccessible to repeated instrumentation and might infect the root canals. The tubules also serve as a bacterial reservoir from which pathogens can recolonize treated periodontal pockets. (Adriaens et al, 1988a, 1988b; Giuliana et al, 1997).

Some periopathogenic species, particularly *Aa* but also *Pg, Pi, P micros*, and some spirochete species, may also invade the soft tissues and thus be inaccessible to nonsurgical subgingival instrumentation (Christersson et al, 1987; Dzink et al, 1989; Fives-Taylor et al, 1999; Lamont and Jenkinson, 2000; Madianos et al, 1996; Pertuiset et al, 1987; Sandros et al, 1994; Sreenivasan et al, 1993). Downgrowth of bacteria from the supragingival area is more important in recolonization of periodontal pockets after periodontal therapy than previously suspected (Socransky and Haffajee, 2002). Subgingival instrumentation followed up with excellent gingival plaque control by self-care and PMTC is very efficient. The effect on the subgingival microflora of gingival plaque control without subgingival instrumentation is more controversial (Petersilka et al, 2002).

The clinical implication of these findings is that standard periodontal treatment of four to six sessions of scaling and root planing at predetermined intervals increases the risk for early recolonization of treated pockets by pathogens migrating from unscaled pockets as well as the tongue, tonsils, saliva, and mucosa. Without proper gingival plaque control, the root surface will be recolonized from the supragingival area within 7 days after a single subgingival instrumentation. However, supplementary complete-mouth disinfection, followed by continued proper gingival plaque control, will delay recolonization and stimulate a shift from periopathogens to a more beneficial microflora. The complete-mouth disinfection protocol, which involves debridement of all periodontal pockets in combination with bactericidal 0.5% iodine solution irrigation, PMTC, scraping the dorsum of the tongue, and rinsing with 0.2% CHX solution, will be discussed in more detail in the next section (Quirynen et al, 2006; for a review, see Quirynen et al, 2001).

Thus, an initial intensive combination of mechanical cleaning and use of chemical antimicrobial agents according to the complete-mouth disinfection concept is recommended for optimal elimination of periopathogens from all the reservoirs of the oral cavity in untreated periodontitis-susceptible patients (particularly those with aggressive periodontitis), in patients with so-called refractory periodontitis, in patients who are to undergo regenerative therapy, and in patients with diabetes or cardiovascular disease. To prevent reinfection, this initial complete-mouth disinfection might be prolonged, based on the individual's needs, and followed up with excellent gingival plaque control by self-care and needs-related intervals of supportive care, including PMTC, debridement, and use of chemical plaque control agents.

Complete-mouth disinfection and one-stage nonsurgical mechanical treatment

As mentioned previously, not only the tooth surfaces but also other specific oral environments, such as the tongue, tonsils, oral mucosa, and periodontal pockets, may serve as a reservoir for bacteria that may colonize tooth surfaces and periodontal pockets. Therefore, oral hygiene procedures in highly infected, at-risk individuals should include more than toothcleaning. In such individuals, an initial intensive complete-mouth disinfection and one-stage nonsurgical mechanical treatment should be the method of choice.

The first study evaluating such principles was carried out in a 30-month randomized controlled caries-preventive study by Axelsson et al (1987b) in a selected group of 187 13-year-old children with more than 1 million mutans streptococci in saliva. Samples were also collected from every approximal surface and the dorsum of the tongue. During an initial intensive period (every second day for a total of three times), PMTC was carried out with needs-related intensity that depended on the levels of mutans streptococci approximally, and the dorsum of the tongue was mechanically cleaned with a tongue scraper. Thereafter, the patient rinsed with a 0.2% CHX solution for 2 minutes, and finally, a 0.5% CHX gel was placed interproximally with a syringe. A dramatic reduction of mutans streptococci had been achieved 2 weeks later. However, a single treatment only every 6 months did not maintain the initial reduction. This indicates that patients who are highly infected with mutans streptococci should be treated more frequently based on their individual needs.

Complete-mouth disinfection principles combined with the so-called one-stage subgingival instrumentation method later were successfully implemented in untreated patients with advanced chronic or aggressive periodontitis (Bollen et al, 1998; De Soete et al, 2001; Mongardini et al, 1999; Quirynen et al, 1999, 2000; Vandekerckhove et al, 1996). For example, Vandekerckhove et al (1996) investigated, over an 8-month period, the clinical benefits of complete-mouth disinfection within a 24-hour period in the control of chronic periodontitis. The control group received the standard regimen of initial periodontal therapy, consisting of scaling and root planing in quadrants at 2-week intervals. In the complete-mouth disinfection group, scaling and root planing of the four quadrants were performed within 24 hours and immediately followed by a thorough supragingival and subgingival application of CHX to limit any transfer of bacteria.

When the Gingival Index to Plaque Index ratio was considered, the ratio was lower in the test group at all follow-up visits. For pockets with probing depths of 7 mm or more, complete-mouth disinfection resulted in a significantly ($P = .01$) greater reduction in probing depth at each follow-up visit; at month 8, the test treatment resulted in an average reduction of 4 mm compared to an average reduction of 3 mm with classic therapy. The gain in clinical attachment level was 3.7 mm for the test group and 1.9 mm for the control group. This pilot study suggests that a complete-mouth disinfection performed in 1 day results in a better clinical outcome in patients with chronic periodontitis than do multiple scalings performed by quadrant at 2-week intervals over several weeks.

This study was followed up by Mongardini et al (1999) in 40 patients with generalized aggressive periodontitis or severe chronic periodontitis. Within 24 hours, the 20 patients in the test group underwent a complete-mouth scaling and root planing in combination with application of different CHX agents for complete-mouth disinfection. The 20 control patients underwent scaling and root planing quadrant by quadrant, resulting in a total of four sessions at 2-week intervals. Except for repeated oral hygiene instructions, the control group received no adjunctive therapy. During the 8-month follow-up, no additional pocket instrumentation was allowed in either the test or the control group so that the ability of the initial treatments to maintain results could be compared.

Generally, the complete-mouth disinfection (test group) resulted in significantly greater reductions of probing depths than did the standard therapy (control group), irrespective of the disease category. In comparison to baseline, significant gains in probing attachment were always recorded in the test group but were only recorded for initially deep pockets (7 mm or greater) in the control group. In addition, mouth malodor was significantly reduced in the test group.

Quirynen et al (1999) evaluated the effect of complete- versus partial-mouth disinfection on the microflora in the treatment of chronic or generalized aggressive periodontitis. The complete-mouth disinfection group showed larger reductions in the proportions of spirochetes and motile organisms in the subgingival flora and more significant reductions in the density of key perio-pathogens, with eradication of *Pg*.

Quirynen et al (2000) later evaluated the relative importance of the use of CHX in the one-stage, complete-mouth disinfection protocol. Patients in a control group received scaling and root planing quadrant per quadrant at 2-week intervals. Two other groups underwent a one-stage complete-mouth scaling and root planing, including mechanical cleaning of the dorsum of the tongue, with or without the adjunctive use of CHX.

All treatment strategies resulted in significant improvements for all clinical variables, but patients in the test groups consistently showed significantly greater probing depth reductions and attachment gains than did those in the control group. This is in agreement with the results of a study by Badersten et al (1984b) that showed that a single well-performed session of scaling, root planing, and debridement was even more successful in the deepest pockets than three instrumentations a 1-month intervals.

From a microbial point of view, both test groups (with or without adjunctive use of CHX) showed greater improvement than the control groups, especially when periopathogens in the periodontal pockets were considered. However,

the differences between the two test groups were negligible. Thus it may be concluded that the initial intensive mechanical removal of supragingival and subgingival biofilms and mechanical cleaning of the dorsum of the tongue are the key factors for success rather than supplementary treatment with CHX.

In another study, De Soete et al (2001) compared the long-term additional microbiologic effect of one-stage complete-mouth disinfections with one-stage scaling, root planing, and debridement alone in patients with advanced chronic periodontitis or aggressive periodontitis. Both treatments resulted in important reductions of the pathogenic species for up to 8 months after therapy, both in their detection level and frequency. In the test groups, an additional improvement was achieved, especially in the chronic periodontitis group, where *Pg* and *Tf (B forsythus)* were reduced below detection level. The number of beneficial species remained nearly unchanged.

Thus, a single subgingival instrumentation without proper subsequent gingival plaque control will allow recolonization of the root surface from the supragingival area within 7 days. On the other hand, subgingival instrumentation in combination with one-stage complete-mouth disinfection, followed by continued excellent gingival plaque control, will prevent or at least delay subgingival recolonization by periopathogens. In addition, a shift to a more beneficial microflora will occur. (For review, see Lang et al, 2008.)

Strategy for initial intensive treatment

During the first appointment, the clinician has the following goals:

- To obtain a brief overview of oral health status through a diagnostic screening supplemented with necessary radiographic examinations
- To gain an impression of the patient's character through an oral and a general history

For the oral history, an evaluation of dental care, oral hygiene habits, fluoride use, dietary and smoking habits, and attitudes toward oral health is of great importance. The most important variables for general history evaluations are level of education, occupation, lifestyle, systemic diseases, use of medicines, attitudes toward general health, and body mass index. The diagnosis reveals the present oral status, but the history discloses the reasons for the status. On the basis of the results of the screening and history, the clinician selects the appropriate detailed supplementary examinations and tests to achieve the following goals:

- To obtain detailed information about the patient's oral health status
- To obtain detailed information about etiologic and modifying factors related to the patient's oral health status

The most important clinical variables related to periodontal diseases are vertical probing attachment loss; horizontal attachment loss (furcation involvement, grades 0 to III); Gingival Index; probing depth; alveolar bone level, shape, and structure, based on conventional or computer-aided complete-mouth radiographs; bleeding on probing; purulent exudate; periodontal pocket temperature; amount and content of gingival crevicular fluid; and subgingival plaque-retentive factors (eg, calculus, rough root surfaces, and restoration overhangs). If retrospective data are available, the incidence of periodontal attachment loss is estimated. From an etiologic point of view, PFRI (Axelsson, 1991), Plaque Index, and the occurrence of subgingival plaque biofilms and specific periopathogens, such as *Aa, Pg, Tf, Td,* and *Pi* (diagnosed via checkerboard DNA-DNA hybridization technique), are of great importance. The most important external and internal modifying factors for periodontal diseases are oral and dental care habits, smoking habits, education level, systemic diseases (particularly type 1 and type 2 diabetes), and genetic susceptibility. Therefore, cessation of smoking and well-controlled diabetes are of great importance for success (for details, see chapter 5 and volume 3 of this series [Axelsson, 2002]).

Based on all data from the diagnosis and history, the patient is classified according to his or her risk for periodontal diseases: no risk (P0), low risk (P1), risk (P2), or high risk (P3). The individ-

ual risk profile (Axelsson, 1998, 2002) is established as a tool for case presentation and communication with the patient (see chapter 5).

The number of visits and the methods and materials used during the initial intensive period will be strictly related to the patient's classification and predicted risk (for details, see Tables 6 and 7 in chapter 5). The clinician performs the initial intensive treatment with the following main goals:

- To establish needs-related self-care habits based on self-diagnosis and education
- To heal diseased periodontal tissues as soon as possible, resulting in a dramatic reduction in PFRI
- To arrest caries without cavitation
- To eliminate plaque-retentive factors such as restoration overhangs, unpolished restorations, calculus, rough root surfaces, and cavitated caries lesions

For nonrisk (P0) and low-risk (P1) patients without any treatment need, the initial preventive treatment will be limited to one or two visits. For risk (P2) and high-risk (P3) patients, the initial intensive treatment may range from three to six visits. These visits will be concentrated in as short a period as possible (7 to 10 days) at about 2-day intervals. However, the first two should take place at exactly a 24-hour interval for evaluation of PFRI and establishment of needs-related oral hygiene habits based on PFRI and education in self-diagnosis (for details, see Axelsson, 2004).

Extraction of untreatable teeth and elimination of plaque-retentive factors

To facilitate mechanical plaque control by self-care as well as PMTC, the clinician must eliminate plaque-retentive factors as early as possible. The most harmful plaque-retentive factors are remaining roots that are untreatable because of caries and teeth that are untreatable because of advanced periodontal disease. Such teeth should be extracted as soon as possible. The increased accessibility for subgingival instrumentation and mechanical plaque control after early extraction of teeth with untreatable advanced periodontitis will result in rapid healing of diseased adjacent approximal pockets.

Adjustment and finishing of ill-fitting restorations will also improve accessibility for mechanical plaque control measures. Overhangs and undercuts of restorations and crowns must be eliminated, and rough surfaces of restorations must be finished and polished. Cavitated caries lesions should be excavated and restored at least semipermanently with glass-ionomer cement or resin-modified glass-ionomer cement. This should be especially beneficial in caries-risk patients because glass-ionomer cement may act as a slow-release fluoride agent that can be recharged with fluoride by daily use of fluoride toothpaste and professional use of fluoride varnishes and gels.

Subgingival and supragingival calculus is eliminated and rough root surfaces are planed with a minimally invasive technique without exposure of the root's dentinal tubules. With these procedures, subgingival biofilms should be removed as well. Recontouring and root resection can reduce the plaque retention in root grooves and furcation-involved teeth (as described in chapter 3). The one-stage complete-mouth disinfection method should be implemented in periodontal-risk (P2 and P3) patients during this initial intensive treatment period.

Reevaluation

Depending on the outcome of the analyses of the subgingival microflora, topical use of doxycycline gels or systemic use of antibiotics (amoxicillin and/or metronidazole) may be indicated in especially susceptible patients with impaired general health (eg, those with severe cardiovascular problems or poorly controlled type 1 or 2 diabetes) (for details, see chapter 3).

Because of this intensive combination of mechanical and chemical plaque control, the periodontal tissues, particularly the free gingivae, will heal. In addition, the PFRI will be dramatically reduced and thus facilitate daily oral hygiene procedures.

In P2 and P3 patients, the effect of this initial intensive treatment should be evaluated within 3 to 6 months. The clinician performs this reevaluation with the following goals:

- To evaluate the results of the initial intensive treatment
- To assess patient compliance
- To evaluate the need for supplementary surgical pocket reduction, treatment of furcation-involved teeth, and regenerative therapy to restore lost periodontal support
- To evaluate if another intensive treatment supplemented with antibiotics is necessary
- To determine the methods and materials needed for the maintenance period and the optimal recall intervals (see Table 7 in chapter 5)

After successful initial intensive treatment, inflamed gingival sites should be healed, and probing depths should be significantly reduced in P2 and P3 patients. Repeated oral microbiology tests may be indicated in P2 and P3 patients who had high levels of periopathogens in deep, diseased pockets at baseline.

At this reevaluation, the dentist decides whether supplementary use of antibiotics, surgical pocket reduction, treatment of furcation-involved teeth, and regenerative periodontal therapy are indicated (see chapters 3 and 4). Through interviews and questionnaires, the patient's knowledge, attitude, and compliance are evaluated. The quality of the patient's self-performed oral hygiene is evaluated by plaque disclosure. It is of great importance to motivate the patient to participate in the evaluation by self-diagnosis at every visit. Based on the outcome of the initial intensive treatment and risk classification, the methods and materials needed for the maintenance period (supportive care) and the optimal recall intervals are determined.

CONCLUSIONS

There is evidence that the periodontal diseases are directly and indirectly caused by microorganisms that colonize the tooth surfaces, forming biofilms, as well as by nonattaching bacteria that invade the periodontal tissues. As a consequence, the soft periodontal tissues will be infected, and the periodontal attachment will gradually be destroyed. However, periodontitis is always preceded by gingivitis. Thus, prevention and treatment of gingivitis (infectious inflamed soft periodontal tissues) will also prevent the development of periodontitis. Three different hypotheses for the etiology of periodontal diseases have been proposed: the nonspecific plaque, ecological plaque, and specific plaque hypotheses. The reality is more likely to be a combination of these three hypotheses. Frequent proper mechanical toothcleaning will prevent the development of gingivitis and prevent recurrence of periodontitis after successful periodontal treatment.

Deep periodontal pockets favor the growth of anaerobic gram-negative microorganisms, among which most periopathogens are found. *Aa* and *Pg* are regarded as specific exogenous transmissible periopathogens, while *Tf* and *Td* in particular are regarded as opportunistic endogenous periopathogens. *Pg*, *Tf*, and *Td* seem to have a synergistic relationship and form the so-called red complex. In addition, research has shown that some herpesviruses may be directly or indirectly involved in the etiology of periodontal diseases.

Several methods and materials are available to promote rapid healing of infectious inflamed periodontal tissues. This initial intensive therapy includes mechanical plaque control by self-care and PMTC, chemical plaque control, and minimally invasive scaling, root planing, and debridement as well as early extraction of untreatable teeth and elimination of plaque-retentive factors. From a cost-effectiveness point of view, the combinations of these methods and materials and their frequency must be based on the individual patient's needs and risk prediction.

The most cost-effective method to prevent infection and inflammation of periodontal tissues and maintain their health after successful initial scaling, root planing, debridement, and PMTC is mechanical plaque control by self-care. Daily toothbrushing is an established habit in industrialized countries as well as some developing countries. However, toothbrushing, particularly self-taught toothbrushing, is not synonymous with complete toothcleaning. Particularly on the wide approximal surfaces of the posterior teeth, the toothbrush has no or very limited accessibility. Therefore, most infectious inflamed sites and deep pockets are located interproximally in the posterior regions in toothbrushing populations.

In contrast to toothbrushing, daily cleaning of the approximal surfaces of the posterior teeth with special oral hygiene aids such as triangular pointed toothpicks, dental tape, and interdental brushes is practiced by less than 10% of the population in most industrialized countries. Thus there is a great potential for improvement of daily gingival plaque control by establishment of interdental cleaning habits. Successful establishment of needs-related self-care habits has to be based on education in self-diagnosis.

True PMTC has to be focused on the key-risk surfaces of the key-risk teeth, where most patients fail to clean properly. That means the approximal surfaces of the posterior teeth and the lingual surfaces of the mandibular posterior teeth. Thus, so-called prophylaxis or polishing with a rotating rubber cup and prophylaxis paste on the buccal and lingual surfaces, which the patients already clean daily with the toothbrush, must not be confused with PMTC. On the other hand, true PMTC will remove plaque biofilms 2 to 3 mm subgingivally from the approximal key-risk surfaces of the posterior teeth. As a consequence, frequent initial PMTC will result in rapid healing of the infectious inflamed gingiva and thus gradually reduce the probing depth and change the ecology of the subgingival microflora. PMTC and self-care education should be continued in a maintenance program on a needs-related basis.

Chemical plaque control may also be performed by the patient as well as by professionals. Daily chemical plaque control is most effectively and inexpensively accomplished with toothpastes that contain plaque control agents. The most common chemical plaque control agents in toothpastes are sodium lauryl sulfate, triclosan with copolymer, and triclosan with zinc citrate.

107

Toothpastes containing triclosan have shown particularly significant effects on plaque and gingivitis in well-controlled long-term clinical studies.

Mouthrinses that contain chemical plaque control agents are also frequently recommended for selected risk patients. However, such products are mostly recommended for daily use intermittently (periods of 2 to 6 weeks), particularly before and after periodontal surgery (regenerative therapy) and during initial intensive periodontal therapy. They are not usually intended for long-term use. The most efficient and best documented chemical plaque control agent in mouthrinses and gels is CHX. However, the oldest product, Listerine, is still in use.

Chemical plaque control by professionals should always be used as a supplement to active nonsurgical periodontal therapy (scaling, root planing, and debridement) and possibly before periodontal surgery (particularly regenerative therapy). The most frequently used solution is iodine, used for irrigation of diseased pockets during nonsurgical instrumentation. After nonsurgical subgingival instrumentation and before regenerative therapy, a controlled, slow-release CHX agent can also be used.

Chemical plaque control products cannot substitute for mechanical plaque control. Such products can only be regarded as a needs-related supplement to mechanical plaque control (for further details on mechanical and chemical plaque control, see Axelsson, 2004).

During the initial treatment of previously untreated periodontitis, minimally invasive scaling, root planing, and debridement, elimination of plaque-retentive factors, and extraction of untreatable teeth are of great importance for rapid healing of infectious inflamed periodontal tissues. At the end of this initial phase, the clinician reevaluates the patient to determine if supplemental therapy is necessary to ensure the complete healing of infectious inflamed periodontal tissues. This additional therapy may include antibiotics, surgical pocket reduction, treatment of furcation-involved teeth, and regenerative periodontal therapy, which will be discussed in chapters 3 and 4.

CHAPTER 3

SUPPLEMENTARY THERAPY FOR HEALING OF INFECTIOUS INFLAMED PERIODONTAL TISSUES

After initial intensive therapy is completed, the clinician performs a thorough reevaluation of the patient's periodontal condition within 3 to 6 months. This evaluation may include measurement of probing depths; assessment of bleeding on probing, periodontal attachment level, furcation involvement, and tooth mobility; determination of the Gingival Index, Plaque Index, and Plaque Formation Rate Index; analyses of the subgingival microflora; and acquisition of radiographs. Based on the results of the reevaluation and the patient's risk profile, the dentist decides whether supplementary use of antibiotics, surgical pocket reduction, treatment of furcation-involved teeth, and regenerative periodontal therapy is indicated to aid in the healing of infectious inflamed periodontal tissues.

The following methods and materials can be a part of supplementary therapy:

- Use of systemic and local antibiotics
- Special treatment of furcation-involved teeth
- Periodontal surgery for accessibility and reduction of deep residual pockets
- Reduction of modifying risk factors (smoking, poorly controlled diabetes, and unhealthy dietary habits)

USE OF LOCAL AND SYSTEMIC ANTIBIOTICS

In contrast to other diseases with a bacterial etiology, most cases of periodontal disease can be successfully prevented, controlled, and treated by mechanical therapy: gingival plaque control by self-care, professional mechanical toothcleaning (PMTC), subgingival scaling, root planing, and debridement, as well as surgical regenerative therapy. However, a limited number of subjects do not respond positively to this mechanical therapy.

In some subjects, a few diseased pockets fail to heal, or the disease recurs despite excellent gingival plaque control, meticulous mechanical periodontal treatment, and a needs-related maintenance program. Most of these susceptible subjects have aggressive periodontitis, are immunocompromised, are heavy smokers, and/or have special subgingival plaque-retentive factors.

In such cases, supplementary antibiotic therapy may be very useful. However, use of antibiotics must always be preceded by comprehensive subgingival debridement, subgingival microbiology sampling, and if possible, sensitivity tests to select the most efficient antibiotic or combination of antibiotics. In periodontal therapy, antibiotics can be used systemically as well as topically.

This combination of mechanical plaque control and antibiotic therapy should be regarded as mechanical and pharmacologic infection control (MPIC). Some manufacturers of local antibiotic preparations have suggested the term *pharmacologic and mechanical infection control (PMIC)*. However, the correct order is *MPIC* because the use of antibiotics always must be preceded by mechanical debridement, as already discussed. The only exceptions may be in patients with acute necrotizing ulcerative gingivitis (ANUG), acute necrotizing ulcerative periodontitis (ANUP), and acute periodontal abscesses, which are very rare, at least in Scandinavia.

Subgingival environment

The effect of antibiotics on subgingival periopathogens is strongly correlated to accessibility, substantivity, and the pharmacokinetic characteristics of the antibiotics in question. The subgingival microflora represents attaching bacteria that form a subgingival plaque biofilm as well as nonattaching motile bacteria.

Mature dental plaque is a microbial biofilm. The growth characteristics have led to the concept of biofilms as ecological communities that evolved to permit survival of the community as a whole (Costerton et al, 1995). Evidence from a variety of sources is consistent with the concept of coevolution of a mixed microbial community to live in proximity to the tooth surface, above and below the gingival margin (Fig 144). This is supported by the presence of a primitive circulatory system and metabolic cooperation, but there are no published mutational and structure-function analyses in vitro or in vivo.

Although the capacity to attach plays a key role in the variety of different microbial species that constitute the dental plaque biofilm, bacterial growth is the primary determinant of the relative proportions of bacteria. Plaque doubling times are rapid in early development and slower in more mature films because of the structure of the biofilms, which contain areas of high and low bacterial biomass interlaced with aqueous channels of different sizes.

It is believed that these channels transport nutrients and metabolic waste products within the colony. For example, dissolved oxygen in living biofilms was measured to be at nearly anoxic values within microcolonies but at significant concentrations at all levels in cell-free aqueous channels (Costerton et al, 1995). This structure provides a means by which the different bacterial species can benefit from their juxtaposition, facilitating a type of physiologic cooperation not seen in mixed populations of planktonic organisms. The unique conditions of physiologic cooperation in biofilms may influence the occurrence of bacterial blooms (periods of rapidly accelerated growth of specific species or groups of species) described in periodontal plaque. In addition, some periopathogens form clusters, for example, the red complex of *Porphyromonas gingivalis (Pg)*, *Tannerella forsythia (Tf)*, and *Treponema denticola (Td)* (Socransky et al, 1998; see also chapter 2).

Thus it may be concluded that microorganisms living in the biofilm are protected and inaccessible to antibiotics as well as phagocytizing leukocytes (the polymorphonuclear leukocytes [PMNLs]), which represent the first line of nonspecific host defense. As a consequence, no or very limited effect will be achieved by the use of antibiotics and antiseptics in the diseased pocket without the first essential step, mechanical disruption and removal of the biofilm by comprehensive debridement. In patients previously receiving inadequate treatment, scaling and root planing may also be necessary before the use of antibiotics because the plaque biofilm covers all plaque-retentive factors, such as rough root cementum, hypoplasia, and calculus.

Some periopathogens, such as *Aggregatibacter actinomycetemcomitans (Aa)*, *Pg*, and some spirochetes, may also invade the soft tissues and multiply and thus be inaccessible to mechanical subgingival instrumentation. This bacterial invasion occurs particularly in patients with ANUP, aggressive periodontitis, and diabetes and in smokers, who often exhibit reduced PMNL function. In such patients, the use of antibiotics should be beneficial as a supplement to subgingival instrumentation.

The subgingival microflora may migrate laterally into local retentive areas such as cementum hypoplasias, iatrogenic grooves, etc, becoming in-

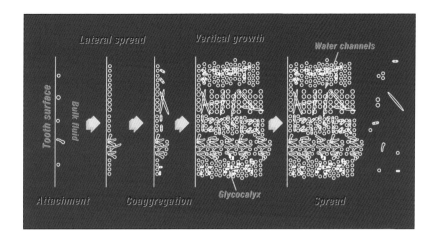

Fig 144 Buildup of the plaque biofilm on the tooth surface. (Courtesy of Dr A. Haffajee.)

accessible for instrumentation. In such cases, supplementary use of antibiotics or open flap surgery may be beneficial. However, periopathogens may also invade dentinal tubules that have been exposed because the protecting root cementum has been removed by invasive scaling and root planing. In such cases, they are protected and inaccessible to mechanical instrumentation as well as antibiotics and may cause recolonization of the root surface and possible infection of the root canal. In the case of root fractures, the bacteria not only migrate apically on the root surface along the fracture but are also inaccessible in the fractured root: Neither instrumentation nor antibiotics can prevent further loss of periodontal support and, finally, loss of the tooth.

It must also be observed that the subgingival environment differs substantially from the supragingival environment. Saliva does not generally penetrate the subgingival environment. The gingival crevicular fluid (GCF) has a composition similar to that of serum. It has a relatively greater host defense capability, with the presence of transiently viable phagocytizing PMNLs, complement, and effective concentrations of most serum antibodies, some of which may be produced locally. Although gingival fluid flow is only approximately 20.0 μL/h, the pocket volume is approximately 0.5 μL. As a result, the total pocket volume is exchanged about 40 times per hour, which limits the time of contact for antibacterial agents placed in the periodontal pocket.

Systemic antibiotics

The systemic environment communicates with the periodontal environment through capillary walls and with the gastrointestinal tract through mucosal walls. It is the ultimate source of most if not all periodontal host defense mechanisms and serves as a diluent for all systemically administered antibacterial agents.

Dilution of systemically administered antibiotics severely limits their effect. An antibiotic agent administered systemically is ultimately dissolved in total body water (42 L), and 50% or more is lost through other compartments (eg, bone, kidney, liver). A typical systemic antibiotic will achieve a peak concentration of 3 μg/mL in blood and gingival fluid (0.0003%). To inhibit the growth of periopathogens, concentrations between 1 and 16 μg/mL must be available. Only agents with high potency and good absorption characteristics can reach the periodontal pocket in therapeutic concentrations, and these agents are then effective only against bacterial strains that are susceptible to the antibiotic at the low concentrations attainable.

Two critical factors should be considered when a systemic antibiotic is selected: gingival fluid concentration and minimum inhibitory concentration. The gingival fluid concentration provides information on the peak levels attained by systemic delivery at the primary ecological niche for periodontal pathogens: the periodontal pocket. The 90% minimum inhibitory concentration is an in vitro determination of the concentration that will inhibit growth of 90% of the bacterial strains of the species tested.

Eight principal antibiotics have been extensively tested for treatment of periodontal diseases: tetracycline, modified tetracyclines (minocycline and doxycycline), erythromycin, clindamycin, ampicillin, amoxicillin, and metronidazole. Each of them has been tested alone or in combination with others. The most frequent and successful combination used during the last decade is amoxicillin and metronidazole.

Antibiotics used systemically in the treatment of periodontal diseases have three different modes of action:

1. Reversible inhibition of protein synthesis
2. Inhibition of cell wall synthesis
3. Inhibition of DNA synthesis

Agents that act by reversible inhibition of protein synthesis

The tetracyclines, clindamycin, and erythromycin act by inhibition of protein synthesis. These agents are broad spectrum and bacteriostatic. To be effective, systemically administered bacteriostatic antibiotics characteristically require longer periods of administration than their bactericidal counterparts.

The tetracyclines have been used extensively in periodontal therapy. They are well absorbed, relatively safe, and after systemic administration appear at higher concentrations in gingival fluid than in serum. As a group, the tetracyclines differ little in their spectrum of antibacterial activity for gram-negative obligate anaerobes. Minocycline, however, appears to be more effective than tetracycline in inhibition of gram-negative facultative anerobes. Minocycline and doxycycline differ substantially from other tetracyclines in having a longer excretion rate, requiring less frequent administration in systemic therapy. Except for the effect of minocycline on actinomycetes, systemic delivery of the tetracyclines does not substantially inhibit the growth of oral gram-positive organisms. The combined effect of increased absorption, higher levels in GCF, and greater effectiveness in the inhibition of gram-negative facultative anaerobes suggests that systemic administration of

minocycline could have unique potential for the treatment of periodontal infections.

Systemic administration of tetracyclines is generally well tolerated. The most common side effect, gastric upset, is less frequent with minocycline and doxycycline because of their superior absorption characteristics. Minocycline has been associated with a high frequency of vertigo, which may be minimized by reducing the dosage to 100 mg per day, taken at bedtime. Tetracycline resistance has been observed in periodontal pathogens. General side effects and precautions for systemic use of tetracyclines have been well described (for reviews, see Slots, 2004 and van Winkelhoff et al, 2000).

Tetracyclines possess several unique non-antibacterial characteristics that may contribute to their efficacy in periodontal therapy. These include collagenase inhibition, inhibition of neutrophil chemotaxis, anti-inflammatory effects, inhibition of microbial attachment, and conditioning of the root surface. Tetracycline solutions bind even more effectively than chlorhexidine gluconate (CHX) to the root surface, providing a slow-release effect.

Clindamycin has been used systemically, with reported success, in the treatment of refractory periodontitis (Gordon et al, 1985, 1990; Magnusson et al, 1994). There is no antibiotic that achieves higher levels of antimicrobial activity than clindamycin for any periopathogen. However, systemic use of this agent is limited because of the risk of development of potentially fatal pseudomembranous enterocolitis, caused by intestinal overgrowth of *Clostridium difficile*.

Erythromycin is a very safe drug, frequently recommended as an alternative to penicillin for allergic patients, but erythromycin has very limited effect on periopathogens because of poor tissue absorption and low concentration in GCF.

Agents that act by inhibition of cell wall synthesis

The penicillins and cephalosporins are antibiotics that act by inhibition of cell wall synthesis. These agents are narrow spectrum and bactericidal. Both are commonly associated with hypersensitivity reactions and may manifest cross-reactivity.

No penicillin can be considered to be broad spectrum. All have major activity in the gram-positive spectrum.

Only the extended-spectrum penicillins, such as ampicillin and amoxicillin, possess substantial antibacterial activity for gram-negative species. Of these, systemic administration of amoxicillin is favored for treatment of periodontal diseases because of the higher concentration achieved in serum and the generally greater susceptibility of periodontal pathogens. At the levels attained in GCF after systemic administration, amoxicillin exhibits high antimicrobial activity for all periodontal pathogens except *Eikenella corrodens*, *Capnocytophaga sputigena*, and *Peptostreptococcus* species. In addition, it inhibits the growth of the gram-positive facultative anaerobes.

Amoxicillin is susceptible to degradation by β-lactamase, which is often found in the periodontal pocket. For this reason, administration of β-lactamase–sensitive penicillin alone, including amoxicillin, is not generally recommended and in some cases may accelerate periodontal destruction. The generally accepted strategy is to administer amoxicillin with a β-lactamase inhibitor such as clavulanic acid, which is commercially available in a single-dose preparation (Augmentin, GlaxoSmithKline). The β-lactamase–producing strains are generally sensitive to this preparation. Some cases of refractory periodontal disease have been successfully treated by adjunctive administration of this preparation (Fine et al, 1998).

Agents that act by inhibition of DNA synthesis

Metronidazole and the quinolone antibiotics (such as ciprofloxacin) inhibit DNA synthesis. Metronidazole is converted to a chemically reactive reduced form that can inhibit DNA synthesis in bacterial species. After about 30 years of clinical testing, metronidazole is generally considered to be safe in humans. Short-term administration of metronidazole is usually well-tolerated, but a unique side effect is a disulfiram (Antabuse, Odyssey Pharmaceuticals) effect: cramps, nausea, and vomiting following alcohol consumption. Metronidazole is also contraindicated in patients who are taking anticoagulants or lithium.

Metronidazole was first tested to treat vaginal trichomonal infections and was serendipitously found to resolve concomitant acute necrotizing gingivitis. In medical practice it is still used for treatment of trichomonal infections as well as many potentially fatal anaerobic infections. Following systemic administration, relatively high peak plasma concentrations are attained within 1 to 3 hours. The concentrations in gingival fluid are generally slightly less than in plasma.

Metronidazole is a synthetic nitroimidazole compound with antibacterial effects primarily on obligate gram-positive and gram-negative anaerobes. The resistance of obligate anaerobes to metronidazole therapy is very low. That means the most important anaerobic periopathogens, and particularly the red complex (*Pg*, *Tf*, and *Td*), could be efficiently treated with metronidazole. However, the facultatively anaerobic *Aa* is less sensitive to metronidazole. On the other hand, the combination of amoxicillin and metronidazole is the most efficient and first choice for antibiotic treatment of *Aa*.

Strategy and recommendations for systemic use of antibiotics

The choice of the most efficient single antibiotic or combination of antibiotics should always be based on subgingival microbial sampling and, if possible, sensitivity tests. Some individuals may harbor species that are less sensitive than do other patients. This may occur more commonly in countries where antibiotics are frequently used. For example, van Winkelhoff et al (2005) recently evaluated the antibiotic resistance of periopathogens isolated in the Netherlands and Spain. This study showed that several antibiotics require higher minimal concentrations to inhibit microbial isolates from Spanish subjects than to inhibit isolates from Dutch subjects.

The authors suspect that severe periodontitis may not be treated everywhere with the same uniform adjunctive antimicrobial regimen (van Winkelhoff et al, 2005). This may indicate the utility of antimicrobial susceptibility testing for a predictable treatment outcome. The issue of susceptibility testing in periodontal practice has been raised previously, but convincing evidence for its clinical benefit has been lacking up to now.

Table 4 Microbial species associated with various clinical forms of periodontitis*					
Species	Localized aggressive periodontitis	Generalized aggressive periodontitis	Progressive (aggressive) adult periodontitis	Refractory periodontitis	Failing guided tissue regeneration
Aggregatibacter actinomycetemcomitans	+++	++	++	++	++
Porphyromonas gingivalis	±	+++	+++	++	++
Prevotella intermedia/nigrescens	++	+++	+++	+++	+++
Tannerella forsythia	±	++	+++	++	++
Fusobacterium species	+	++	+++	++	+++
Peptostreptococcus micros	±	++	+++	++	+++
Eubacterium species	–	+	++	+	+
Campylobacter rectus	+	++	++	+	+++
Treponema species	++	+++	+++	++	++
Enteric rods and *Pseudomonas* species	–	–	±	+	±
β-Hemolytic streptococci	?	++	++	++	+
Candida species	–	–	–	±	–

*Modified from van Winkelhoff et al (1996).

– = Not elevated in comparison to health; ± = occasionally isolated; + = up to 10% of patients positive; ++ = between 10% and 50% of patients positive; +++ = more than 50% of patients positive; ? = unknown.

Because chronic periodontitis can successfully be treated by mechanical instrumentation and mechanical gingival plaque control, this study indicates that the optimal use of antibiotics must be restricted to patients with special severe periodontal status after subgingival microbial sampling and sensitivity tests. Such selective periodontal conditions are:

- Aggressive periodontitis:
  - Localized aggressive (early-onset) periodontitis (particularly in patients with high levels of *Aa*)
  - Generalized aggressive (early-onset) periodontitis
  - Aggressive periodontitis in adults
- Refractory periodontitis (particularly in patients with diabetes and in smokers)
- Periodontitis in patients with immunodeficiency (eg, AIDS, use of cytostatics) or severe cardiovascular disease
- ANUP

Table 4 (van Winkelhoff et al, 1996) shows the relative proportion of microbial species associated with various clinical forms of periodontitis.

The aim of supplementary systemic antibiotic therapy in periodontics is to eliminate or markedly suppress the most potent periopathogens from the diseased pockets and other reservoirs in the oral cavity (particularly the dorsum of the tongue) in susceptible individuals with the aforementioned conditions. Patients with peri-implantitis may also benefit from antibiotic therapy. In addition, antibiotics should be used prophylactically before extractions and surgical as well as nonsurgical treatment, particularly in patients with some cardiovascular disease conditions. It also seems reasonable to assume that elimination of periopathogens (in particular the exogenous *Aa* and *Pg*) by systemic or topical use of antibiotics prior to regenerative therapy could be critical for optimal regeneration.

Except for prophylaxis and maybe for ANUP and acute periodontal abscesses, use of antibiotics should be preceded by bacterial sampling and, if possible, sensitivity tests. In particular, the study by van Winkelhoff et al (2005) highlighted the need of sensitivity tests for evaluation of the most suitable antibiotic therapy. In this study, significantly higher minimum inhibitory concentration values were noted in Spanish strains of *Fusobacterium nucleatum* for penicillin and iprofloxacin; of *Prevotella in-*

termedia (Pi) for penicillin, amoxicillin, and tetracycline; of *Peptostreptococcus micros* for tetracycline, amoxicillin, and azithro-mycin; and of *Pg* for tetracycline and ciprofloxacin. Based on breakpoint concentrations, a higher number of resistant strains in Spain were found in *F nucleatum* for penicillin, amoxicillin, and metronidazole; in *Pi* for tetracycline and amoxicillin; and in *Aa* for amoxicillin and azithromycin. On the other hand, resistance of *Pg* strains was not observed for any of the antibiotics tested either in Spain or the Netherlands.

These observations are important because antibiotic therapy should primarily be focused on elimination of the exogenous periopathogens *Aa* (particularly associated with the etiology of localized aggressive early-onset periodontitis) and *Pg* and secondary suppression of the other species of the red complex (*Tf* and *Td*).

From this point of view, Winkel et al (2001) performed an interesting double-blind placebo clinical study with the combination of amoxicillin and metronidazole and included microbial analysis of the subgingival microflora. In their study of patients with chronic periodontitis, the researchers found that the significantly better clinical outcome in the test group could be attributed to patients infected with *Pg*. Patients in the test group who did not have this pathogen did not derive greater benefit from the combined antibiotic regimen than patients in the control group derived from a placebo. These observations indicate that not all patients benefit equally from systemic administration of metronidazole plus amoxicillin. Microbial testing may separate patients who will benefit from adjunct antibiotic therapy from patients who will not, suggesting that selective use of potent antimicrobial therapies is prudent.

At the 2nd European Workshop on Periodontology, the following questions related to systemic use of antibiotics in periodontal therapy were addressed (Lang et al, 1996):

- Which groups of patients benefit from systemic administration of antibiotics during periodontal therapy?
  - A number of studies indicate that localized aggressive early-onset periodontitis and other forms of aggressive early-onset periodontitis can be treated successfully by me-

chanical treatment alone (Wennström et al, 1986). However, several studies show a more predictable positive outcome with the use of adjunctive systemic antimicrobial therapy (Guerrero et al, 2005; Kaner et al, 2007; van Winkelhoff et al, 1989; Winkel et al, 1998, 1999; Xajigeorgiou et al, 2006). There is evidence to support the use of systemic antibiotic therapy in cases of *Pg-* and/or *Aa-* associated aggressive early-onset periodontitis. The high susceptibility of aggressive early-onset patients to continued periodontal breakdown, together with data indicating that elimination of *Pg* and *Aa* by mechanical means is not predictable (Quirynen et al, 2001; Renvert et al, 1990), makes a strong case for systemic antimicrobial therapy. Maximal suppression of these organisms seems to be a reasonable therapeutic approach.
  - Patients with generalized refractory periodontitis who have evidence of ongoing disease despite optimal mechanical therapy may benefit from systemic administration of antibiotics.
  - Patients with acute conditions such as abscess formation or necrotizing periodontitis may also benefit from systemic antibiotics.
  - Microbiologic evaluation may facilitate the choice of therapy. It is biologically sound and good medical practice to base systemic antimicrobial therapy on appropriate microbiologic data. However, further research is needed to determine the utility of microbiologic testing.
- In which phase of treatment is systemic antibiotic administration most beneficial?
  - With the exception of acute conditions such as abscesses or necrotizing periodontitis, systemic antimicrobial therapy should not be administered without prior mechanical therapy.
- Based on scientific evidence, which antibiotic treatment regimens can be recommended?
  - Several regimens have been tested for the treatment of *Aa-*associated localized aggressive early-onset periodontitis, including tetracyclines, metronidazole, and metronidazole in combination with amoxicillin. Although no direct comparisons are available, substantial evidence indicates that metro-

Box 2 Recommended systemic antibiotic periodontal therapy after microbial diagnosis of specific microbes*†

- *Aggregatibacter actinomycetemcomitans:*
  - Amoxicillin plus metronidazole
  - Amoxicillin plus clavulanic acid
  - Doxycycline/minocycline or azithromycin (in case of penicillin allergy)
- *Porphyromonas gingivalis, Tannerella forsythia, Treponema denticola* (the red complex):
  - Metronidazole
- Enterobacteria (for example, *Escherichia coli, Enterobacter* species, and *Klebsiella* species):
  - Ciprofloxacin (preceded by sensitivity tests)

*More than 5% of the total cultivable microflora or more than 106 by paperpoint sampling and checkerboard hybridization DNA-DNA analyses.

†Modified from Asikainen et al (2002).

Box 3 Recommended systemic therapy based on clinical periodontal diagnoses*

- Acute periodontal conditions (ANUP and periodontal abscesses):
  - Metronidazole, 250 mg, 3 times per day for 7 to 10 days (in smokers, 400 mg, 3 times per day)
- ANUG and acute mucosal infection:
  - Selection of antibiotics based on microbial analysis and sensitivity testing (in case of enterobacterial infection, see Box 2)
- Localized and generalized aggressive early-onset periodontitis and aggressive periodontitis in adults with confirmed *Aggregatibacter actinomycetemcomitans* infection:
  - Amoxicillin, 250 mg, 3 times per day plus metronidazole, 250 mg, 3 times per day for 7 to 10 days
  - Amoxicillin, 500 mg, 2 times per day plus ciprofloxacin, 500 mg, 2 times per day for 7 to 10 days
  - Amoxicillin plus clavulanic acid, 500 mg, 2 times per day for 7 to 10 days
- Aggressive periodontitis in adults with confirmed periopathogenic infection (for example, the red complex *Porphyromonas gingivalis, Tannerella forsythia,* and *Treponema denticola*) and *Prevotella intermedia:*
  - Metronidazole, 250 mg, 3 times per day for 7 to 10 days (in smokers, 400 mg, 3 times per day for 10 days)
- Refractory periodontitis and immunodeficient patients:
  - Probing depth reduction by nonsurgical or supplementary surgery (and possibly regenerative therapy) and use of metronidazole or metronidazole combined with amoxicillin, 250 mg, 3 times per day for 7 to 10 days
  - Selection of antibiotics based on microbial diagnosis and sensitivity testing

*Modified from Asikainen et al (2002).

nidazole in combination with amoxicillin is more efficacious than metronidazole alone (Guerrero et al, 2005; van Winkelhoff et al, 1989; Xajigeorgiou et al, 2006). By implication, other *Aa*-associated periodontal diseases in need of systemic antimicrobial therapy can be treated with a similar regimen.

- Aggressive early-onset periodontitis associated with both *Pg* and/or *Aa* has been treated with tetracyclines, metronidazole, metronidazole in combination with amoxicillin, and amoxicillin in combination with clavulanic acid. The data are inadequate for definite recommendation of any one option.
- Various antibiotic regimens have been tested for generalized refractory periodontitis; although the short-term effects have been promising, treatment response among patients has varied greatly. Recurrence of disease has been attributed to the observed reemergence of putative pathogens. There are few comparative studies of the efficacy of these regimens.

More than 10 years after the workshop, the answers developed for these questions are still valid, with minor additions.

Boxes 2 and 3 show recommendations for systemic use of antibiotics in Scandinavia (Asikainen et al, 2002).

In addition, screening for eradication of the exogenous periopathogens *Aa* and *Pg* in family members might be indicated, to reduce the risk of reinfection and possible recurrence of disease in patients who have been treated for infection by these microbes.

Based on a systematic review of 20 years of dental literature, Walker and Karpinia (2002) concluded that, in particular, treatment of *Aa*-associated localized aggressive early-onset periodontitis and aggressive refractory periodontitis may be more successful if systemic antibiotics are used as a supplement to nonsurgical or surgical therapy. Because of the emergence of tetracycline-resistant *Aa* (prevalence about 25%), the combination of amoxicillin and metronidazole is recommended for treatment of *Aa*-associated localized aggressive early-onset periodontitis. The most efficient antibiotic for treatment of aggressive refractory periodontitis was not as clear, and the authors recommended that the selection be case dependent based on microbiologic analyses and sensitivity tests. Depending on the outcome of the analyses, metronidazole, metronidazole plus amoxicillin, amoxicillin plus clavulanic acid, or clindamycin can be used.

To assess the need for additional antibiotic treatment, completion of conventional mechanical therapy should be followed by microbiologic testing comprehensive enough to allow selection of the optimal drug regimen in cases where antibiotic therapy is warranted. The tests should be repeated 1 to 3 months after antimicrobial therapy to verify elimination or marked suppression of the pathogens and to screen for possible superinfection. Ideally, the posttreatment composition of the subgingival microbiota should be similar to that found in periodontally healthy individuals.

Separate microbial samples may be taken from individual pockets with recent disease activity, or samples from several subgingival sites may be pooled: Pooled samples provide useful information on the range of periodontal pathogens to be targeted by antibiotic therapy. A representative subgingival sample may be obtained by pooling specimens from one deep bleeding or suppurating periodontal pocket in each quadrant.

The oral microbiology test should be supplemented by a susceptibility test in order to select the most effective drug or combination of drugs and to prevent the development of antimicrobial resistance (for details on oral microbiology tests and periodontal sampling techniques, see volume 3 [Axelsson, 2002]).

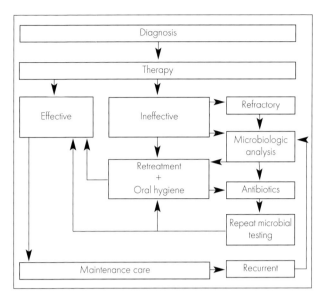

Fig 145 Flow chart of periodontal systemic antibiotic therapy. (Modified from van Winkelhoff et al, 1996, with permission.)

As discussed earlier, potent antibiotics should not be used without prior thorough mechanical debridement, excellent gingival plaque control, adequate clinical diagnosis, microbial analysis, and, if possible, susceptibility testing of target organisms. The flow chart in Fig 145 (van Winkelhoff et al, 1996) presents a practical approach to antibiotic therapy for patients with untreated adult periodontitis.

Clinical and microbial effects of systemic antibiotics

The effectiveness of antibiotic therapy in periodontics can best be demonstrated in randomized controlled clinical studies. Many existing studies are difficult to interpret because of their use of clinically different patient groups, failure to assess periodontitis disease activity, varying antimicrobial regimens, limited and varied evaluation periods (often not exceeding 1 year), major differences in baseline subgingival microbial composition, lack of randomization and double-blind evaluation, and inadequate gingival plaque control.

The most commonly used study design evaluates systemic antibiotics as an adjunct to scaling and root planing. This is in agreement with good medical practice: The bacterial load should be reduced as much as possible before antibiotic therapy. This type of study compares possible additional clinical and/or microbial effects of the antibiotic drug with those of a placebo medication or no control medication (see Guerrero et al, 2005; Winkel et al, 1999).

A second model examines the effectiveness of antimicrobial therapy in patients with refractory periodontitis or with recurrent abscess formation. The subjects have experienced further loss of periodontal attachment after thorough conventional mechanical treatment, with or without periodontal surgery.

The optimal study design for evaluation of antimicrobial periodontal therapy is a prospective, randomized, placebo-controlled, double-blind investigation. Uncontrolled longitudinal, retrospective, and case-report studies are less reliable.

To date, most clinical studies have evaluated the supplementary effect on mechanical periodontal therapy of a single antibiotic agent, but the current trend is to combine antibiotics to control the mixed subgingival periopathogens and eliminate the exogenous pathogens *Aa* and *Pg*, which are responsible for true periodontal infection.

The most common single antibiotics tested in periodontal therapy are tetracyclines, metronidazole, clindamycin, and Augmentin. During the last decade, the combination of amoxicillin and metronidazole has most frequently been tested, particularly in *Aa*-associated localized aggressive early-onset disease. Metronidazole and amoxicillin combined seem to exert synergistic activity against *Aa*. Studies by van Winkelhoff et al (1989, 1992) have shown that amoxicillin (375 mg, three times daily) plus metronidazole (250 mg, three times daily) for 10 days following scaling and root planing eliminated *Aa* in 97% or more of patients with *Aa*-associated localized aggressive early-onset periodontitis and resulted in improved clinical status. In a randomized placebo-controlled clinical trial, Guerrero et al (2005) also showed that amoxicillin (500 mg, three times daily) plus metronidazole (500 mg, three times daily) for 7 days following complete-mouth nonsurgical subgingival instrumentation resulted in significantly greater reduction of deep pockets and attachment gain after 6 months than did placebo controls in a selected group of patients with generalized aggressive early-onset periodontitis.

In another recent study, Xajigeorgiou et al (2006) also showed that scaling and root planing plus amoxicillin plus metronidazole resulted in significantly greater reductions of deep pockets (greater than 6 mm) and suppressed the red complex species and *Aa* better than did scaling and root planing alone in patients with generalized aggressive periodontitis after 6 months.

In a 24-month randomized controlled study in adult periodontitis patients, Haffajee et al (2006) evaluated the long-term effect of nonsurgical therapy, periodontal surgery, amoxicillin plus metronidazole, and placebo on probing depth, attachment level, and the red complex of periopathogens (*Pg*, *Tf*, and *Td*) as well as *Eubacterium nodatum* following initial complete-mouth scaling, root planing, debridement, and oral hygiene education. The combination of amoxicillin plus metronidazole resulted in the greatest gain of periodontal attachment, while there were only minor differences in probing depth reduction among the four groups.

Amoxicillin plus metronidazole also resulted in the most significant reduction of periopathogens. The aggressive *Pg* and *Tf* were almost eliminated, while, in the placebo group, *E nodatum* and *Td* had increased almost to baseline values after 24 months. Even in the nonsurgical and surgical groups, *Pg* and *Tf* in particular were consistently reduced, while the counts of *E nodatum* and *Td* increased during the last 6 months of the study. There was almost no difference between the nonsurgical and surgical groups.

In another study, Haffajee et al (2006) randomly assigned adult periodontitis patients to one of four different treatment groups:

1. Initial scaling, root planing, and oral hygiene education (positive control)
2. Initial scaling, root planing, and oral hygiene education plus metronidazole, 250 mg, three times daily for 14 days

3. Initial scaling, root planing, and oral hygiene education plus PMTC once a week for 3 months
4. Initial scaling, root planing, and oral hygiene education plus metronidazole, 250 mg, three times daily, plus PMTC once a week for 3 months

The greatest probing depth reductions compared to the positive control group (0.15 mm) were achieved by metronidazole plus professional mechanical toothcleaning (0.32 mm), followed by metronidazole alone (0.28 mm). The combination of metronidazole and PMTC once per week also resulted in the most significant reduction of red complex periopathogens in initially deep diseased pockets. That means frequent PMTC continuously reduced probing depth (thereby changing the ecology) and prevented recolonization by periopathogens subgingivally after the successful initial treatment by scaling, root planing, and systemic administration of metronidazole (MPIC). The results of this study confirmed the important role of initial intensive treatment followed by excellent gingival plaque control.

In a randomized 12-month clinical study, the same research group (Haffajee et al, 2006) also compared the effect of mechanical debridement with and without initial systemic administration of antibiotics (amoxicillin plus metronidazole) in adult periodontitis patients. Supplementary initial use of systemic antibiotics resulted in 0.8-mm probing depth reduction and 0.4-mm attachment gain compared to 0.5-mm and 0.0-mm, respectively, without antibiotics.

In a selected group of subjects with refractory periodontitis, Haffajee et al also evaluated the effect of a comprehensive MPIC program during a 24-month period (unpublished data, Haffajee A, 2006). Initially, all the subjects received complete-mouth scaling, root planing, and debridement under local anesthesia and comprehensive education in proper self-care procedures. Directly after subgingival instrumentation, controlled slow-release tetracycline fibers (Actisite, Alza) were placed in all pockets of 4 mm or more. In addition, systemic antibiotics (amoxicillin, 500 mg, three times daily plus metronidazole, 250 mg, three times daily) were prescribed

for 14 days. PMTC was carried out once a week during the first 3 months. Maintenance subgingival debridement, PMTC, and self-care education as well as clinical and microbial evaluations were performed every 3 months during the 24-month study.

At 24 months, there were significant reductions in plaque scores, bleeding on probing, pocket suppuration, and probing depths as well as significant gains in periodontal attachment compared to the baseline values. The median counts of subgingival microbial taxa were also substantially reduced from baseline. Thus it may be concluded that such an MPIC program can successfully heal infectious inflamed periodontal tissues and prevent further progression, even in refractory patients.

As discussed earlier, it is difficult to compare the effect of systemic antibiotics on periodontal disease in many published studies because of the enormous variations in clinical and microbial variables, sample size, periodontal status at baseline, lengths of the study, study design, and so on. Of 158 published articles on the supplementary effect of systemic antibiotics to scaling and root planing, only 25 were eligible for inclusion in a systematic review by Herrera et al (2002).

Overall, groups treated with scaling and root planing in combination with systemic antibiotics demonstrated better results in clinical attachment level and periodontal probing depth than did those treated with scaling and root planing alone or a placebo. Only limited meta-analyses could be performed because of the difficulties in pooling the studies and the lack of appropriate data. The analysis revealed a statistically significant additional benefit for spiramycin (change in probing depth) and amoxicillin plus metronidazole (change in clinical attachment level) in deep pockets. Herrera et al (2002) concluded:

Systemic antimicrobials, in conjunction with SRP [scaling and root planing], can offer an additional benefit over SRP alone in the treatment of periodontitis, in terms of CAL [clinical attachment level] and PPD [periodontal pocket depth] change, and reduced risk of additional CAL loss. However, differences in study methodology and lack of data precluded an adequate and complete pooling of data for a more comprehensive analysis. It was difficult to establish definitive conclusions, although patients with deep pockets, progressive or 'active' disease, or specific microbiological profile, can benefit more from this adjunctive therapy.

(For reviews on systemic use of antibiotics, see Herrera et al, 2002, 2008; Mombelli, 2008; Slots and Ting, 2002; Slots, 2004; and van Winkelhoff et al, 1996.)

Local antibiotics

During the last 15 to 20 years, a wide range of delivery systems have been developed for local application of antibiotics for treatment of periodontal diseases: hollow fibers, acrylic resin strips, dialysis tubes, monolithic fibers, polypropylene fibers, resorbable cellulose, biodegradable gel, and resorbable collagen. Specific advantages and disadvantages are associated with local application. Local delivery of antibiotics in the subgingival area can provide much higher concentrations than the systemic route. For example, due to the substantivity of tetracycline on root surfaces, concentrations of 600 $\mu g/mL$ or more have been reported for 10 days after application on monolithic fibers (Goodson et al 1983, 1991a; Mombelli et al, 1997): The maximum concentration of tetracycline in crevicular fluid after systemic administration is approximately 8 $\mu g/mL$. Local application causes fewer side effects than systemic administration and reduces problems of patient compliance.

Disadvantages of topical therapy are the costs, the relatively time-consuming application procedures, the difficulty in accessing the deeper parts of the lesions, the inability to kill key pathogens at mucosal sites, and the failure of the antibiotic to penetrate the deeper parts of the tissues. Furthermore, in patients with localized aggressive periodontitis, *Aa* is detectable not only at sites with periodontal destruction but also at subgingival sites without measurable periodontal breakdown (van Winkelhoff et al, 1994). These sites will be unaffected by application of topical antibiotics to the active disease sites and may serve as foci for recurrent infection. The same

kind of reinfection can occur from other sites or oral niches (dorsum of the tongue) harboring the other exogenous periopathogen, *Pg*.

Local application of antibiotics in the treatment of periodontitis has, however, several important advantages over systemic use, and both approaches should be regarded as different measures for treatment of destructive periodontal diseases. Particularly in maintenance patients who exhibit a few sites that do not heal in spite of comprehensive subgingival debridement and excellent gingival plaque control (so-called refractory periodontitis) or a few sites with recurrence of active lesions, local delivery of efficient, controlled slow-release antibiotics should be very attractive.

However, local delivery of antibiotics has to be preceded by site-specific subgingival microbial analyses for selection of the most efficient antibiotic and by one-stage complete-mouth disinfection to improve accessibility of the antibiotic by mechanical removal of the plaque biofilms and to prevent reinfection by periopathogens (in particular *Aa, Pg,* and *Tf*).

Local delivery systems

The objective of local delivery devices is to establish a drug reservoir in the periodontal pocket, prolonging effective concentrations at the site of action despite loss by crevicular fluid clearance. In principle, a local delivery device consists of a drug reservoir and a mechanism to regulate the rate of drug release.

Local delivery devices offer either sustained or controlled drug release: By definition, the duration of sustained drug release is less than 24 hours, while the duration of drug release for controlled slow-release delivery systems is 3 to 11 days.

Sustained slow-release delivery uses formulations that expose the antibiotic reservoir to removal mechanisms (GCF washout) and exhibit first-order drug release kinetics: The agent is dissipated exponentially at a rate directly proportional to its concentration. Most such delivery systems are biodegradable (eg, cellulose, collagen, gels). In controlled slow-release drug delivery, the antimicrobial reservoir is protected from local removal mechanisms after placement, enabling zero-order drug release kinetics that maintain consistently elevated pocket concentrations of the agent during its application, for example, monolithic fibers (Actisite, 25% tetracycline).

Topical antibiotics

A limited number of antibiotics have been used in delivery devices for local use in periodontal therapy: tetracycline, minocycline, doxycycline, metronidazole, clindamycin, amoxicillin plus clavulanic acid, and ofloxacin.

These antibiotics differ in mode of action and spectrum of susceptible microorganisms. Because all have been shown to be generally effective against bacteria associated with periodontitis, rational selection can be based only on the unique characteristics of the microflora of the individual patient and site. Potential side effects and, in particular, the risk of inducing bacterial resistance, should be evaluated. Nonantibiotic effects, such as the anticollagenase effect of tetracyclines, should also be considered. It would therefore be practical to have more than one antimicrobial agent available in local delivery systems.

Several investigations have evaluated the microbiologic effects of sustained or controlled local delivery of antibiotics using a variety of microbiologic methods: predominant cultivable microbiota, selective media identification of target organisms, darkfield microscopy, and DNA probe analysis. Data have also been expressed using different clinical outcome variables. The results indicate that significant suppression of the subgingival microbiota can be achieved (Hanes and Purvis, 2003; Kinane and Radvar, 1999; Rams and Slots, 1996).

In several studies, moreover, the application of the local delivery device was accompanied by mechanical plaque removal by scaling and root planing. The observed microbial suppression in such studies should therefore be ascribed to a combination of mechanical and chemotherapeutic effects. In this context, it is important to note that a 10-fold decrease in total cultivable bacteria can be expected from mechanical debridement alone (Haffajee et al, 1997).

Also of interest is the observation that even very high concentrations of antibiotics in controlled slow-release delivery systems maintained over a therapeutic period of at least 7 days failed to completely eliminate the periodontal pathogenic microflora from all treated sites (Mombelli et al, 2002).

To date, four commercial products have received regulatory approval in the European Union:

1. *Actisite:* 25.0% tetracycline fiber, nonresorbable controlled-delivery system
2. *Elyzol:* 25.0% metronidazole gel, resorbable sustained-delivery system (Colgate)
3. *Dentomycin:* 2.0% minocycline lipid gel, resorbable sustained-delivery system (Blackwell Supplies)
4. *Atridox:* 8.5% doxycycline polymer gel, resorbable controlled-delivery system (Tolmar)

Except for Elyzol, the same commercial products have been cleared by the US Food and Drug Administration. Table 5 presents pharmacokinetic variables of the four different products.

Tetracycline fibers (Actisite). The vehicle comprises cylindrical, nonresorbable fibers of biologically inert (ethylene-vinyl acetate) plastic copolymer, generally considered safe. The active agent is 25% w/w tetracycline hydrochloride powder. The delivery device is supplied individually packaged as a thread 0.5 mm in diameter and 23.0 cm in length, containing 12.7 mg (approximately 0.5 mg/cm) of tetracycline.

On average, Actisite provides gingival fluid concentrations of tetracycline exceeding 1,300 μm/mL by controlled slow release for 10 days. This is of great importance because tetracycline is bacteriostatic and requires longer exposure time than do bactericidal antibiotics. This concentration is more than 100 times higher than that provided by systemic tetracycline.

The main indications for use of Actisite fibers are localized sites that remain diseased or exhibit recurrent disease despite thorough scaling, root planing, and debridement and excellent gingival plaque control as well as infected sites prior to regenerative therapy. The criteria for diseased pockets may be bleeding on probing, increased probing depth, attachment loss, increased pocket temperature (fever), exudate, and infection by

Table 5 Pharmacokinetic variables of most relevant sustained-release or controlled-delivery devices for subgingival application of antimicrobial agents*

Drug	Concentration (%)	Composition of delivery device	Type	Decay	Duration of reservoir	MIC_{90}[†] ($\mu g/mL$)	Observation time (h)
Tetracycline fibers	25.0	Ethylene-vinyl acetate monolytic fiber	Controlled-delivery	Pseudo-zero	> 240 h	50	264
Metronidazole gel	25.0	Glycerol monooleate + sesame oil gel	Sustained-release	Exponential	< 12 h	32	16
Minocycline lipid gel	2.0	LS-007 gel	Sustained-release	2× exponential	< 24 h	16	21
Doxycycline polymer gel	8.5	Polymer	Controlled-delivery	Unknown	> 7 d	Unknown	Unknown

*Modified from Quirynen et al (2002).

[†]MIC_{90} = Minimum inhibitory concentration for 90% of the strains; based on data from Mombelli and Van Winkelhoff (1997) and Tonetti (1997).

exogenous *Aa* and *Pg* and/or endogenous periopathogens, such as *Tf* and *Td*.

However, *Aa* may be resistant against tetracycline. In addition, *Aa* may be inaccessible to topical delivery of tetracycline because it invades the soft periodontal tissues. Therefore, *Aa*-infected sites should not be treated with tetracycline fibers.

Prior to placement of the Actisite fibers, the selected pockets are mechanically cleaned by debridement and PMTC and irrigated by a pulsated jet device or a syringe with 0.5% iodine or 0.1% CHX solutions.

Actisite placement is not difficult but requires some initial practice. The manufacturer recommends the following technique: Actisite is removed from the pouch and the protective sheath. A piece no shorter than 7.5 cm is cut (shorter fibers may be difficult to handle). For a deep pocket, a longer segment of fiber is used (13.0 to 17.0 cm). Unused fiber cannot be stored for later use because of photosensitivity and degradation. The local authority on medical waste should be consulted to determine proper disposal procedures for any unused fiber.

Although most practitioners use a gingival retraction cord packer to place Actisite because the serrations facilitate placement, a smooth instrument may also be used. In the mandibular anterior region, pockets are tight and narrow, and the smaller diameter of the periodontal probe can be useful. With deep pockets or a furcation, the longer length of a probe may facilitate placement at the base of the pocket. The universal curette, shaped to fit around the tooth, can also be used for fiber placement. In a furcation area, the narrow diameter and long neck of an amalgam plugger is useful for placement of fibers.

Actisite placement is easier if moisture and bleeding are controlled. Assistance is recommended during the procedure.

Figures 146a to 146d show the technique for placement of the tetracycline fiber in the diseased pockets of a maxillary central incisor. For maximum effect, the pocket should be completely filled. If fiber protrudes above the gingival margin, the excess should be cut off. The pocket should not be overfilled because the fiber may become dislodged. Tissue blanching can be an indication of overfill.

Figs 146a to 146d Application of Actisite fiber around a maxillary central incisor. (Courtesy of Dr M. Tonetti.)

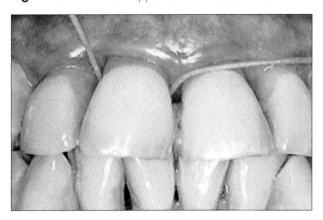

Fig 146a The fiber is passed through the interproximal contacts and wrapped loosely around the tooth.

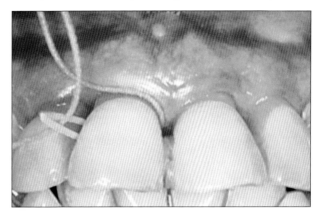

Fig 146b The fiber will not pass through a tight contact without breaking. A floss threader or dental floss in the form of a loop is used to pass the fiber under the contact.

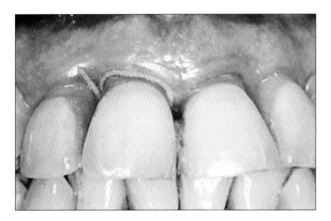

Fig 146c The fiber is wrapped completely around the tooth at least once, and the pocket is filled entirely.

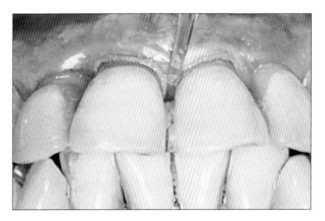

Fig 146d A gingival retraction cord packer is used to gently place the fiber under the gingival margin around the entire tooth. One end of the fiber will be placed at the base of the deepest part of the pocket.

A cyanoacrylate adhesive keeps Actisite in place. A disposable applicator is used to apply the adhesive. To maximize infection control, an applicator should be used only once and then discarded. A used applicator should not be inserted in the adhesive bottle. Before adhesive is applied, excess moisture is removed from the treated surface with cotton rolls or gauze; however, the site should not be completely dry because moisture is the catalyst that causes the adhesive to set. The adhesive is applied sparingly to the tooth surface because the adhesive tends to flow readily to other areas of the mouth.

If the fiber protrudes, for example, from a shallow sulcus, any exposed fiber and the tooth surface should be covered with adhesive. The adhesive sets in approximately 1 minute. Immediately after application, the adhesive should be covered with a thin layer of petroleum jelly to prevent the adhesive from sticking to the mucosa or tongue.

Placement techniques may have to be varied in different situations. For tight interproximal contacts, the entire tooth can be treated without passing the fiber through the contacts: A gingival retraction cord packer is used to gently place the fiber in the interproximal area, from the buccal or lingual direction, until it protrudes on the other side. A double strand of fiber, twisted, can facilitate filling of deep pockets, particularly in the pos-

Box 4 Instructions for patients after placement of Actisite controlled slow-release tetracycline fibers

- Do not brush or floss the treated area.
- Do not eat hard or crunchy foods.
- Do not chew gum or eat sticky foods.
- Avoid touching the area with the tongue or fingers.
- Do not push a loose fiber back in place.
- Contact the clinician if the fiber is dislodged within a week or if there are other concerns.

terior region, where access is more difficult. To treat a tooth with many deep pockets, the fiber is wrapped around the tooth multiple times and, where necessary, layered. To aid retention in a furcation, a separate segment of fiber is placed in this region, and the rest of the tooth is then treated as described earlier.

Special precautions are necessary for treatment of a highly inflamed site and in cases of suppuration. The following procedures are recommended: The fiber is loosely inserted in the pocket to avoid formation of a lateral fistula, and the adhesive is applied. Ten days later, the fiber is removed. At this stage, there should be no persistent suppuration. For optimal effect, any fiber lost in the first 7 days must be replaced.

The time required for Actisite placement will vary with probing depth, location of the tooth, and the operator's experience. As with any dental procedure, maxillary teeth, unobstructed by tongue and saliva, are easier to treat than mandibular teeth, and anterior teeth are easier to treat than posterior teeth because they are more accessible. Most patients do not experience pain during the Actisite procedure, and fiber placement itself does not require local anesthesia, but this may be necessary for the preceding debridement.

Patient education will improve the success of Actisite therapy. Verbal instructions will reinforce the information provided in the patient education materials and increase the patient's compliance (Box 4). Patients must maintain good oral hygiene in the untreated areas of the dentition. To help keep the fiber-treated area clean, an antimicrobial rinse may be recommended (eg, 0.1% CHX twice daily). The appointment for fiber re-

moval should be scheduled to allow a total of 10 days of therapy.

Because neither the adhesive nor the fiber is biodegradable, both must be completely removed. This is a simple procedure and takes only a few minutes. The adhesive and fiber are removed with a curette or cotton pliers. Subsequently, the pocket is flushed with water to check for any remaining fiber and adhesive.

After fiber removal, the gingiva is often distended for a few hours, providing good visibility of the root surface and an opportunity to remove any residual calculus. To avoid accumulation of food debris in the distended pocket, patients should be instructed not to chew on the treated area for 24 hours and to continue with the antimicrobial rinse (0.1% CHX) for a further 2 weeks to help maintain good oral hygiene.

Actisite is contraindicated in patients known to be sensitive to tetracycline. As with other antibiotic preparations, Actisite therapy may result in overgrowth of nonsusceptible organisms, including fungi. Therefore, Actisite should be used cautiously in patients with a history of oral candidiasis. The most common adverse reactions are limited to discomfort on placement (in 10% of patients) and local erythema following removal (in 11% of patients).

The clinical application of Actisite in two patients will be described. The first, a 51-year-old woman with severe generalized periodontitis, was treated by initial therapy and complete-mouth surgery. After completion of active therapy, she was enrolled in a 3-month recall program and maintained a very good level of oral hygiene over 5 years. At a recall appointment, a 6-mm suppurating pocket with evidence of recent 4-mm attachment loss was observed mesial to the maxillary right central incisor (Fig 147a). The pocket was loosely filled with tetracycline fiber (Figs 147b and 147c).

Ten days later, the fiber was removed, and the acute suppuration had resolved. At 2- and 6-month follow-up examinations, a 2-mm gain in probing attachment level was observed, along with a 2-mm recession of the gingival margin. The probing depth stabilized at about 2 mm without bleeding on probing. The patient then reentered the regular maintenance program (Fig 147d).

Figs 147a to 147d Application of Actisite in a patient with a 6-mm suppurating pocket. (Courtesy of Dr M. Tonetti.)

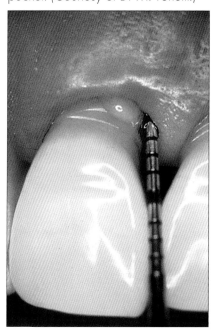

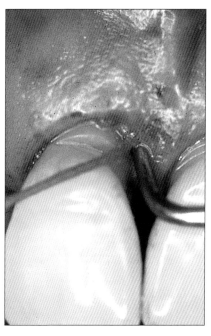

Fig 147a A 6-mm pocket with purulence and bleeding on probing is present at the mesial aspect of a right maxillary central incisor.

Fig 147b After subgingival debridement, an Actisite fiber is applied.

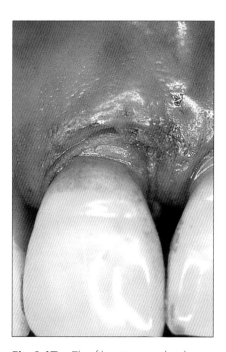

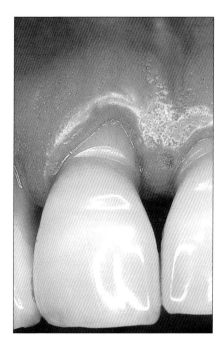

Fig 147c The fiber is completely positioned. A superficial layer of the fiber is visible circumferentially around the tooth.

Fig 147d Six months after treatment, the recession at the gingival margin has increased. Bleeding on probing and purulence are absent. The probing depth has been reduced to 2 mm.

Figs 148a to 148d Application of Actisite in a patient with grade II furcation involvement. (Courtesy of Dr M. Tonetti.)

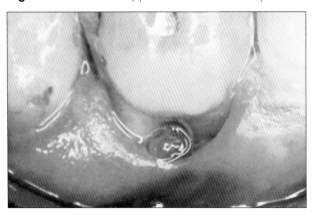

Fig 148a Grade II furcation involvement is present on the buccal surface of a mandibular right first molar following initial nonsurgical debridement.

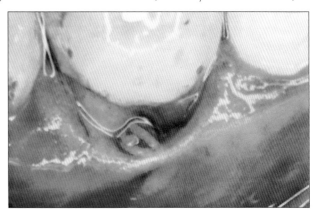

Fig 148b An Actisite fiber is applied to the furcation area.

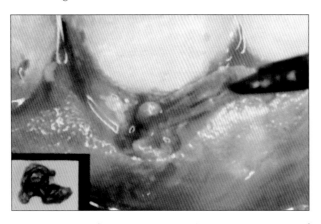

Fig 148c The fiber is removed. *(inset)* Appearance of used fiber.

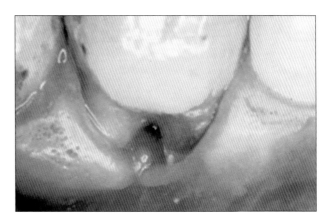

Fig 148d At the 2-month follow-up, the soft tissues are healed, and some gingival recession has occurred. After microbial sampling was performed, the site was treated with regenerative therapy.

Another patient, a 30-year-old man, presented with mild generalized periodontitis and grade II furcation involvement on the buccal aspect of the mandibular right first molar. After initial therapy, no bleeding on probing was detectable in most of the dentition. Probing depths were 3 mm or less. However, on the buccal aspect of the mandibular right first molar, bleeding on probing persisted, along with severe edema of the interradicular papilla (Fig 148a). On the mesial aspect of the distal root, vertical probing depths reached 7 mm; horizontal probing was 6 mm. Tetracycline fibers were inserted in an attempt to fill both the vertical and horizontal components of the defect (Fig 148b). Fiber removal (Fig 148c)

was followed by supplementary scaling, root planing, and debridement.

The reduction in inflammation after tetracycline treatment resulted in resolution of the edema and control of the bleeding on probing. Slight recession of the gingival margin was also observed (Fig 148d). Residual vertical and horizontal components were subsequently treated by regenerative therapy.

In multicenter studies, the effect of tetracycline fibers on probing depth reduction and attachment level has been similar to that of scaling, root planing, and debridement (Goodson et al, 1991a). In addition, a study in maintenance patients with persistently infected deep pockets showed that

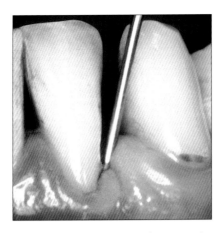

Fig 149a Application of metronidazole gel commences from the bottom of the pocket.

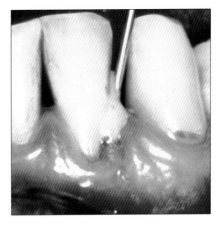

Fig 149b Application of the gel continues until the pocket is filled with some supragingival excess.

scaling and root planing combined with tetracycline fibers had a significantly better effect than scaling and root planing alone on probing depth and periopathogens after 12 months (Aimetti et al, 2004; for reviews on the effect of tetracycline fibers, see Greenstein and Rethman, 1996; Pavia et al, 2003; and Tonetti, 1998).

Metronidazole gel (Elyzol). Elyzol metronidazole gel is a sustained-release bioresorbable delivery device loaded with 40% metronidazole benzoate, corresponding to 25% metronidazole (250 mg/g). The matrix consists of a mixture of glycerol monooleate and sesame oil, formulated to obtain a reserve hexagonal phase in contact with an aqueous environment. The product is supplied in amber glass cartridges, each containing 1 g of gel, corresponding to 250 mg of metronidazole. The cartridges are preloaded into a specially designed disposable applicator. Stored at or below room temperature, the gel has a shelf life of 3 years.

The innovative feature is the gel itself: Its specific structure and subsequent degradation ensure a sustained slow release of the drug. Enzymes in the GCF play an essential role in the release process. With its pharmacokinetics and phase transfer properties, the gel is formulated specifically to meet the demands of an antimicrobial product for local administration.

The system allows the active substance to be placed at the sites of infection, in the dental pockets. The gel melts at just below body temperature, spreading freely in the liquid state to all parts of the gingival pocket. Contact with GCF transforms the liquid to a solid, which then slowly dissolves, gradually releasing metronidazole in adequate concentration, and for sufficient duration, to be effective against infection.

After systemic administration of metronidazole, concentrations similar to plasma levels (5 to 20 µg/mL) have been found in periodontal pockets. In contrast, local application of Elyzol in periodontal pockets results in initial concentrations ranging from 100 to 1,000 µg/mL, about 100 times the minimum inhibitory concentration of most anaerobic periopathogens (Stoltze and Stellfeld, 1992). Because conventional susceptibility determinations are performed at drug concentration levels of less than 64 µg/mL, it is suspected that bacteria normally considered nonsusceptible to metronidazole (such as *Aa*) may be reduced after local application of Elyzol.

The device is applied so that the pocket is filled to excess (Figs 149a and 149b). No specific data are available on the size and the stability of the drug reservoir established a few minutes after application.

Based on the assumption of a single-compartment open model, a half-time elimination of 3.4 hours is expected. The duration of effective antimicrobial concentrations is less than 1 day. In most cases, the delivery device is completely resorbed in less than 12 hours. In this context, it should be noted that planktonic bacterial cultures in vitro have shown the bactericidal activity of metronidazole to be time independent (Stoltze and Stellfeld, 1992).

Hence, metronidazole is active against the predominant gram-negative and gram-positive anaerobic subgingival microflora associated with periodontal diseases. In contrast to the broad-spectrum antibiotic tetracycline, however, metronidazole does not interfere with strepto-coccal species associated with periodontal health, and resistance will not develop.

Although the manufacturer recommends two applications within a week, the effective antimi-crobial concentrations last only 24 hours after ap-plication, and the clinical effect could therefore be enhanced by application on 2 successive days or by three applications within a week.

Indications for use of Elyzol are similar to those for Actisite: *(1)* at localized sites of persis-tent or recurrent infection after initial thorough scaling, root planing, and debridement, supple-mented with a tailored maintenance program, and *(2)* at infected sites prior to regenerative ther-apy. In contrast to Actisite, Elyzol gel is resorbable and can be used not only during the week prior to guided tissue regeneration and guided bone regeneration in cases of peri-implantitis but also during the surgical procedures to prevent direct infection of the biodegradable barriers during initial wound healing.

In a review of the use of metronidazole gel, Magnusson (1998) concluded that metronida-zole gel has shown clinical effects similar to those of scaling and root planing in both initially treat-ed and maintenance patients, in long-term stud-ies (up to 24 months). However, metronidazole gel cannot be recommended as a substitute for scaling and root planing because of unknown side effects. The supplementary effect to scaling and root planing in patients exhibiting chronic periodontitis seems to be negligible (Jansson et al, 2003; Leiknes et al, 2007).

The supplementary effect of Elyzol gel to sub-gingival scaling, root planing, and debridement has yet to be evaluated in a double-blind, split-mouth study. In clinical practice, topical use of antibiotics should always be preceded by me-chanical debridement to improve accessibility (for review, see Magnusson, 1998).

Minocycline gel (Dentomycin). Dentomycin minocycline gel is also available in Japan under the name Periocline (Sunstar). Minocycline oint-ment is a bioresorbable system, comprising 2% minocycline hydrochloride in a matrix: a mixture of hydroxyethyl cellulose, aminoalkyl methacry-late, triacetine, and glycerin. Magnesium chloride is used to modify the release properties.

The somewhat viscous gel (0.5 g, containing 10.0 mg of minocycline) is loaded in a disposable polypropylene syringe with a plastic contra-angle tip, to be applied four times at 14-day in-tervals. The tip of the applicator is inserted to the base of the periodontal pocket, and the pocket is filled to the gingival margin as the applicator is slowly withdrawn. The patient may resume brushing, flossing, eating, and drinking 2 hours after treatment.

Dentomycin is unstable at room temperature and must be refrigerated. The product informa-tion provided by the manufacturer states that peak plasma concentrations of approximately 0.1 µg/mL occur during administration and a peak concentration of 0.2 µg/mL occurs after the entire contents of the syringe (10.0 mg) are in-gested. These data suggest that 50% or more of the material is lost from the periodontal pocket when the patient swallows.

Concentrations of minocycline in the cre-vicular fluid decrease according to a double-exponential process. The half-time elimination, based on the assumption of a single-compart-ment open model, is estimated at about 4 hours, and the duration of effective antimicrobial activi-ty is expected to be about 1 day. Minocycline pos-sesses good substantivity, and this may partly ex-plain the sustained-delivery profile. No explicit data are available on the establishment of a sub-gingival drug reservoir after application.

The indications for use are similar to those for metronidazole gel, that is, in localized dis-eased pockets of 5-mm depth or more in main-tenance patients with refractory or recurrent periodontitis. The application of the gel must always be preceded by subgingival debridement and PMTC.

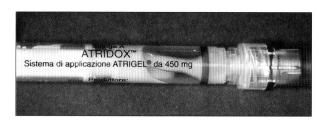

Fig 150 Atridox consists of doxycycline granulate and a delivery vehicle, which are mixed together by 100 to 150 pumping movements.

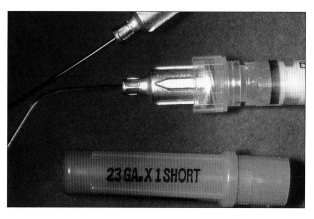

Fig 151 Mixed Atridox gel is kept in the vehicle syringe and applied to the diseased pocket via a curved cannula. (Courtesy of Dr G. Heden.)

The gel is contraindicated for patients with known hypersensitivity to tetracyclines, patients with complete renal failure, pregnant women, and children.

In a multicenter study involving about 500 patients with moderate to advanced chronic periodontitis, scaling and root planing followed by the application of minocycline gel resulted in significantly more sites with less than 5-mm probing depth than did scaling and root planing alone after 3 months (Paquette et al, 2004). In a 15-month double-blind, randomized, parallel, comparative study, scaling and root planing plus minocycline resulted in greater reductions of probing depth and suppression of periopathogens than scaling and root planing plus placebo gel (van Steenberghe et al, 1999; for review, see Vandekerckhove et al, 1998).

Doxycycline (Atridox). Atridox is a two-syringe mixing system for controlled release of doxycycline for up to 7 days (Fig 150). One syringe contains the delivery vehicle, which is a bioresorbable, flowable polymeric formulation. The second syringe contains 50 mg of doxycycline hyclate. The delivery vehicle and the doxycyline granulate are mixed together, and a curved cannula is attached for delivery of the gel (Fig 151). The cannula is placed to the bottom of the pocket and slowly withdrawn coronally while the pocket is filled with some excess of the gel (Figs 152a and 152b). A plane instrument is used to distribute the excess in

the pocket (Fig 152c), and supragingival excess is removed (Fig 152d). In contact with GCF and saliva, the gel will harden to a bioresorbable material for controlled slow release of doxycycline for about 7 days.

Normally, doxycycline is bacteriostatic. However, with the high concentration of doxycycline achieved with this local delivery system, it should also be bactericidal for most periopathogens in the pocket.

The indications for use of Atridox are similar to those for the other local antibiotic delivery systems, primarily in localized persistent diseased deep pockets (greater than 5 mm) or in localized recurrent diseased deep pockets in refractory and maintenance patients. However, subgingival microbial sampling and sensitivity tests and mechanical subgingival debridement should always precede selection of the antibiotic system to ensure that the most suitable antibiotic is used.

Atridox is contraindicated for children up to 12 years of age, pregnant women, patients who need prophylactic systemic antibiotics before surgery, and patients with reduced renal or hepatic function.

Multicenter studies have shown that scaling and root planing in combination with Atridox results in greater clinical improvement than either scaling and root planing alone (Eickholz et al, 2002; Garrett et al, 1999; Wennström et al, 2001) or reduction of subgingival periopathogens alone (Ratka-Krüger et al, 2005). Particularly in smokers,

Figs 152a to 152d Application of Atridox doxycycline gel. (Courtesy of Dr G. Heden.)

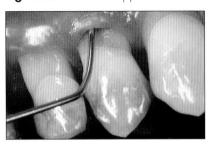

Fig 152a Atridox doxycycline gel is applied from the bottom of a deep diseased pocket on the buccal surface of a maxillary first premolar after subgingival debridement.

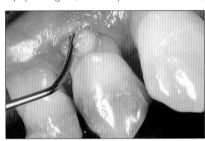

Fig 152b The doxycycline gel is applied with some supragingival excess.

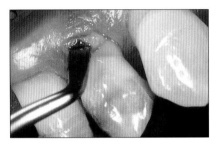

Fig 152c Excess gel is pressed down in the pocket with a plane instrument.

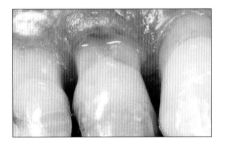

Fig 152d Clinical status after removal of excess gel.

the adjunctive effect of Atridox to scaling and root planing seems to be important (Machion et al, 2004; Ryder et al, 1999; Tomasi and Wennström, 2004). However, in maintenance patients with diseased pockets, topical use of locally delivered doxycycline did not achieve any additional effect when used with nonsurgical periodontal therapy (Bogren et al, 2008; Tomasi et al, 2008).

Comparison of available delivery devices

Most studies on the effect of locally delivered antibiotics have compared the effect of a single antibiotic to that of scaling and root planing or compared the effect of scaling and root planing plus an antibiotic to that of scaling and root planing alone. To date there is only one study of the relative efficacies of Actisite, Elyzol, and Dentomycin as adjuncts to scaling and root planing in the treatment of sites with persistent periodontal lesions following a course of initial mechanical periodontal therapy. In this controlled, randomized, single-blind,

parallel group study, 67 patients were randomly assigned to one of four treatment groups: *(1)* scaling and root planing (positive control), or *(2)* scaling and root planing plus a single application of tetracycline fibers, *(3)* scaling and root planing plus two applications of metronidazole gel, *(4)* scaling and root planing plus 3 applications of minocycline ointment (Radvar et al, 1996).

All treatments resulted in significant improvements in the outcome variables, but in terms of probing depth reductions and decrease in gingival inflammation, only the group treated with the combination of tetracycline fibers and scaling and root planing was significantly better than the positive control. There were no significant differences among the four treatment modalities in terms of clinical attachment level. The authors concluded that, while all three local antimicrobial delivery systems seemed to offer some benefit over scaling and root planing alone, tetracycline fibers demonstrated a significantly greater advantage in the treatment of persistent periodontal lesions (Radvar et al, 1996). More studies are needed to evaluate the relative efficacies of all these systems in the treatment of all clinical variables related to periodontal diseases.

Adverse reactions and side effects

The same precautions that apply to systemic administration of antibiotics also apply to local application. In particular, local delivery devices should not be used in subjects with known allergy to the active drug, components of the drug delivery device, or its breakdown products.

In general, however, a major advantage of local application is the minimal incidence of side effects frequently associated with systemic administration, such as gastrointestinal and vaginal complications. Local delivery, however, does not preclude the selection of resistant bacterial strains or the overgrowth of intrinsically resistant organisms at the site of administration or elsewhere. To date, no data are available on the possible effects of local delivery on the gastrointestinal microflora, prompting speculation and concern about the spread of bacterial resistance and even of a potential increase in the risk of transfer of multidrug resistance. This important issue warrants more thorough investigation. With respect to the oral microflora, the few available studies on the increase in bacterial resistance following local delivery of tetracycline and minocycline show, in an extremely limited number of cases, a significant increase in the proportions of resistant strains immediately after application and a return to baseline levels after a few months (Madinier et al, 1999; Walker et al, 1981).

Apart from the possible selection of resistant bacterial strains, other concerns are the potential for overgrowth or oral candida, local side effects such as pain on application, the development of abscesses, and tooth sensitivity. Furthermore, patient acceptability, taste disturbances, and other subjective aspects have not been adequately documented.

In patients with a history of immunodeficiency or frequent courses of antibiotics, it is generally recognized that local delivery devices should be used with caution, and possibly following additional testing, to avoid overgrowth of commensal organisms such as candida and to avoid selection of resistant enteric microorganisms.

Also of importance is the variability in the propensity of antibiotics to induce bacterial resistance. In this respect, metronidazole or some of the antiseptics could have particular advantages over tetracycline and minocycline. Given the increasing problems of bacterial resistance, the use of antibiotics for the treatment of periodontal disease should be highly selective, based on microbiology susceptibility tests and avoiding the indiscriminate, repeated use advocated by some manufacturers. Such selective use implies the definition of clear, possibly narrow indications.

Strategies for local slow-release delivery of antibiotics

Comprehensive nonsurgical scaling, root planing, and debridement, supplemented by high standards of gingival plaque control, will heal most diseased sites. However, complete removal of subgingival plaque biofilm cannot always be achieved, even by open flap surgery, because of plaque-retentive factors such as calculus, cementum hypoplasia, and iatrogenic defects that result in grooves and exposed dentinal tubules.

Observations that some periodontal bacteria (*Pg* and *Aa*) may penetrate the surrounding periodontal soft tissue have given new impetus to the evaluation of systemic antimicrobial therapy, on the assumption that local antimicrobial drug delivery systems in the periodontal pocket cannot achieve effective concentrations within the surrounding soft tissue. Variable responses of *Aa*-associated periodontal disease have been attributed to failure of the locally delivered drug to reach to the depths of soft tissue penetration.

It has been proposed that bacteria observed in dentinal tubules on exposed root dentin surfaces could serve as reservoirs for reinfection of periodontal pockets. Local drug delivery is the only therapy known to penetrate the root surface. It is not known whether reinfection from dentinal tubules is a serious problem or whether antibiotic penetration would be effective in reducing the risk.

Considering the overall efficacy data—the fact that even the controlled-delivery system with the best pharmacokinetic profile, which effects substantial depression of the subgingival microbiota, is unable to completely disinfect a periodontal pocket—and concerns about the implications of widespread use of antibiotics in dentistry, the first conclusion to be drawn from the available evidence is that local delivery should be used only after meticulous comprehensive mechanical removal of subgingival biofilms to optimize accessibility of the antibiotic to the remaining periopathogens. At present, this can be achieved by a combination of mechanical root debridement, PMTC, and local delivery of the selected antimicrobial agent. Several approaches could be attempted to increase the efficacy of locally delivered drugs against biofilm bacteria and avoid the side effects associated with invasive mechanical instrumentation of the root surface, eg, concurrent use of surface-active agents, enzymes, electric fields, or ultrasonics.

Another factor in determining the optimal therapeutic strategy is the predicted duration of microbial suppression. Several investigations using mechanical debridement alone, local delivery alone, or a combination of the two have shown initial suppression of pathogens (associated with drug and/or mechanical treatment) to be followed by a rebound toward pretreatment levels. Therefore, the initial professionally performed MPIC has to be combined with optimal gingival plaque control by self-care and PMTC at needs-related intervals for maintenance of successful therapy (for details, see chapter 5 and volume 4 [Axelsson, 2004]).

A key issue requiring clarification is the choice of local or systemic administration. The additional component in systemic antibiotic therapy is its effect on invasive bacteria beyond the scope of the local delivery system. At present, it is premature to evaluate the effectiveness of this strategy. The clinical and microbiologic diagnosis (eg, localized or generalized aggressive *Aa*-associated periodontitis, refractory disease with persistence of localized nonresponsive sites, recurrent localized periodontitis), the treatment objective, and the overall oral ecology are key factors for the selection of the most appropriate delivery route (for reviews on local delivery of antibiotics, see Bonito et al, 2005; Greenstein, 2006; Greenstein

and Polson, 1998; Greenstein and Tonetti, 2000; Quirynen et al, 2002; Rams and Slots, 1996; and Tonetti, 1997; for a review on locally delivered and systemically used antibiotics, see Walker and Karpinia, 2002).

SPECIAL TREATMENT OF FURCATION-INVOLVED TEETH

Healing of infectious inflamed tissues in the furcation areas is very difficult because of the limited accessibility for gingival plaque control by self-care, PMTC, and subgingival debridement. Therefore, periodontal support is lost faster in furcation sites than in other sites.

When the furcation areas of multirooted teeth are involved, treatment is very complex. Various treatment modalities have been described, and selection of the appropriate form of treatment requires a proper understanding of problems posed by the anatomy and pathology of the furcation. The basic rationale for therapy is to arrest the progression of periodontal disease, to promote regeneration of periodontal tissues, and to establish conditions that facilitate adequate gingival plaque control.

Treatment may be limited to periodontal therapy or may comprise a complex, multidisciplinary approach that includes restorative therapy, endodontics, and/or orthodontics. The different treatment modalities are broadly correlated with the classification of furcation lesions.

Treatment of periodontal disease around a multirooted tooth should not be initiated until the presence of a furcation involvement has been investigated, that is, after examination comprising both clinical probing and radiographic analysis. Graduated curved periodontal probes, explorers, or slim curettes should be used for the clinical examination. Methods and materials for diagnosis of furcation involvement at different sites are described later in this chapter (also see Axelsson, 2002). The vitality of the affected tooth must also be tested in order to differentiate between a plaque-associated lesion and a lesion of pulpal origin in the furcation area.

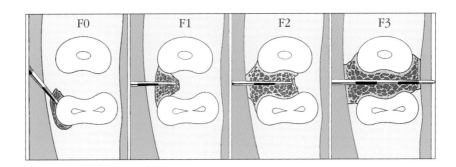

Fig 153 Furcation involvement, grades 0 to III (F0 to F3). (Courtesy of Dr K. Rateitschak.)

Classification

Furcation involvement may be classified according to the severity of horizontal destruction in the interradicular area (Fig 153):

- Grade 0: No furcation involvement
- Grade I: Horizontal loss of supporting tissues not exceeding one-third the width of the tooth
- Grade II: Horizontal loss of supporting tissues exceeding one-third the width of the tooth but not encompassing the total width of the furcation area
- Grade III: Horizontal through-and-through destruction of the supporting tissues in the furcation

Epidemiological data in randomized samples of 50-, 65-, and 75-year-old individuals in the county of Värmland, Sweden (Axelsson, 1998, 2002, 2004; Axelsson et al, 1990, 2000), showed that the highest prevalence of grade II and III furcation involvement was on the distal surfaces of the maxillary first molars, while grade I was most common on the buccal surfaces of the mandibular first molars in 50-year-olds.

Predisposing factors

These analytic epidemiologic data as well as data from the classic study on the "natural history of periodontal disease" (Löe et al, 1978) indicate that the distal surfaces of the maxillary first molars are the key-risk surfaces for vertical as well as horizontal loss of attachment because of insufficient gingival plaque control interproximally between the maxillary first and second molars. There are several predisposing factors for progression of periodontal disease in the furcation areas:

- Complicated internal furcation root surface morphology
- Cervical enamel projections (CEPs)
- Accessory pulp canals
- Bifurcation ridges
- Location of the furcation relative to the cementoenamel junction (CEJ)
- Location and diameter of the furcation entrance

Almost 100% of all mandibular molar roots and 90% of maxillary mesiobuccal roots exhibit concave surfaces. These concave surfaces limit accessibility to plaque control, scaling, root planing, and debridement, thus favoring maintenance of infections and progression of attachment loss. However, the furcation concavities are covered by thicker cementum than the adjacent convexities. This may have some clinical importance during instrumentation.

The CEP into the furcation areas is an anatomic anomaly, usually covered by a junctional epithelial attachment instead of a connective tissue attachment. Masters and Hoskins (1964) studied the prevalence of CEPs on 474 extracted molars. CEPs occur primarily on the buccal surfaces of mandibular molars (about 30%) and on maxillary molars (about 20%); the highest prevalence is on the buccal surface of mandibular second molars. CEPs may be classified into the following grades according to severity:

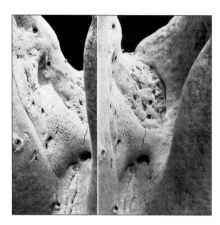

Fig 154 Detail of the furcation area. Perforations indicate accessory canals from the pulp, confirming the need to perform a pulp test for all teeth with furcation involvement.

- Grade I: Short CEP from CEJ
- Grade II: Longer CEP, approaching the furcation area
- Grade III: CEP extending directly into the furcation area

There is general agreement that *(1)* grade I projections are most common, *(2)* buccal surfaces are most often affected, and *(3)* CEPs as a group are found in decreasing order of prevalence on mandibular second molars, maxillary second molars, mandibular first molars, and maxillary first molars. The presence of a CEP is a risk factor for development of isolated furcation lesions.

Histologic and gross anatomic studies in animals and on extracted human molars have demonstrated the presence of accessory canals, especially in the region of furcations. Other studies on extracted molar teeth, utilizing radiopaque dyes injected under pressure, have reported accessory canals in the furcation region in more than 50% of specimens (Gutmann, 1978; Lowman et al, 1973). About 75% of the maxillary and mandibular furcations exhibit accessory foramina (Vertucci and Williams, 1974). Figure 154 shows several accessory canals with foramina in the furcation areas of two maxillary molars. The high incidence of accessory canal foramina opening at the furcation region suggests that pulpal disease could be a cofactor in the pathogenesis of furcation involvement. There is a fairly high association between periodontal inflammation resulting from pulpal lesions and the presence of accessory canals. Thus, furcation involvement may arise from pulpal pathosis. After endodon-

tic therapy, regeneration of attachment may be achieved. Therefore, on the bases of clinical reports and the high prevalence of accessory canal foramina opening at the furcation regions, all furcation lesions should be monitored for the possible presence of contributory pulpal disease by vitality testing of the pulp.

Bifurcation ridges from the mesial surface of the distal root to the distal surface of the mesial root may occur frequently in mandibular molars (in more than 50%). The ridge is mostly formed of cementum. The presence of an intermediate bifurcation ridge in a mandibular molar may demand special consideration when the method of treatment for a periodontal lesion is selected because this anatomic structure creates niches where plaque can accumulate undisturbed when the furcation is exposed to the oral environment.

The closer the position of the furcation relative to the CEJ, the greater the chance of furcation involvement. If the furcation becomes diseased in a tooth with a long trunk and a short root, the remaining roots have relatively little surface area embedded in surrounding osseous structure; as a result, the prognosis is often poor. Conversely, a tooth with a short trunk is more likely to develop early furcation involvement but often has longer remaining roots, giving the tooth greater potential for corrective therapy. For example, the entrance to the furcation area on the distal surfaces of maxillary first molars is located at the center of the surface and relatively close to the CEJ, in contrast to the entrance to the furcation on the mesial surface, which is located mesiolingually and more apically. This may explain the high

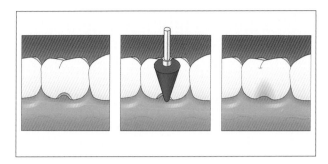

Fig 155 Odontoplasty on the buccal surface of a mandibular first molar with grade I furcation involvement.

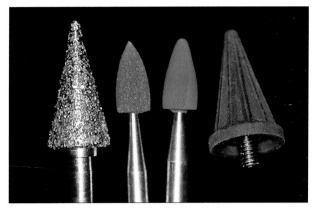

Fig 156 Rotating instruments suitable for odontoplasty. *(left to right)* Rough, pointed diamond tip (Dentatus); brown rubber polishing tip (Shofu); green extrafine rubber polishing tip (Shofu); and pointed rubber tip for prophylaxis paste (Young Dental).

prevalence of grade II and grade III furcation involvement distally in maxillary first molars.

The mandibular furcation entrance is usually located midway between the mesial and distal surfaces of the tooth. The buccal furcation entrance diameter of the mandibular and maxillary first molar ranges between 0.50 and 1.75 mm. The buccal furcation entrance diameter of the maxillary first molars is smaller than either the mesiopalatal or distal diameter. Similarly, the buccal entrance diameter of the mandibular first molars is smaller than the lingual. There is a low correlation between the mesiodistal widths at the CEJ of both maxillary and mandibular first molars and their furcation entrance diameters. Therefore, large teeth do not necessarily have large furcation entrance diameters.

Treatment of grade I furcation involvement

Early diagnosis is essential for successful management of the furcation problem. Although effective mechanical plaque control by self-care may remove subgingival plaque as far as 1 mm buccally and 2 to 3 mm interproximally below the gingival margin, subgingival plaque control is a total failure in furcation areas. This residual plaque may lead to a total loss of attachment between the roots rather than on the outer surface.

Depending on the probing depth, the fibrosity of the tissue, and the amount of attached gingiva, the treatment of a grade I furcation may involve scaling, root planing, debridement, selective grinding, and/or odontoplasty. Grade I and some shallow grade II lesions may also respond quite well to surgery, such as a modified Widman flap procedure, without osseous contouring. In shallow grade II lesions, thorough pocket elimination procedures with odontoplasty may also produce predictable long-term results.

Odontoplasty, "the reshaping of a portion of a tooth" (American Academy of Periodontology, 2001), may be incorporated into the management of some grade I and shallow grade II lesions in order to widen the narrower furcation entrances, allowing more effective debridement, PMTC, and gingival plaque removal by self-care (Fig 155). Odontoplasty in grade I furcation involvement is most frequently performed nonsurgically on the buccal surfaces of maxillary and mandibular molars and the lingual surfaces of mandibular molars. Because of limitations of access and difficulty in achieving optimal plaque control, such recontouring is difficult in proximally located furcations, that is, in maxillary molars and premolars when adjacent teeth have approximal contact. Exceptions are when the teeth are prepared for complete-coverage crowns.

The following instruments are useful for odontoplasty procedures (Fig 156):

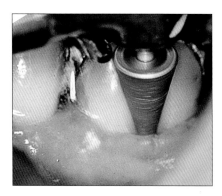

Fig 157a Use of a rough diamond tip to recontour the buccal surface of a mandibular first molar with grade I furcation involvement.

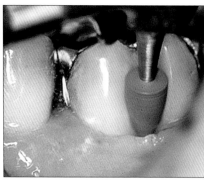

Fig 157b Finishing of the recontoured surface with a rubber tip.

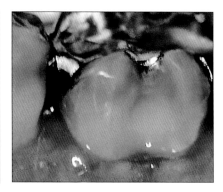

Fig 157c Clinical result immediately after treatment.

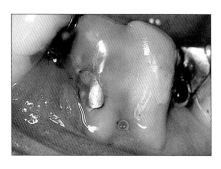

Fig 158 Stable, healthy periodontal status 33 years after odontoplasty was performed to eliminate grade I furcation involvement in a mandibular molar.

- One rough, pointed diamond tip for recontouring the tooth.
- Two rubber polishing tips (fine and extrafine)
- One pointed rubber tip

Odontoplasty for treatment of grade I furcation involvement on the buccal surface of a mandibular first molar is shown in Figs 157a to 157c. The deepest portion of the furcation defect is located with the tip of the rough diamond instrument. The area of involvement is eliminated by the diamond, which is used with copious water spray in a gradually more vertical position (see Fig 157a). Finally, the instrument is used laterally in a vertical position to flatten the vertical groove.

The recontoured surface is finished with rubber tips and copious water spray (see Fig 157b). The recontoured surface is then polished with the rubber prophylaxis tip and a fluoride prophylaxis paste. Alternatively, calcium hydroxide paste could be applied to block exposed, sensitive dentinal tubules. For caries prevention, the recontoured surface may be coated with CHX var-

nish and fluoride varnish, applied with a pointed bristle brush. Figure 157c shows the clinical result immediately after treatment. In 3 weeks, a healthy buccal papilla will fill the cervical concavity of the recontoured surface if the patient maintains excellent gingival plaque control.

Figure 158 shows the long-term stable clinical result 33 years after odontoplasty on the buccal surface of another mandibular molar. The gingivae were healthy, and the vertical and horizontal probing depths were only 1 mm.

Figure 159a shows exceptionally deep odontoplasties performed on the buccal surfaces of the maxillary left molars because of grade I to II furcation involvement. This case is an exception and was carried out because the patient was well educated in needs-related self-care methods of plaque control (Fig 159b). Figure 159c shows the long-term result 36 years after treatment. No further progression of the furcation involvement had occurred, and plaque disclosure revealed that the patient had maintained a high standard of plaque control in spite of the deep recontouring.

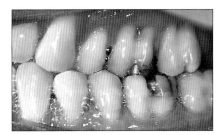 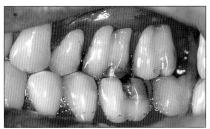 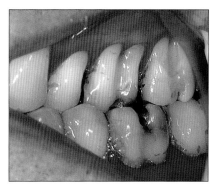

Fig 159a Clinical status directly after extraordinarily deep odontoplasty on the buccal surfaces of the maxillary first and second molars because of grade I to II furcation involvement and limited odontoplasty on the mandibular first molar.

Fig 159b Plaque disclosure at the first recall examination reveals the excellent standard of plaque control by the patient after systematic education in self-care.

Fig 159c The periodontal status is excellent 36 years after treatment because of the maintenance program and the patient's high standard of oral hygiene, as shown after plaque disclosure.

Even furcation-involved molars with old complete-coverage crowns can be successfully recontoured (Fig 160). In nonvital molars, grade II involvement can also be treated successfully by recontouring (Fig 161).

The progression of periodontitis is more rapid in furcation defects (horizontal pockets) than in vertical pockets because of more limited access during plaque control procedures. When crowns and fixed partial dentures for multirooted teeth are planned, careful examination for possible furcation involvement is therefore most important. On the other hand, there is unique access for recontouring of grade I and initial grade II furcation involvement during preparation. To ensure adequate access for hygiene, the technician has to design crowns that resemble a recontoured natural crown (Figs 162a to 162d).

The long-term outcome of odontoplasty is closely related to the quality of gingival plaque control obtained through self-care as well as PMTC. For self-care, the use of a double-ended interspace brush (Lactona 27, Lactona) or an electric toothbrush with a pointed brush (Rotadent, Pro-Dentec) together with the most efficient fluoride toothpaste is recommended.

Treatment of grade II and grade III furcation involvement

Mandibular molars

Furcation involvement in mandibular molars is diagnosed and confirmed by the combination of clinical probing and radiographs (conventional apical and vertical bitewing radiographs or computer-aided digitized radiographs). Because of the vertically curved entrance of the furcation area, a slim double-ended universal curette (Goldman-Fox 3) seems to be tailored for probing in the furcation area (Fig 163). There are also specially designed curved furcation probes (Fig 164). The probe can also be used in situ to provide an indicator of the furcation lesions on the radiograph (Fig 165).

Figure 166a shows heavy amounts of calculus on the root surfaces in an advanced (grade III) furcation lesion affecting a mandibular second molar. The findings were confirmed clinically after extraction of the tooth (Fig 166b). Figure 167a also shows a mandibular second molar without a maxillary opposing tooth. Grade III furcation involvement was confirmed clinically after

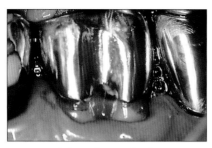

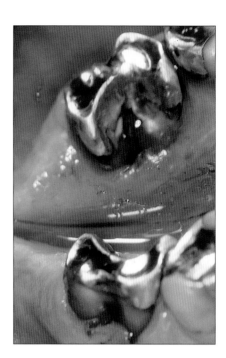

Fig 160 *(above)* Grade I furcation involvement has been eliminated by recontouring of an existing complete-coverage gold crown.

Fig 161 *(right)* In this nonvital tooth with an old amalgam crown, grade I to II furcation involvement buccally *(bottom)* and deep grade II involvement lingually *(top, mirror view)* has been eliminated by extremely deep recontouring, particularly lingually, almost to the level of a hemisection.

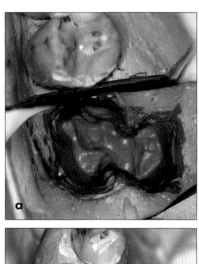

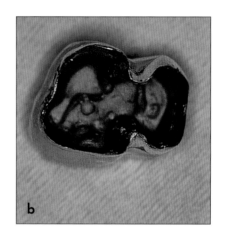

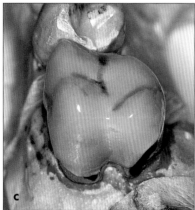

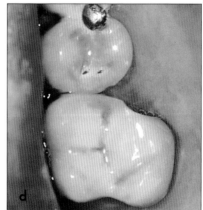

Figs 162a to 162d Grade I furcation involvement has been eliminated through mesial and distal recontouring during preparation of a permanent crown for a maxillary first molar. Note how the design of the crown allows optimal accessibility for hygiene procedures.

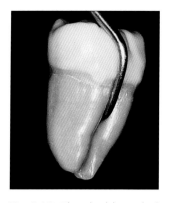

Fig 163 The double-ended Goldman-Fox No 3 (Hu-Friedy) is a long, slim curette used for diagnosis of furcation involvement in maxillary and mandibular molars.

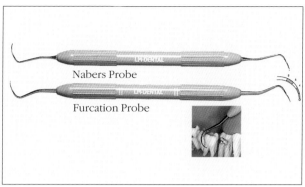

Fig 164 Curved furcation probes (LM-Instruments).

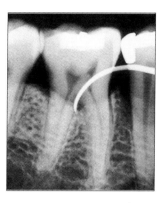

Fig 165 Furcation probe in situ at a mandibular first molar with furcation involvement.

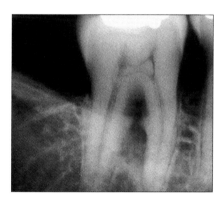

Fig 166a Radiograph of a mandibular molar with grade III furcation involvement. There is no maxillary opposing tooth. Interradicular alveolar bone loss extends to about 50% of the root length.

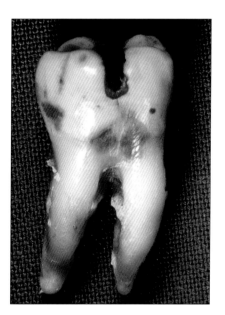

Fig 166b The presence of heavy amounts of calculus is confirmed clinically after tooth extraction.

extraction of the tooth (Fig 167b). The tooth exhibited extensive granulation tissue in the furcation area. The large, overcontoured, rough amalgam restoration demonstrated the important role of local plaque-retentive factors.

Nonsurgical scaling, root planing, and debridement are extremely complicated for mandibular molars with grade II or III furcation involvement because of limited accessibility to the concave distal surface of the mesial root and mesial surface of the distal root (Figs 168 and 169). Particularly thick, fibrous gingiva located coronal to the entrance to the furcation area limits the accessibility during nonsurgical instrumentation. This was confirmed in a study by Matia et al (1986), who evaluated the efficiency of curettes and ultrasonic scalers for scaling the molar furcation area with and without surgical access.

Postscaling examinations revealed that the mean percentage of calculus present on the dome surface of the furcations was 49.7% in the untreated control group, 37.7% in the closed curettage group, and 34.1% in the closed ultrasonic scaling group. In groups scaled after surgical exposure, the dome surface had the lowest mean percentage of remaining calculus, 2.7% for the opened curettage group and 1.0% for the opened ultrasonic scaling group. The results demonstrated the inadequacy of calculus removal utilizing a closed, nonsurgical approach to grade II and grade III furcation involvement, regardless of whether curettes or ultrasonic instruments are used.

The ideal treatment of grade II furcation defects, particularly on the buccal surfaces of mandibular molars, would be elimination of the defect by regeneration of the alveolar bone, periodontal ligament, and root cementum. However, although positive results of such therapy are predictable under special conditions, it is not realistic to expect regenerative therapy to be generally successful. At present, the profession is still awaiting evidence of successful regenerative therapy for grade III furcation defects, and the results to date for grade II defects on approximal surfaces of maxillary molars have been limited (Jepsen et al, 2004; Meyle et al, 2004; Pontoriero and Lindhe, 1995a and 1995b; Pontoriero et al, 1988, 1989; for details, see chapter 4).

Advanced grade II and grade III furcation lesions require a more complex approach to therapy than odontoplasty, including sectioning through the furcation. Before tooth-sectioning procedures are discussed, it is important to define certain terms as specified by the *Glossary of Periodontal Terms* (American Academy of Periodontology, 2001):

- *Root resection (amputation):* "Surgical removal of all or a portion of a root"
- *Root hemisection:* "The surgical separation of a multirooted tooth, especially a mandibular molar, through the furcation in such a way that a root and the associated portion of the crown may be removed or restored"

Root hemisection can usually be performed nonsurgically, without an open flap procedure. In cases where there is a risk that overhangs of tooth substance may be overlooked during tooth hemisection and root resection, flap elevation is indicated. This allows direct inspection of the surgically cut dentinal surface. A radiograph should also be obtained of the area immediately after the hemisection to verify that such overhangs do not persist.

As a rule, endodontic treatment of the root to be retained following tooth hemisection and root resection should be performed prior to treatment. That means the outcome of the endodontic treatment is known before extraction of the roots. In multirooted teeth with advanced destruction of the supporting tissues, it may not always be possible to decide until surgery which root or roots it is possible or most favorable to preserve. As an alternative to permanent obturation of all root canals before treatment, pulpectomy can be performed, and the canals can be filled with calcium hydroxide. Each of the openings to the root canals is sealed with glass-ionomer cement. Root hemisection or resection can thus be carried out without risk of bacterial contamination of the root canal. Permanent obturation of the roots in such cases is performed after hemisection or resection.

When the root or roots to be retained following root separation are being selected, the following factors should be considered:

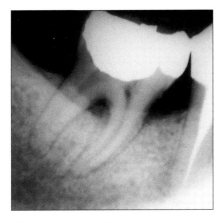

Fig 167a Mandibular second molar with grade III furcation involvement.

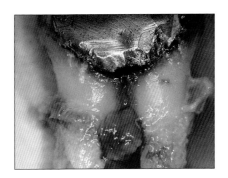

Fig 167b Extraction of the tooth reveals clinically extensive granulation tissue in the furcation area and a large, overcontoured amalgam restoration.

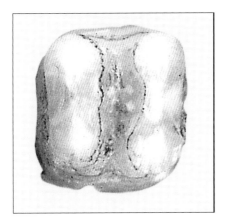

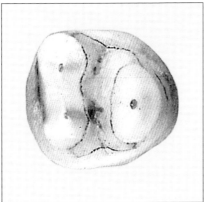

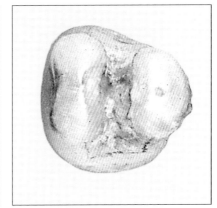

Fig 168 Cross section of the mesial and distal roots of the *(left to right)* mandibular first, second, and third molars.

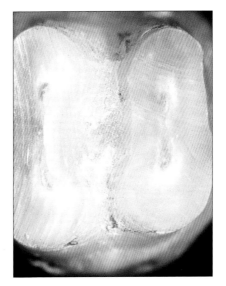

Fig 169 Cross section of the mesial *(left)* and distal *(right)* roots of an extracted mandibular first molar close to the furcation area.

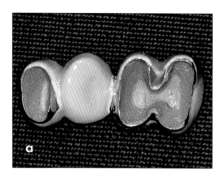
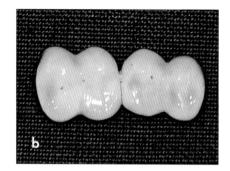

Figs 170a and 170b A permanent reconstruction is fabricated after recontouring of a mandibular first molar, which had exhibited grade II furcation involvement buccally and grade I involvement lingually. The second molar was hemisectioned, and the mesial root was extracted because of grade III furcation involvement.

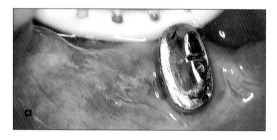
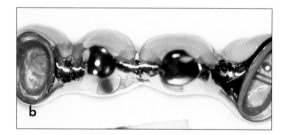

Figs 171a and 171b Because the mandibular first molar was missing and the second molar exhibited grade III furcation involvement, the mesial root of the second molar was extracted, and a permanent reconstruction extending from the second premolar to the distal root of the second molar was fabricated.

- The amount of supporting tissue remaining around the various roots
- The stability of the individual roots
- The root and root canal anatomy with respect to endodontic and restorative treatment procedures
- The periodontal condition
- The position of the various roots in the alveolar process in relation to adjacent and opposing teeth

In cases where, for example, the furcation of a mandibular first molar is involved to an extent that calls for tooth separation, it is usually easy to decide which root should preferably be retained on periodontal grounds. If the amount of remaining periodontium around the two roots is similar, it is often preferable for endodontic purposes to retain the distal root. This root has generally only one, wide root canal and is therefore easily accessible to endodontic treatment. However, after loss of the mesial portion of the tooth, prosthetic re-

placement by means of a fixed partial denture is often necessary (Figs 170a and 170b).

Figures 171a and 171b show a case in which a remaining distal root of a mandibular left second molar was hemisectioned because of grade III furcation involvement. The left first molar was already missing. After healing, a permanent reconstruction was made, consisting of a cast abutment with a post for the hemisectioned root, and a prosthesis from the second premolar to the distal root of second molar (see Fig 171a). To minimize the risk of root fracture, the abutment was designed with a separately cemented post and core, with a cervical collar (see Fig 171b). For extra retention of the prosthesis, the abutment preparation included a parapulpal pin. On the other hand, provided that the mesial root of a mandibular molar has a root canal anatomy that allows proper root obturation and insertion of a post, the root can be preserved and used as an abutment for a single crown, avoiding extensive bridge therapy.

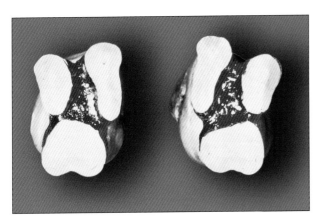

Fig 172 Cross section of the furcation regions of the maxillary left and right first molars.

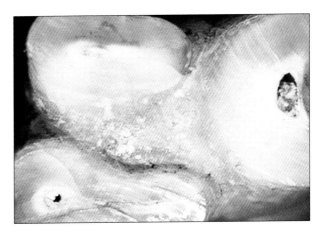

Fig 173 Furcation region of the maxillary right first molar.

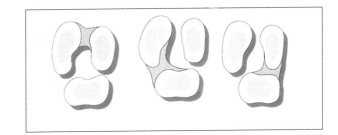

Fig 174 Different variations of fusion of divergent roots in maxillary molars.

In some cases of furcation therapy, it is important to note the proximity of the roots involved. If sectioning is planned and multiple roots are to be retained, it may be necessary to separate the roots orthodontically to achieve an embrasure that is adequate for gingival plaque control. The two tooth segments may be united in a single metallic restoration or separated and restored as single-rooted teeth with separate crowns. This procedure is sometimes called *bicuspidization* or *premolarization* and is most frequently performed on mandibular molars. A single isolated retained root of a formerly multirooted tooth has the same periodontal prognosis as any other single-rooted tooth after periodontal therapy, provided that gingival plaque control is well maintained.

Maxillary molars

Root resection or hemisection in maxillary molars presents greater difficulties. Because these teeth usually have three roots, one or two roots can be preserved after separation. The mesiobuccal roots of the first and second molars are comparatively wider buccopalatally than the distobuccal roots. The palatal roots are often wider mesiodistally than buccopalatally. The oval mesiobuccal roots often have marked invaginations, while the distobuccal roots generally have a more rounded outline and less frequently exhibit distinct invaginations (Figs 172 and 173).

Another morphologic variation that influences the diagnosis and treatment of furcation involvement in maxillary molars is fusion of divergent roots (Fig 174).

The clinical examination of furcations on the approximal tooth surfaces may be more difficult when adjacent teeth are present, especially if the contact area between the teeth is large. This is particularly the case in maxillary molars. As a rule, however, the furcation on the mesial surface of a maxillary molar should be probed from the mesiopalatal aspect of the tooth (Fig 175). The furcation on the distal surface is probed from the distobuccal aspect in a slightly apical direction (Fig 176).

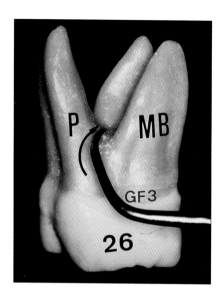 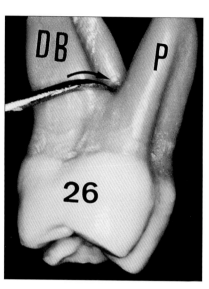 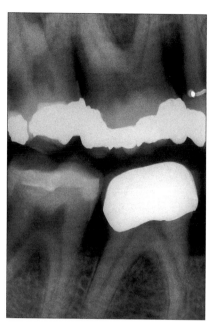

Fig 175 Mesial furcation involvement of the maxillary left first molar (tooth 26). This must be diagnosed in a mesiolingual-apical direction. (MB) Mesiobuccal root; (P) palatal root; (GF3) Goldman-Fox 3 curette.

Fig 176 Distal furcation involvement of the maxillary left first molar (tooth 26). This must be diagnosed in a distobuccal-apical direction. (DB) Distobuccal root; (P) palatal root.

Fig 177 Vertical bitewing radiographs offer the best projection for diagnosis of the alveolar bone level and localization of the furcation areas.

Radiographic analysis should supplement clinical examination of possible furcation involvement. The information obtained should be related to findings from the clinical examination. Vertical bitewing radiographs achieve the best projection and information about the alveolar bone level and location of the furcation entrance (Fig 177).

Although radiographs are necessary to determine the presence of bone loss in the furcation area, they cannot be used alone because they may be imprecise and inadequate to detect furcation involvement with any predictable accuracy. However, taking several radiographs from different angles can be valuable in evaluating root divergence or proximity and root configuration as well as in observing the height and width of the furcation chamber relative to the alveolar bone. For a more accurate assessment of the extent of the lesion, radiographs may be taken with probe, explorers, or curettes in place.

In cases of advanced destruction of the supporting apparatus in the maxillary molars, the oc-

currence of furcation involvement mesially and distally may be suspected when the image of the interdental alveolar bone crest in the radiograph is located apical to the normal level of the furcations. The diagnosis has to be confirmed by probing. In this context, it should be observed that even extensive loss of alveolar bone in the interradicular area of maxillary molars is often not disclosed on the radiograph because of the superimposition of remaining bone structure and the palatal root.

Even with careful clinical and radiographic examination, it is often impossible to determine the extent of the furcation defect without raising a flap to allow direct inspection. In cases of advanced periodontal disease around maxillary molars, separation of all three roots is often necessary to obtain access to the interradicular area, for assessment of the height of the remaining bone at the buccal surface of the palatal root and the palatal surfaces of the buccal roots, for example.

In most cases of deep grade II or III furcation involvement, resection may be the treatment of choice. Whether endodontics should be per-

Figs 178a to 178g Technique for resection of the distobuccal root. (Courtesy of Dr K. Rateitschak.)

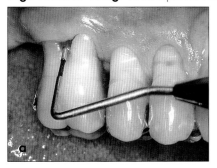
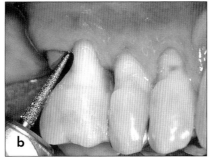
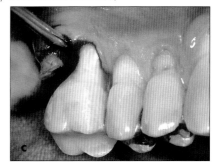

Figs 178a to 178c The mesiobuccal and palatal roots were already obturated, and the distobuccal root was resected using a pointed diamond bur.

Figs 178d and 178e After resection, the tooth is recontoured distobuccally for optimal accessibility for oral hygiene procedures.

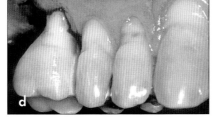
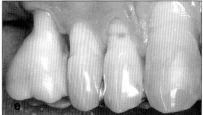

Fig 178f After resection, the distobuccal opening into the cavum is restored.
Fig 178g The contra-angled interspace toothbrush is the most suitable oral hygiene aid for cleaning this particular surface.

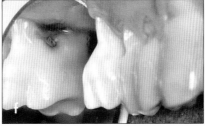
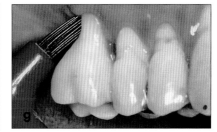

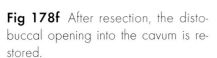

formed before or after resection has been a subject of great controversy, with some authors claiming that endodontic procedures should be done prior to root resection and others advocating vital root resection (Rosenberg, 1988; Smukler and Tagger, 1976). If it is possible to determine preoperatively which root or roots are to be removed, then endodontic therapy should precede root resection. However, occasionally the prognosis for individual roots cannot be determined until hemisection, with or without raising a flap, and the root or roots with poor prognosis are then removed at the time of hemisection. When a vital root is involved, a pulpotomy is performed; this will generally provide comfort for the patient for 2 weeks, after which endodontic treatment can be completed.

Resection. When a maxillary molar exhibits furcation involvement on the buccal aspect only or

when the buccal furcation and one of the proximal furcations are periodontally involved (eg, the buccal and the distal furcations), the tooth may be treated by resection of the distobuccal root (Figs 178a to 178g). Such a root resection can often be performed without the removal of excessive coronal tooth substance, avoiding the need for a cast crown. It can also be carried out successfully in maxillary molars to prolong the survival of existing crowns and bridges (Fig 179).

Resection of the palatal root might be an unusual way to solve a furcation problem. However, if the buccal furcation is intact, or the buccal roots are fused (see Fig 174), and a mesial and/or distal furcation involvement is combined with advanced loss of attachment around the palatal root, then the removal of this root and the maintenance of the buccal portion of the tooth, including the two buccal roots, may be the procedure of choice.

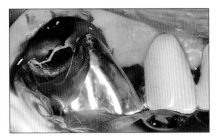

Fig 179 Clinical status directly after resection of the distobuccal root of a maxillary first molar and recontouring of the existing prosthetic abutment.

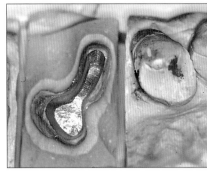

Fig 180a Hemisection and extraction of the distobuccal root of a maxillary left first molar because of grade II distal furcation involvement. Grade I mesial furcation involvement has been eliminated by recontouring.

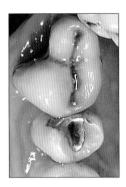

Fig 180b Hygienic design of the permanent crown.

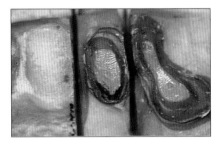

Fig 181a After extraction of the furcation-involved maxillary left first premolar and hemisection of the distobuccal root of the furcation-involved maxillary left first molar, the remaining part of the tooth has been recontoured and prepared. A cast gold post and core restoration has been cemented.

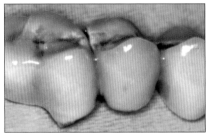

Fig 181b The hemisectioned first molar is used as an abutment in the permanent fixed partial denture that also replaces the extracted maxillary first premolar.

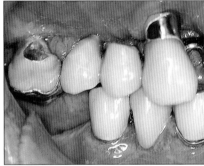

Fig 182 The buccal roots of a maxillary first molar with mesial and distal grade III furcation involvement have been resected to preserve a 30-year-old fixed partial denture in a woman who is more than 80 years old.

Hemisection. As discussed earlier, the distal surfaces of the maxillary first and second molars have the highest prevalence of grade II or III furcation involvement. Therefore, resection or hemisection of the distobuccal root is by far the most frequent treatment performed for furcation involvement in maxillary molars. If the tooth is to receive a crown or be used as a prosthetic abutment, hemisection of the distobuccal root and recontouring of the remaining tooth are the methods of choice (Figs 180 and 181).

It is important for the final crown to have a hygienic design that facilitates self-care procedures for gingival plaque control (see Fig 180b). Use of an electric toothbrush with a rotating pointed brush (Rotadent) or a double-ended interspace brush (Lactona 27) may be recommended to the patient.

Resection of teeth with furcation involvement can sometimes be used to preserve an existing prosthesis (Fig 182). When the roots that can or should be retained are being selected in cases of multiple furcation involvements in the maxillary molars, the position of the various roots in the jaw in relation to adjacent teeth must be considered. Provided the endodontic prognosis is favorable, the buccal roots may be retained in preference to a palatal root. For example, if the maxillary second premolar is present, then one or several of the buccal roots of the molars should be preserved as potential distal abutments in a complete prosthesis. Their position in the dental arch is more favorable than that of the

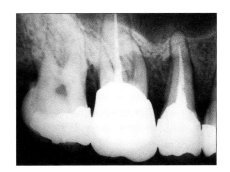

Fig 183a Advanced loss of alveolar bone around the maxillary right posterior teeth in a 40-year-old smoker. There were grade III furcation involvements on the mesial, buccal, and distal aspects of the first and second molars.

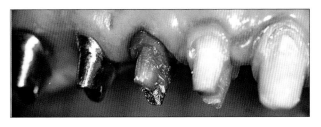

Fig 183b After initial nonsurgical scaling, root planing, debridement, PMTC, and oral hygiene education, the first and second molars were hemisectioned without flap surgery. The distobuccal and palatal roots of the molars were extracted, and the mesiobuccal roots received endodontic treatment. Cast gold post and core restorations with collars were made for the mesiobuccal roots of the molars, and the canine and premolars were prepared as abutments for a fixed partial denture.

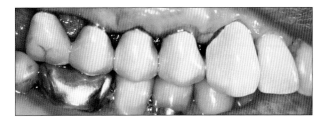

Fig 183c Definitive fixed partial denture in the same patient. The margins were placed supragingivally to enhance plaque control and eliminate any visible gold margin anteriorly.

Fig 183d Radiograph taken 2 years after treatment.

Fig 183e Radiograph taken 17 years after treatment, revealing further improvement in alveolar bone support as a result of an effective maintenance program.

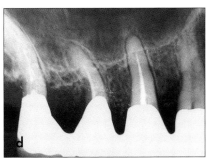
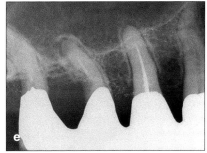

palatal roots in relation to the premolar. The mesiobuccal root is particularly stable because it is relatively wide in the buccolingual direction, similar to that of the premolars (see Fig 172). The case shown in Figs 183a to 183e illustrates this principle.

Maxillary premolars

Particularly in the maxillary first premolars, the root anatomy often varies. In addition, the roots harbor irregularities such as longitudinal grooves,

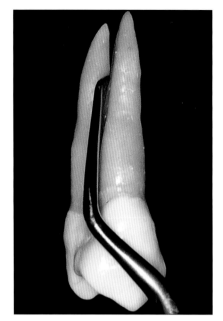

Fig 184 Goldman-Fox 4, a thin curette with an elongated neck, is used for diagnosis of furcation involvement in maxillary first premolars.

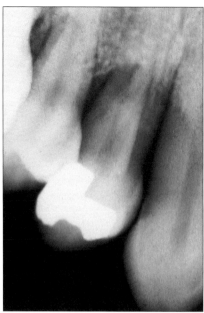

Fig 185a Eccentric radiograph of a maxillary first premolar for the diagnosis of furcation involvement. The level of the furcation area should be compared with the most coronal margin of the alveolar bone. The obvious furcation involvement of the maxillary first premolar was confirmed by probing with a curette.

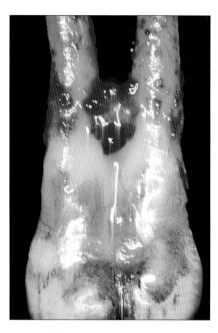

Fig 185b The maxillary first premolar has been extracted because of grade III furcation involvement. Attached granulation tissue is visible in the furcation area.

invaginations, or true furcations that may open at varying distances from the CEJ. Clinical examination of maxillary premolars is often difficult, because access for probing is limited. It may not always be possible to identify the presence and severity of furcation involvement in such teeth until a flap is raised for exploratory surgery.

For clinical diagnosis of furcation involvement on the mesial and distal surfaces, a slim, extended double-ended universal curette such as the Goldman-Fox 4 is suitable (Fig 184). The furcation area of the maxillary premolars may be best identified on radiographs obtained by directing the radiographic beam toward the canine (Figs 185a and 185b). Comprehensive radiographic examination should include both paralleling periapical and bitewing radiographs.

Maxillary premolars may have three roots. Maxillary first premolars with furcation involvement are usually extracted if distal teeth that are suitable as prosthetic abutments are present. An alternative to a fixed partial denture could be a single osseointegrated implant.

Resection and hemisection. Root resection of maxillary first premolars is rarely possible because of the anatomy of the tooth. The furcation is often located so far apically that the maintenance of one root serves no meaningful purpose. In most cases, therefore, a grade III furcation involvement in a maxillary first premolar dictates tooth extraction. Figures 186a and 186b show a rare exception in which a maxillary left first premolar with grade III furcation involvement was hemisectioned nonsurgically, although a second premolar remained.

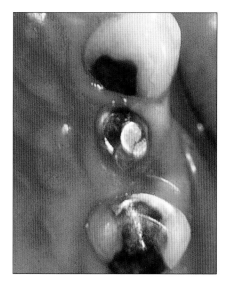

Fig 186a The buccal root of a maxillary first premolar with grade III furcation involvement has been extracted after hemisection.

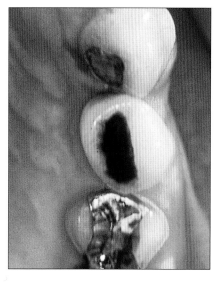

Fig 186b After preparation of the palatal root, a permanent crown is made.

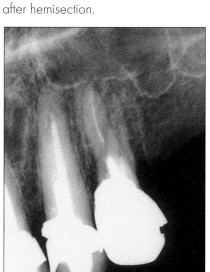

Fig 187a The eccentric radiograph reveals that the furcation involvement affecting the maxillary first premolar is located relatively coronally.

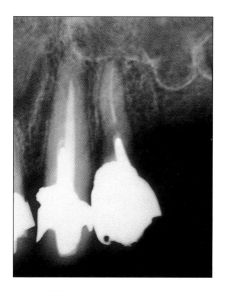

Fig 187b The buccal root has been removed by resection during open flap surgery.

In this case, there was advanced recession of the buccal root, and the furcation area was located much more coronally than usual. The first molar had previously been hemisectioned, and the distobuccal and palatal roots had been extracted because of grade II to III furcation involvement mesially, distally, and buccally.

If the affected maxillary first premolar is the most posterior remaining tooth, resection or hemisection should be attempted so that the tooth can serve as an abutment (Figs 187 and 188).

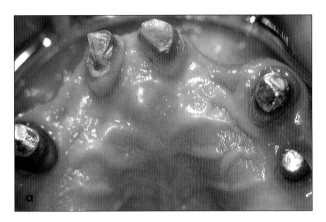
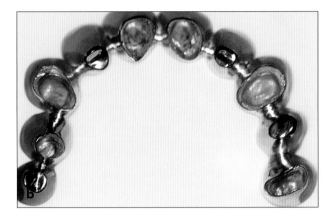

Figs 188a and 188b The maxillary left first premolar, the most posterior tooth remaining in the quadrant, is hemisectioned and used as an abutment for a permanent complete prosthesis.

Tunnel preparation

As discussed earlier, Matia et al (1986) demonstrated the very limited effect of nonsurgical scaling, root planing, and debridement in mandibular molars with grade II or III furcation involvement. The choice of instrument—hand instrument or ultrasonic scaler—made no difference.

To date, there is very limited information available on the effect of regenerative therapy in grade III furcation defects. Therefore, the so-called tunnel preparation is an alternative to hemisection, especially in mandibular first molars with coronally located grade III furcation involvement, divergent roots, and substantial vertical loss of alveolar bone in the furcation area. Under certain circumstances, the tunnel preparation may also be used in maxillary molars (Figs 189a to 189d).

A tunnel preparation may be attempted to provide access for cleaning. The teeth to be tunneled must have sufficient root divergence to accommodate cleaning devices, but the procedure may jeopardize the tooth by removing too much supporting bone. The prognosis for a tunnel preparation may be more predictable for grade III furcation involvement than for grade II involvement because much less bone will have to be removed to provide access to the furcation for cleaning devices. The major advantage of the tunnel preparation is that it does not involve endodontics or fixed restorative procedures.

Tunneling involves surgical exposure of the entire furcation area. Following elevation of mucoperiosteal flaps on the buccal and lingual aspects of the affected tooth, the root surfaces are scaled and planed, and any irregularities in the alveolar bone crest are recontoured. The flaps are repositioned at the interradicular sutures. Surgical packs may be applied to prevent excessive growth of granulation tissue in the tunnel space during healing.

Unless the patient maintains excellent plaque control, there is a major risk for caries on the root surfaces denuded by tunneling. Tunneling should be restricted to conditions where there is enough space between roots to allow interradicular cleaning. Minimally invasive instruments are recommended for scaling, root planing, and debridement in the furcation area to prevent iatrogenic removal of cementum and exposure of root dentin and dentinal tubules. For caries prevention, the exposed interradicular root surface should be frequently treated with CHX varnish and fluoride varnish (for details, see Axelsson, 2004).

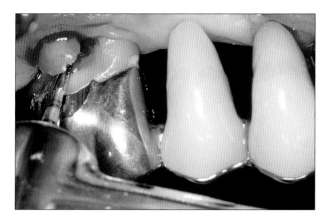

Fig 189a The distobuccal root of a maxillary first molar with an extremely advanced grade III furcation involvement (open furcation area) and very thin, divergent roots is resected. The tooth has served for more than 30 years as the most posterior abutment of a fixed complete prosthesis in an 82-year-old woman.

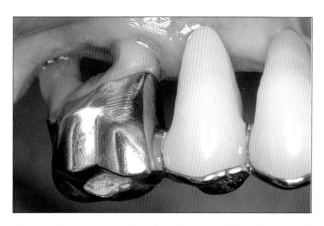

Fig 189b Because of tooth mobility and the absence of the first and second premolars, after the resection, a wide tunnel is prepared between the mesiobuccal and palatal roots.

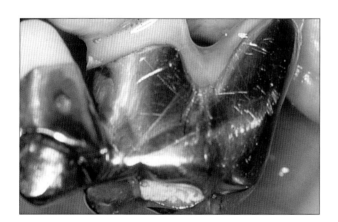

Fig 189c Lingual view of the tunnel preparation.

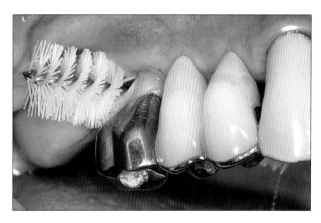

Fig 189d For proper cleaning between the roots, an interdental brush and fluoride toothpaste are used.

Tooth extraction

Extraction of a periodontally involved multirooted tooth will predictably eliminate the disease in the area and is indicated when destruction of the periodontium has progressed to such a level that no root can be preserved. Teeth with untreatable furcation involvement should be extracted as early as possible to improve access for nonsurgical scaling, root planing, and debridement of the approximal root surfaces of adjacent teeth. The result is dramatic healing at these sites (Figs 190a to 190c). Extraction is also indicated when the maintenance of the affected tooth will not improve the overall treatment or when treatment of the tooth with furcation involvement will not result in conditions that allow adequate plaque control by the patient.

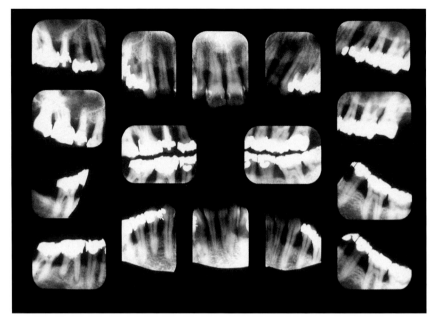

Fig 190a Complete-mouth radiographs showing relatively advanced loss of periodontal support for a patient of this age (a 42-year-old smoker). Both maxillary first molars, the maxillary left second molar, and the mandibular right second molar were hemisectioned because of grade III mesial, buccal, and distal furcation involvement. The furcation-involved mandibular right first molar, both maxillary first premolars, the maxillary lateral incisors, and the maxillary left second premolar were extracted as early as possible. Provisional prostheses were made for the 4-month healing period. Subsequently, a permanent maxillary fixed complete prosthesis and a fixed mandibular right partial prosthesis were made.

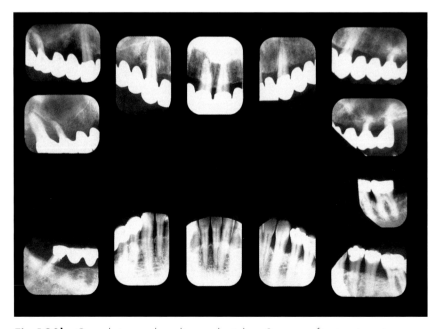

Fig 190b Complete-mouth radiographs taken 3 years after treatment.

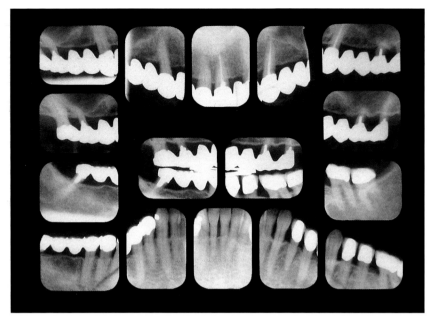

Fig 190c Complete-mouth radiographs taken 25 years after initial treatment. Because of a maintenance program based on excellent gingival plaque control, accomplished through self-care as well as through PMTC and debridement at needs-related intervals, there has been no further loss of teeth or periodontal support. The well-mineralized margin of the alveolar bone indicates that the remaining periodontal support is healthy.

It is generally agreed that the need to extract a tooth with grade II to III furcation involvement is highly individual, but some guidelines may be proposed. Extraction of a tooth with a grade III furcation defect is suggested under the following conditions:

- The affected tooth is an unopposed molar that is the terminal tooth in the arch.
- The affected tooth is a first molar with adjacent second premolar and second molar, each with adequate bone support.
- The affected tooth is mobile and is a solitary distal abutment tooth.

(For review on treatment of furcation-involved teeth, see Cattabriga et al, 2000; DeSanctis and Murphy, 2000; McClain and Schallhorn, 2000; Sanz and Giovannoli, 2000; Svärdström, 2001.)

PERIODONTAL SURGERY FOR ACCESSIBILITY AND REDUCTION OF DEEP RESIDUAL POCKETS

Four decades ago, probing depths greater than 3 mm were usually an indication for periodontal surgery. At that time, comprehensive nonsurgical periodontal treatment, frequent PMTC, and establishment of needs-related oral hygiene habits did not always precede periodontal surgery. Therefore, many sites, particularly interproximal sites, exhibited probing depths greater than 3 mm. As a consequence, too many patients received four complete-quadrant gingivectomies or flap surgery.

Gingivectomy and large-flap surgery have been out of fashion for more than three decades in Scandinavia, however, because of a large-scale focus on nonsurgical periodontal treatment, PMTC, education in proper self-care, and needs-related maintenance care by dentists and dental hygienists. Nevertheless, in spite of comprehensive nonsurgical periodontal treatment and excellent gingival plaque control, some deep infectious pockets will not be reduced and healthy. Thus, only mini-flap surgery is indicated for visible inspection, cleaning and planing of the root surfaces, and probing depth reduction.

The decision as to whether periodontal surgery is necessary in a new patient with untreated advanced periodontal disease always has to be preceded by history taking, detailed examination, prediction of periodontal risk, and initial intensive therapy, as well as all other secondary measures, including extraction of untreatable teeth, excavation of cavitated caries lesions, elimination of plaque-retentive factors in the gingival region, and chemical plaque control. The effect of this initial intensive treatment has to be evaluated before any decision about surgery is made. In a maintenance patient, the indications for periodontal surgical therapy should be limited to:

- Single, deep infectious sites with refractory loss of periodontal support despite excellent mechanical gingival plaque control by self-care, professional debridement, and chemical plaque control.
- Regenerative periodontal therapy (see chapter 4).

The main goal of all prevention and treatment of periodontal diseases is to control infectious disease by facilitating gingival plaque control. Supplementary periodontal surgery should therefore fulfill the following main goals:

- Improvement of accessibility and visibility for correct diagnosis and proper root surface instrumentation
- Establishment of clinical conditions that facilitate the patient's efforts at gingival plaque control, as well as PMTC, by elimination of subgingival plaque-retentive factors and reduction of probing depths
- Regeneration of lost periodontal tissues destroyed by periodontal disease (see chapter 4)

Periodontal surgical techniques

Despite the many surgical techniques and subsequent modifications described over the years, two basic main approaches have involved *(1)* pocket elimination (or pocket reduction) procedures, with the ultimate objective of eliminating the pocket as a physical entity, and *(2)* reattachment, new attachment, or readaptation procedures aimed at closing the periodontal pocket space, with the ultimate goal of regenerating lost periodontal support. The classification of surgical procedures is based on the elimination or the reduction of the soft tissue component of the pocket, while maintaining the facility for any osseous therapy:

- Pocket elimination procedures:
  - Apically repositioned flap
  - Resection (internal/external bevel gingivectomy)
- Pocket reduction procedures (access flaps for debridement):
  - Modified Widman flap
  - Other procedures (eg, regenerative therapy and gingival curettage)

In 1989, the consensus of the World Workshop on Clinical Periodontics (Nevins et al, 1989) was that gingival curettage has limited, if any, current application in the treatment of chronic adult periodontitis. It offers no supplementary clinical effect to scaling and root planing alone (Figs 191 and 192; for details on surgical techniques related to regenerative therapy, see chapter 4).

Pocket elimination procedures

The aim of resective periodontal surgery is the establishment of a morphologically normal dentogingival relationship. This is accomplished by apical repositioning or sacrifice of the detached wall tissue.

Apically repositioned flap. A full-thickness, mucoperiosteal flap, prepared with an internal bevel incision, is repositioned at the level of the bony crest. Thus, the entire mucogingival complex is displaced apically, eliminating the pocket but preserving the entire zone of keratinized gingiva and providing access for root surface instrumentation and osseous surgery.

A reverse bevel incision is made from the gingival margin to the alveolar crest but may be located at varying distances from the gingival margin, depending on the thickness of the gingiva. Thus, in patients with thick gingiva, the incision is made further away. The beveled incision is also scalloped to ensure maximal coverage of the crestal alveolar bone when the flap is repositioned. Where necessary, vertical releasing incisions extending into the alveolar mucosa are made at the borders of the surgical field to allow apical repositioning of the flap over the crestal bone. This technique cannot be performed in the palate because the flap cannot be displaced apically.

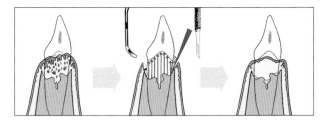

Fig 191 Gingival curettage includes removal of the pocket epithelium with a sharp curette as well as scaling, root planing, and debridement. (Courtesy of Dr K. Rateitschak.)

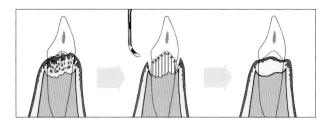

Fig 192 Subgingival scaling, root planing, and debridement are performed to remove biofilms and calculus and to plane the outer surface of the root cementum. (Courtesy of Dr K. Rateitschak.)

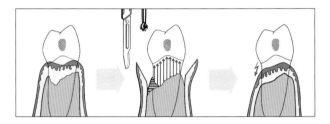

Fig 193 Resective therapy and the apically repositioned flap include elimination of intrabony pockets by osteoplasty. (Courtesy of Dr K. Rateitschak.)

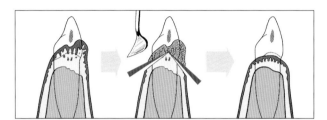

Fig 194 Gingivectomy and gingivoplasty are mainly performed for elimination of pseudopockets. The *red lines* indicate the location and direction of incisions. (Courtesy of Dr K. Rateitschak.)

Resection.

1. *Internal bevel gingivectomy:* In the inverse bevel resection, the location of the insertion is designed to provide a gingival tissue margin that will follow the outline of the bony crest. A full mucoperiosteal flap is raised, the marginal collar of tissue is removed, and scaling, root planing, and debridement are performed. Bone recontouring may be necessary to reestablish physiologic contours, albeit at a reduced, more apical level. The flaps are then sutured into position over the alveolar bony crest (Fig 193).

2. *External bevel gingivectomy:* This so-called gingivectomy procedure represents the oldest surgical technique in periodontics. The objectives include the elimination of supracrestal pockets to allow root instrumentation and the creation of soft tissue and tooth anatomy that the patient can easily maintain. The technique is carried out with a continuous incision directed coronally at a 45-degree angle to the long axis of the tooth, ending on the tooth at the base of the pocket. The buccal and lingual incisions are then ex-

tended interproximally, and the incised tissues are removed. The wound and adjacent intact tissue are trimmed further to obtain a physiologic contour of the gingival tissue. The exposed roots are carefully scaled, planed, and debrided. A periodontal dressing is placed over the entire surgical area and retained for 7 to 14 days (Fig 194).

Wound epithelialization commences within a few days, reaching completion within approximately 2 weeks. Epithelial cells proliferate from the wound margins, migrating toward the root at a constant rate of 0.5 mm per day. Regeneration of the supracrestal connective tissue then occurs, and a free gingival unit with all the characteristics of the normal free gingiva is reestablished. This coronal regrowth of tissue from the original incision level appears clinically as a gain in marginal height of the gingiva. Complete soft tissue healing takes place in about 4 to 5 weeks, after which some additional remodeling of the alveolar bony crest may occur.

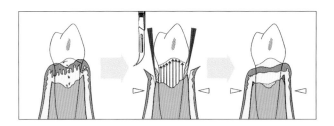

Fig 195 The modified Widman flap technique is used for pocket reduction. The *red lines* indicate the location and direction of incisions. (Courtesy of Dr K. Rateitschak.)

Today, the only indications for gingivectomy should be the elimination of hyperplastic gingival tissues and the creation of access to the subgingival margins of caries lesions before restorative treatment.

Pocket reduction procedures

Access flaps for debridement. Flap debridement surgery may be defined as surgical scaling, planing, and debridement of the root surface and the removal of granulation tissue after the reflection of the soft tissue flap. The most commonly practiced technique is based on the modified Widman flap, although not always performed as originally described by Ramfjord and Nissle (1974; Fig 195).

The original Widman flap (Widman, 1918) was a mucoperiosteal flap that followed a scalloped gingival incision that separated the pocket epithelium and inflamed connective tissue from the noninflamed gingiva and was bordered by two vertical releasing incisions extending to the alveolar mucosa. The flap was elevated to expose 2 to 3 mm of the alveolar bone. The soft tissue collar incorporating the pocket epithelium and connective tissue was removed, the exposed root surfaces were scaled, planed, and debrided, and the bone was recontoured to reestablish a physiologic alveolar form. The flap margins were placed at the level of the bony crest to achieve optimal pocket reduction.

The main advantages of this technique over gingivectomy were claimed to be a reduction in postoperative discomfort, because healing was by primary intention, and the reestablishment of a physiologic bony contour at sites with angular bony defects.

The term *modified Widman flap* was adopted for the flap procedure designed to obtain access to the root surface and close postoperative adaptation of healthy collagenous connective tissue and normal epithelium to the root surface (Ramfjord and Nissle, 1974; Ramfjord et al, 1987; Fig 196). Unlike its predecessor, this procedure did not aim at surgical pocket elimination and apical displacement of the flap. Therefore, the interproximal bone was not exposed, and infrabony defects were not eliminated by osseous recontouring. The initial inverse bevel incision, which passed down to bone, commenced approximately 1 mm from the gingival margin and extended as far as possible between the teeth to ensure optimal flap adaptation and complete coverage of the interdental bone. However, when esthetic considerations are paramount, intracrevicular incisions starting at the free gingival margins are used to minimize postsurgical gingival shrinkage (Ramfjord et al, 1987; Smith et al, 1987). Vertical releasing incisions are usually not required for the mucoperiosteal flap elevation for access to the root surfaces and interproximal bone.

The collar of soft tissue around each tooth is excised by a combination of vertical incisions from the bottom of the pocket to the subjacent bony crest and a horizontal incision following the contour of the alveolar bone. Following careful scaling, root planing, and debridement, all soft tissues are removed from the bony surfaces of intrabony defects, and the flaps are joined to meet interproximally. To achieve a good interproximal junction, the flaps can be trimmed, and bone can be removed from the outer aspect of the alveolar process. The flaps are secured with individual interproximal sutures.

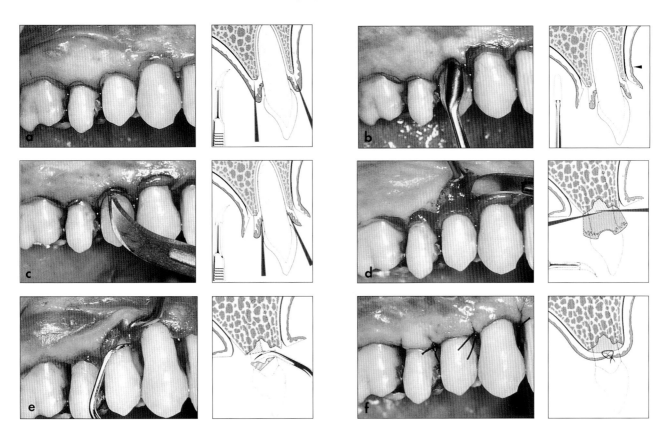

Fig 196 Clinical and schematic illustrations of the modified Widman flap technique. The *red lines* indicate the location and direction of incisions. *(a)* First incision, a scalloping inverse bevel. *(b)* Flap reflection. *Black arrow* indicates mucogingival junction. *(c)* Second incision, an intrasulcular incision. *(d)* Third incision. *(e)* Root instrumentation with direct vision. *(f)* Tight coverage of interdental defects by interdental suturing. (Courtesy of Dr K. Rateitschak.)

Although the chief aim of the modified Widman flap surgery is, according to Ramfjord and Nissle (1974), healing and reattachment of periodontal pockets with minimum loss of periodontal tissues during and after surgery, reduction in probing depth by shrinkage occurs in some individuals.

Other techniques. Reduction of probing depths distal to the maxillary second molars is complicated because of the thick fibrous tissues. Figures 197 to 200 show three different techniques to solve this problem: the modified incision, the classic distal wedge incision, and the wedge incision. Special periodontal surgery techniques such as the simplified papilla preservation flap and the modified papilla preservation flap will be discussed in chapter 4.

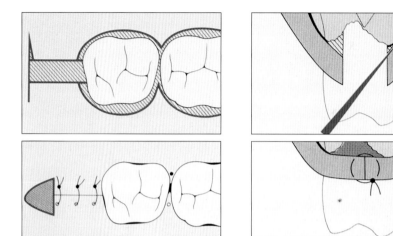

Fig 197 Modified incision technique for pocket reduction distal to the maxillary second molars. (Courtesy of Dr K. Rateitschak.)

Figs 198a to 198f Modified incision technique. (Courtesy of Dr K. Rateitschak.)

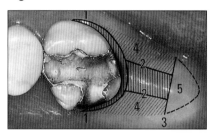

Fig 198a Sequence of incisions (1 to 5) during the surgical procedure.

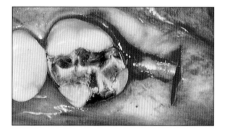

Fig 198b Clinical view following modified incision technique.

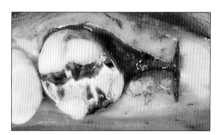

Fig 198c After removal of tissue wedge, reflection of undermined buccal and lingual flaps, and root surface debridement.

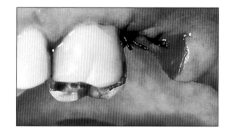

Fig 198d The flaps have been sutured.

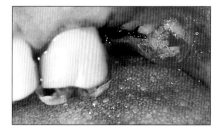

Fig 198e The unnecessary distal tissue has been removed by gingivectomy.

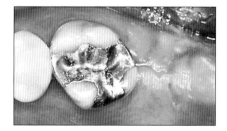

Fig 198f Healed result after pocket reduction with the modified incision technique.

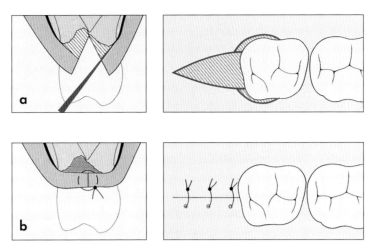

Fig 199 Classic distal wedge incision for pocket reduction. *(a)* The first incisions delineate the excision. The second incision *(red line)* undermines and thins the buccal and lingual flaps. *(b)* The repositioned and sutured flaps will result in elimination of the deep pocket distally. (Courtesy of Dr K. Rateitschak.)

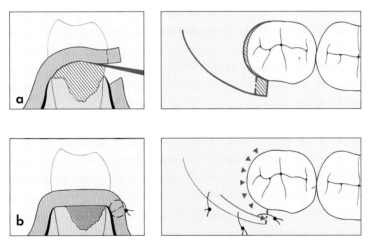

Fig 200 Wedge incision for pocket reduction. *(a)* The curved facial incision is made distal to the mandibular second molar. After flap reflection, subjacent tissue is removed, and the tip of the flap is shortened. *(b)* After root surface debridement, the flap is sutured to the primary incision site. *Arrowheads* indicate close fit of the flap to the distal surface of the tooth. (Courtesy of Dr K. Rateitschak.)

Nonsurgical versus surgical periodontal treatment

Randomized, controlled split-mouth longitudinal studies (of 1 year or more) should be the best method for comparing the effects of nonsurgical and surgical periodontal therapy. In this way, the role of internal modifying factors (such as genetic factors and diabetes) and external modifying factors (such as smoking and oral hygiene habits) may be similar for the two therapies. However, for ethical reasons, untreated negative control quadrants are unacceptable longitudinally in patients who are susceptible to periodontitis.

This split-mouth design was initiated in the early 1970s in pioneering longitudinal studies (Knowles et al, 1979, 1980; Ramfjord et al, 1975) that evaluated the long-term effects of three different treatment procedures:

1. *Subgingival curettage:* Closed subgingival scaling, root planing, and debridement (ie, nonsurgical treatment)
2. *Modified Widman flap surgery:* Pocket reduction procedures without bone removal and repositioning of the flap but with interdental coverage and suturing
3. *Pocket elimination surgery:* Reversed bevel flap, bone contouring, and apical positioning of the flap (or gingivectomy if no bone removal was needed for pocket elimination)

The effects on probing depth and probing attachment level were analyzed after 5 years (Ramfjord et al, 1975) and 8 years (Knowles et al, 1979, 1980). Figure 201 shows the effect of the three different procedures on probing attachment level at sites with different initial probing depths.

The authors drew the following conclusions:

- The magnitude of pocket reduction following periodontal therapy is positively related to the magnitude of the original pocket.
- Changes in attachment levels also have a direct relationship to the original probing depth.
- All four probed surfaces of the teeth respond similarly to treatment when pockets of equal initial depth are compared.

- Moderate and deep periodontal pockets can be reduced in depth and do not deepen over 8 years following subgingival curettage, modified Widman flap surgery, and pocket elimination surgery.
- Attachment levels in both moderate and deep pockets can be improved clinically.
- Pocket reduction in moderately deep pockets is greater after modified Widman procedures and pocket elimination surgery than after curettage, but the total reduction is significant for all three methods.
- Although all three methods result in gain of attachment in moderately deep pockets, the long-term gain is significant only after curettage and modified Widman flap surgery.
- For deep pockets (7 mm or more), pocket reduction is also significant and well sustained for all three methods. However, the reduction obtained after curettage tends to be smaller than that obtained with the other two methods.
- The greatest significant gain of attachment in deep pockets over time was achieved with modified Widman flap surgery.

These conclusions still seem to be relevant, as shown in later reviews of similar split-mouth studies (Claffey et al, 2004; Heitz-Mayfield et al, 2002).

In another split-mouth study, Pihlström et al (1983, 1984) compared the effects of nonsurgical and surgical therapy. Their results showed that in sites with initially moderate and deep pockets (7 mm or more), a single initial nonsurgical treatment (scaling, root planing, and debridement) was at least as successful as supplementary surgery (modified Widman flap) on probing attachment level gain.

Lindhe et al (1982, 1984) compared the effects of nonsurgical and surgical treatment, after 2 and 5 years, in 15 patients with advanced periodontal disease. The results after 2 years (Lindhe et al, 1982) showed that scaling and root planing used alone were almost as effective in restoring clinically healthy gingiva and preventing further loss of attachment as their use in combination with the modified Widman flap procedure. Both treatment modalities prevented recurrence of periodontal disease for the 24 months of observation. Analysis of probing depth data revealed that both

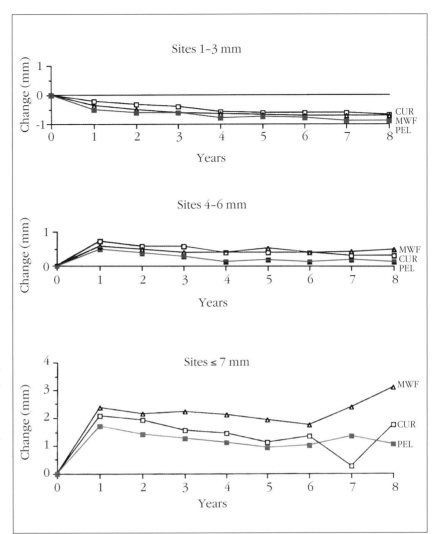

Fig 201 Change of probing attachment levels during 8 years of supportive care at sites with initial probing depths of 1 to 3 mm, 4 to 6 mm, or 7 mm or more. (CUR) Curettage (nonsurgical treatment); (MWF) modified Widman flap; (PEL) pocket elimination surgery with reversed bevel flap and osteoplasty. (Modified from Knowles et al, 1979, with permission.)

methods of treatment resulted in a high frequency of probing depths of less than 4 mm. The reduction was more pronounced in initially deep than in initially shallow pockets and more marked in initially deep sites subjected to surgery than in sites treated by scaling and root planing alone. The deep sites also had a more pronounced gain of clinical attachment than did sites with initially shallow pockets. Significant loss of attachment did not occur in sites treated by scaling and root planing alone, but in sites with initial probing depths of less than 4 mm, attachment loss did occur after Widman flap surgery. After 5 years, little difference was observed between the two methods at individual sites (Lindhe et al, 1984).

In a 5-year study, Isidor and Karring (1986) compared the effects of nonsurgical treatment and two different surgical methods in a split-mouth design:

1. Nonsurgical scaling, root planing, and debridement with hand instruments under local anesthesia and no intentional curettage
2. Reversed bevel, full-thickness, apically positioned flap, and no osseous recontouring
3. Modified Widman, full-thickness replaced flap, without osseous recontouring

During the first year after treatment, PMTC was carried out every second week. The patient received oral hygiene education, PMTC, and debridement four times during the second year and twice yearly during the third through fifth years.

After 5 years, the results for probing depths as well as probing attachment levels, including proximal sites with angular osseous defects, were similar, regardless of treatment method. At 5 years, compared to 1 year, a slight relapse of probing depths and probing attachment levels was observed. This could be due to the fact that somewhat lower plaque scores were observed at 1 year than at 5 years, because of the high quality of gingival plaque control obtained through PMTC performed every second week during the first year.

In a 5-year study, Ramfjord et al (1987) compared the effect of four different periodontal treatments: pocket elimination or reduction surgery, modified Widman flap surgery, subgingival curettage, and nonsurgical scaling, root planing, and debridement. For probing depths of 1 to 3 mm, nonsurgical scaling, root planing, and debridement as well as subgingival curettage led to significantly less attachment loss than pocket elimination and modified Widman flap surgery. For 4- to 6-mm pockets, nonsurgical scaling, root planing, and debridement and curettage had better attachment results than pocket elimination surgery. For the 7- to 12-mm pockets, there were no statistically significant differences among the various procedures. The authors concluded that a protocol of nonsurgical scaling, root planing, and debridement was the treatment of choice for periodontal pockets of 6 mm or less, provided that proper access to the root surface could be obtained. For pockets of 7 mm or more, the results were similar for all four methods of treatment. There was no additional benefit from curettage over nonsurgical scaling, root planing, and debridement.

In addition, the authors found that maintenance care should include re-treatment of pockets with persistent pus and/or bleeding. Regardless of the modality of treatment, furcation involvement was the greatest hazard in the prognosis. Re-treatment was needed more often after nonsurgical scaling, root planing, and debridement than after the other procedures, but with additional scaling and debridement, the results were as good as those for any other procedure (Ramfjord et al, 1987; for further review, see Becker et al, 2001; Kaldahl et al, 1988; Lindhe and Nyman, 1985; Schroer et al, 1991).

All the aforementioned studies have been carried out in adult patients, mostly exhibiting moderate or severe chronic periodontitis. However, Wennström et al (1986) carried out a 5-year longitudinal split-mouth study of aggressive localized (early-onset) periodontitis in youths (juvenile group) or aggressive periodontitis in young adults (postjuvenile group) to evaluate the healing following surgical or nonsurgical therapy.

The patients, referred for treatment of advanced aggressive periodontal disease, were divided into groups based on their age and the location of the diseased sites, a juvenile group (n = 11) and a postjuvenile group (n = 5). The patients in the juvenile group had periodontal lesions only on first molars and incisors. The diseased sites on one side of the jaws were randomly treated by scaling, root planing, and debridement in conjunction with a modified Widman flap procedure, while in the contralateral quadrants, treatment was restricted to scaling, root planing, and debridement. The patients were subjected to PMTC once every 4 weeks during the first 6 months following active therapy and subsequently at 3-month intervals. Two years after treatment, this maintenance care program was terminated. A final examination was performed 5 years after therapy. None of the patients involved in the trial received antibiotic treatment during the 5 years of observation.

The response to therapy, in both the juvenile and the postjuvenile groups, was almost identical to that in patients with adult periodontitis given similar treatment. Examinations 6, 24, and 60 months after active treatment of juvenile and postjuvenile lesions showed that excision of granulation tissue after flap elevation did not increase the degree of probing depth reduction, probing attachment gain, or bone fill over that achieved with meticulous nonsurgical root surface instrumentation.

For both patient groups and for both treatments, some relapse of the initial improvements in probing depth and probing attachment level was noted between 2 and 5 years. The lack of supervised, professional maintenance during this period may explain the relapse. However, at 5 years, there were no sites in either of the patient groups or either of the treatment groups that exhibited probing attachment loss of 2 mm or more compared to baseline data.

Heitz-Mayfield et al (2002) presented a systematic review of the effect of surgical debridement versus nonsurgical debridement for the treatment of chronic periodontitis. They searched for randomized controlled trials of at least 12 months' duration. Of almost 600 abstracts, only 6 randomized controlled trials could be included in a meta-analysis (Isidor and Karring, 1986; Kaldahl et al, 1988, 1996; Lindhe and Nyman, 1985; Lindhe et al, 1982, 1984; Pihlström et al, 1981, 1983, 1984; Ramfjord et al, 1987). The meta-analysis indicated that, 12 months following treatment, surgical therapy resulted in 0.6 mm more of probing depth reduction and 0.2 mm more of clinical attachment level gain than nonsurgical therapy in deep pockets (of more than 6 mm). However, in 4- to 6-mm pockets, nonsurgical therapy resulted in a 0.4-mm greater gain of clinical attachment level and a 0.4-mm lesser reduction of probing depth than surgical therapy. In shallow pockets (of 1 to 3 mm), nonsurgical therapy resulted in 0.5 mm less attachment loss than surgical therapy.

There are many reasons why there is loss of attachment after treatment in shallow pockets in spite of proper gingival plaque control:

- Most shallow sites are located buccally and lingually.
- Instrumentation during initial treatment and maintenance treatment may result in trauma.
- Toothbrushing and other self-care procedures may result in trauma.
- The marginal periodontal tissues may remodel as an effect of the improved and changed conditions after treatment, particularly after surgery.

- The periodontal tissues undergo gradual recession related to the aging process.
- The periodontal structures can remodel in association with a process of continuous eruption of the teeth because of abrasion.

In another overview of nonsurgical and surgical therapy, Claffey et al (2004) discussed some problems that can affect the interpretation of results of split-mouth studies. Some of these problems included: *(1)* designs in which initial therapy, including complete-mouth root planing, was performed at the outset so that what was actually studied was an adjunctive effect of either further root planing or a surgical procedure; *(2)* results of probing measurements expressed as means of subgroups of sites, possibly masking individual site deterioration; *(3)* short-term clinical results that may reflect improvements that are changes in inflammation rather than changes in attachment loss; *(4)* lack of untreated control subjects, dictated by ethical considerations; and *(5)* assignment of quadrants to certain treatment modalities, inevitably resulting in the application of clinically inappropriate techniques at some individual sites, for example, treatment of shallow pockets with pocket elimination procedures.

The overall recommendations for the sequencing of nonsurgical and surgical treatment of periodontal diseases are:

- Establishment of needs-related oral hygiene habits (for details, see Axelsson, 2004)
- An initial single, thorough session of nonsurgical scaling, root planing, and debridement that results in clean and smooth root surfaces without exposure of root dentin and dentinal tubules and elimination of supragingival and subgingival plaque-retentive factors in the gingival region
- Supplementary selective open flap surgery, limited to:
  - Single sites with deep pockets that are inaccessible to complete nonsurgical treatment
  - Exploratory surgery on teeth or surfaces with possible root grooves, root resorptions, furcation involvement, root fractures, or other plaque-retentive factors

— Sites with refractory loss of probing attachment and deep diseased pockets with suppuration, despite initial adequate nonsurgical treatment and meticulous gingival plaque control
— Regenerative therapy by guided tissue regeneration or growth factors or a combination of these two methods (see chapter 4)

Traditional procedures, such as initial general pocket elimination by gingivectomy or major flap surgery with osseous contouring and apically positioned flaps, are no longer considered to be the state of the art but rather maltreatment.

Effect of combined therapies

Recently, Haffajee et al (2006) evaluated the effect of different therapies and combinations of therapies on attachment level changes in periodontitis subjects with different microbial profiles in a 12-month study. After initial scaling, root planing, and debridement, 493 subjects were randomly assigned to 1 of 17 different treatment groups for modified Widman flap surgery, apically repositioned flap (pocket elimination), systemic amoxicillin plus metronidazole, systemic amoxicillin, systemic metronidazole, local delivery of tetracycline, systemic doxycycline, systemic azithromycin, PMTC, low-dose doxycycline, or different combinations of these therapies. The greatest gain of attachment level was achieved in a group that received a combination of modified Widman flap surgery, systemic amoxicillin plus metronidazole, and local delivery of tetracycline. The group that had the next greatest gain received the combination of systemic amoxicillin plus metronidazole and local delivery of tetracycline. A group that underwent apically repositioned flap surgery exhibited the greatest loss of attachment level; the next greatest loss was seen in the group that did not receive any additional therapy.

In a meta-analysis, Hung and Douglass (2002) evaluated the effect of scaling and root planing, surgical treatment, and antibiotic therapies on periodontal probing depth and attachment loss. Scaling and root planing alone was one of the primary treatment arms for inclusion. Patients or quadrants of each patient were randomly assigned to study groups. Sample size was used to weigh the relative contribution of each study.

The meta-analysis showed that periodontal probing depth and gain of attachment level did not improve significantly following scaling and root planing for patients with shallow initial periodontal probing depths. However, there was about a 1.0-mm reduction for medium initial periodontal probing depths and a 2.0-mm reduction for deep initial periodontal probing depths. Similarly, there was about a 0.5-mm gain in attachment for medium initial periodontal probing depths and slightly more than a 1.0-mm gain in attachment for deep initial periodontal probing depths. Surgical therapy for patients with deep initial probing depths provided better results than did scaling and root planing in reducing probing depths, thus confirming the results from the previously discussed split-mouth studies. When patients were followed up over 3 years or more, these differences were reduced to less than 0.4 mm. Antibiotic therapy showed results similar to those of scaling and root planing. However, a consistent improvement in periodontal probing depth and gain of attachment was demonstrated when local antibiotic therapy was combined with scaling and root planing.

REDUCTION OF MODIFYING RISK FACTORS

There are several external and internal factors that may modify the outcome of periodontal therapy in individual patients. The American Academy of Periodontology (1996) defines these factors as follows:

• *Risk factor:* An environmental, behavioral, or biologic factor that, if present, directly increases the probability that a disease will occur and that, if absent or removed, reduces that probability. Risk factors are part of the causal chain.
• *Risk indicator:* A probable or putative risk factor, often detected in cross-sectional studies, that has not yet been confirmed by longitudinal studies.

- *Risk predictor:* A characteristic that is associated with elevated disease but may not be part of the causal chain. Predictors are useful for identifying who is at risk but not for identifying likely interventions.
- *Prognostic risk factor:* An environmental, behavioral, or biologic factor that, when present, directly affects the probability of a positive outcome of a therapy rendered for the disease.

However, in the literature, such factors are usually termed *risk factors* (for details, see chapter 5 and volume 3 of this series [Axelsson, 2002]). Important external modifying risk factors are:

- Use of tobacco products (particularly cigarette smoking)
- Low socioeconomic status (particularly low educational level)
- Poor compliance (particularly poor oral hygiene) and irregular dental care
- Acquired systemic and infectious diseases (particularly infection with human immunodeficiency virus)
- Stress
- Local plaque-retentive factors

Most of these factors can be eliminated or controlled and thus improve the outcome of periodontal treatment. Smoking is regarded as the most important external modifying risk factor. Therefore, smoking cessation is of greatest importance for successful periodontal therapy. However, establishment of needs-related self-care and dental care habits and early elimination of plaque-retentive factors are also very important.

The most important internal modifying risk factors are:

- Genetic factors (particularly polymorphism of proinflammatory cytokines)
- Impaired host factors (particularly reduced PMNL function)
- Systemic diseases (particularly type 1 and type 2 diabetes)

Studies have shown that there seems to be a synergistic negative effect of smoking in patients who exhibit genetic polymorphism of the proinflammatory cytokines interleukin 1α and interleukin 1β (Axelsson, 2002). Therefore, it is of greatest importance that such individuals stop smoking. In addition, anti-inflammatory drugs could be useful for those patients, at least during the initial periodontal treatment.

In addition, several studies have shown that there is a two-way negative relationship between diabetes and periodontal diseases. Therefore, control of diabetes and efficient periodontal treatment are of greatest importance in such patients (for review, see Axelsson, 2002; Ramseier, 2005).

Conclusions

The importance of initial needs-related combinations of mechanical and chemical plaque control, one-stage complete-mouth disinfection, nonsurgical periodontal therapy, and elimination of plaque-retentive factors during an intense, 1-week-maximum phase cannot be overstated. This initial intense therapy can be supplemented with antibiotics, surgical pocket reduction, treatment of furcation-involved teeth, and regenerative periodontal therapy, as needed, in high-risk maintenance patients with recurrent periodontal disease and in so-called refractory patients.

Antibiotics can be delivered systemically or locally. Similar to chemical plaque control agents, antibiotics cannot substitute for mechanical plaque control and nonsurgical scaling, root planing, and debridement. Use of antibiotics always has to be preceded by mechanical removal of supragingival and subgingival plaque biofilms because antibiotics have no access to microbes protected in well-matured biofilms.

Only patients with ANUG or ANUP and acute periodontal abscesses may initially need antibiotics. Selection of a single antibiotic or combinations of antibiotics should always be based on subgingival microbial analysis. Sensitivity tests should also be carried out because some periopathogens may have developed resistance to a certain antibiotic.

Antibiotics will only be used selectively as a supplement to nonsurgical periodontal therapy and regenerative therapy. Such selective periodontal conditions are aggressive periodontitis (particularly in patients with high levels of *Aa*), refractory periodontitis (particularly in diabetic patients and smokers), and ANUP. Antibiotics may also be used in patients with immunoinsufficiency or severe cardiovascular disease.

According to systematic reviews, there is consensus that systemic use of antibiotics has a positive supplementary effect to nonsurgical periodontal therapy. In particular, the combination of amoxicillin and metronidazole seems to be the most efficient antibiotic supplement to nonsurgical periodontal therapy in patients with high levels of *Aa* and the red complex (*Tf, Pg,* and *Td*).

Tetracycline, metronidazole, minocycline, and doxycycline are available in local delivery systems. Locally delivered antibiotics may be most useful in refractory patients with a few persistent diseased deep pockets and as a supplement to debridement in a few sites before regenerative therapy. According to systematic reviews, tetracycline fiber seems to be the most efficient locally delivered antibiotic as a supplement to nonsurgical periodontal therapy.

Healing of infectious inflamed periodontal tissues in furcation areas is very complicated because of limited accessibility (particularly on the approximal sites of the maxillary molars and first premolars) to methods of gingival plaque control. Therefore, loss of periodontal support is faster in sites exhibiting furcation involvement than in other sites. The distal surfaces of the maxillary first molars have the highest prevalence of furcation involvement, followed by the buccal and lingual surfaces of the mandibular first molars.

Grade I furcation involvement on the buccal surfaces of the molars and the lingual surfaces of the mandibular molars can successfully be treated by improved gingival plaque control, PMTC, subgingival instrumentation, and possibly supplementary recontouring (odontoplasty) to reduce the horizontal pocket and thus increase the accessibility for gingival plaque control. Grade II and particularly grade III furcation involvement in mandibular molars frequently necessitates hemisection or extraction, depending on how useful the tooth is. Grade II involvement can also be successfully treated by regenerative therapy. Grade II furcation involvement is most frequently found at distal sites of the maxillary first molars, which mostly require elimination of the distobuccal root by resection or hemisection. A hygienic design of the reconstruction after hemisection is very important to improve the accessibility for plaque control. Grade III involvement may be treated with hemisection, tunneling, or extraction.

After initial nonsurgical periodontal therapy, mini-flap periodontal surgery may be necessary in a few persistent deep pockets to improve visibility for diagnoses, to achieve root instrumentation, to achieve probing depth reduction, and to perform regenerative therapy. Gingivectomy and large, quadrant-sized flaps have been out of fashion for many years.

To improve the effect of mechanical and pharmacologic infection control on healing infectious inflamed periodontal tissues, as many modifying risk factors as possible should be eliminated or reduced. In particular, cessation of smoking and well-controlled diabetes are of great importance.

CHAPTER 4

REPAIR AND REGENERATION OF
LOST PERIODONTAL TISSUES

Successful healing of infectious inflamed periodontal tissues can be achieved by needs-related combinations of efficient methods and materials that are aimed at the causative factors. Successful healing is characterized by, among other things, reduced probing depth and formation of a new junctional epithelium attached to the root surface. This epithelium prevents exposure of the connective tissue and alveolar bone and direct contact with the root surface, which could result in root resorption or ankylosis.

Occasionally, healing after conventional periodontal therapy—nonsurgical as well as surgical—will result in minor formation of new periodontal support in the most apical part of the periodontal defect, but not at a magnitude that could be considered clinically important (for review, see Polimeni et al, 2006). However, even sites with healthy deep periodontal pockets and long junctional epithelia should be regarded as risk sites for recurrence of periodontal destruction. In particular, sites with remaining intrabony defects and furcation involvement must be regarded as high-risk sites.

Therefore, successful periodontal therapy must include regeneration or at least repair of lost periodontal tissues after healing of infectious inflamed periodontal tissues.

In addition, a needs-related maintenance (supportive) care program must be introduced to prevent recurrence of periodontal disease and thus maintain the long-term outcome of successful periodontal therapy (see chapter 5).

DEFINITION OF TERMS

The most recent *Glossary of Periodontal Terms* (American Academy of Periodontology, 2001) provides the following definitions for these terms related to repair and regeneration of lost periodontal tissues:

- *Repair:* Healing of a wound by tissue that does not fully restore the architecture or function of the part (Fig 202).
- *Regeneration:* Reproduction or reconstitution of a lost or injured part. Histologically, periodontal regeneration is defined as regeneration of all tissues that represent the periodontal support, including alveolar bone, periodontal ligament, and cementum, over a previously diseased root surface (see Fig 202).
- *Bone fill:* Clinical restoration of bone tissue in a treated periodontal defect. Such bone fill in intrabony defects or furcation involvements without re-formation of periodontal ligament and cementum should be regarded as repair of alveolar bone.
- *New attachment:* Union of connective tissue or epithelium with a root surface that has been deprived of its original attachment apparatus. This new attachment may be epithelial adhesion and/or connective adaptation or attachment and may include new cementum (Fig 203).
- *Clinical attachment level (CAL):* Distance from the cementoenamel junction to the tip of a periodontal probe during periodontal diagnostic probing.

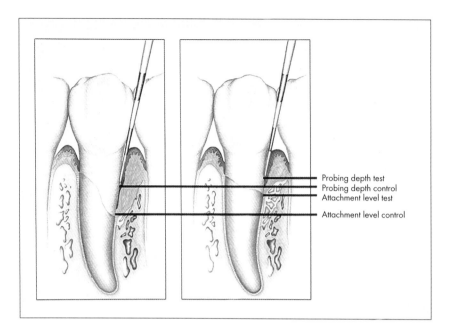

Fig 202 Difference between repair *(left)* and regeneration *(right)*. (Courtesy of Biora.)

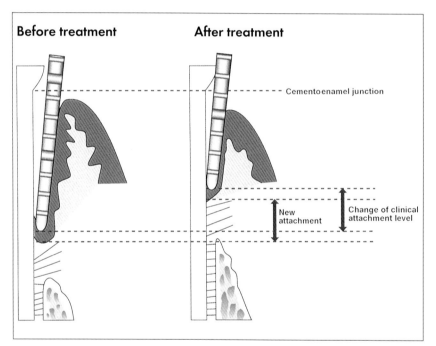

Fig 203 New attachment and regeneration after regenerative therapy of a diseased periodontal pocket. In contrast to true regeneration of the periodontal tissues, no alveolar bone was regenerated in the new attachment area. (Courtesy of Dr K. Rateitschak.)

- *Open probing clinical attachment:* CAL measured at surgery after regenerative procedures.
- *Guided tissue regeneration (GTR):* Procedures attempting to regenerate lost periodontal structures through differential tissue responses. *Guided bone regeneration* typically refers to ridge augmentation or bone-regenerative procedures; *guided tissue regeneration* typically refers to regeneration of periodontal attachment. Barrier techniques, using materials such as expanded polytetrafluoroethylene (e-PTFE), polyglactin, polylactic acid, calcium sulfate, and collagen, are employed in the hope of excluding the epithelium and the gingival corium from the root or existing bone surface, in the belief that they interfere with regeneration (Fig 204).

Fig 204 Regeneration of an intraosseous periodontal defect by GTR with a barrier membrane *(blue outline)* during open flap surgery. *(left)* After surgical elevation, the root surface is carefully mechanically cleaned using minimally invasive instrumentation *(red arrows)* then chemically conditioned. *(middle)* Placement of custom-designed membrane. *(right)* The flaps are tightly sutured. (Courtesy of Dr K. Rateitschak.)

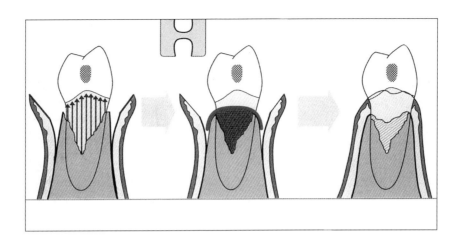

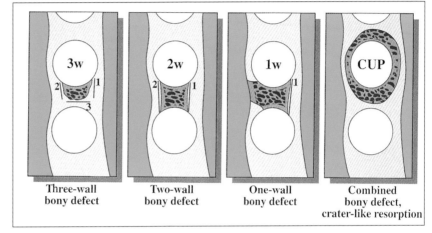

Fig 205 Through a combination of radiographs, probing depths, and attachment level data, different types of bony defects (three-, two-, and one-wall and combined bony defects [CUP]) may be diagnosed.

INDICATIONS

Intrabony defects

The accessibility for efficient nonsurgical instrumentation in narrow two- and three-wall intrabony defects is very limited (Fig 205). As a consequence, the infected and diseased pocket will not heal. In addition, the effect of gingival plaque control by professional mechanical toothcleaning (PMTC) and self-care is limited as long as deeper localized subgingival periopathogens remain. The risk of further periodontal destruction is increased in such defects. Thus, regenerative periodontal therapy should be a priority in two- and three-wall intrabony defects. Fortunately, regenerative therapy has been most successful in such defects (for review, see Needleman et al, 2005; Trombelli, 2005).

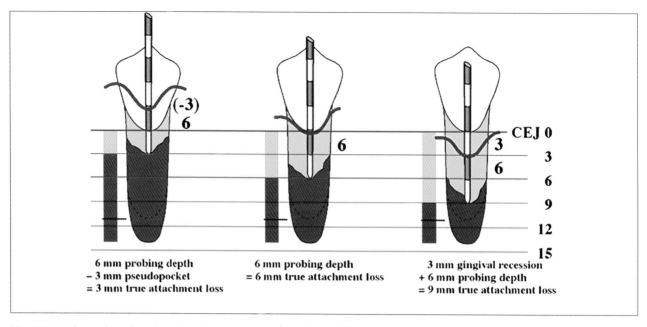

Fig 206 Relationship of probing depth to attachment loss. Three different clinical attachment levels (3, 6, and 9 mm) can result in the same probing depth (6 mm). (CEJ) Cementoenamel junction. (Modified from Rateitschak et al, 1989, with permission.)

Furcation involvement

Furcation-involved teeth represent the most complicated accessibility problems for nonsurgical instrumentation. In particular, grade II and grade III furcation involvement on the mesial and distal surfaces of the maxillary molars and first premolars is usually inaccessible to complete nonsurgical as well as surgical therapy (see chapter 3). On the other hand, grade II furcation involvement can successfully be eliminated by regenerative therapy on buccal and lingual sites of mandibular molars and buccal sites of maxillary molars (for review, see Jepsen et al, 2002).

Recession and sensitive exposed root surfaces

Progressive periodontitis will result in exposed root surfaces, particularly in smokers. Successful nonsurgical and surgical periodontal therapy will reduce probing depths and, as a consequence, expose the root surfaces. An incorrect toothbrushing technique (horizontal scrubbing) can also result in excessive recession, particularly on the buccal surfaces of the canines and first premolars.

Exposed root surfaces on the buccal surfaces of the maxillary incisors and first premolars may be a severe esthetic problem, especially in patients with a low lip line. In addition, the root surfaces of vital teeth that exhibit exposed root dentin due to invasive scaling may be very sensitive. The sensitivity may inhibit the patient's attempts at plaque control, sooner or later leading to root caries. Coronally positioned flap surgery in combination with regenerative therapy is indicated to cover the exposed root surfaces, especially in the maxillary anterior region. Such therapy has been proven successful (Al-Hamdan et al, 2003).

ASSESSMENT OF PERIODONTAL REPAIR AND REGENERATION

Clinical probing of attachment level, radiographs, and reentry observations are the most common means of evaluating the effect of regenerative therapy. However, none of these methods can differentiate between repair and true regeneration because repair of intrabony defects and furcations results in new bone formation close to the root surface. A very thin epithelium separates the root surface from the new bone. Neither the periodontal probe nor radiographs and reentry can distinguish such a thin epithelium from a true regenerated periodontal ligament. True regeneration can only be proven by histologic analyses (American Academy of Periodontology, 1996), which are not clinically practical. Therefore, probing of alterations in CAL and assessment of bone level changes on radiographs are frequently used to evaluate the short- and long-term outcomes of regenerative therapy.

Clinical probing

Deep diseased periodontal pockets (of 5 mm or more) are a local risk factor for further periodontal destruction. However, probing depth does not disclose the true loss of periodontal attachment. Teeth with different CALs can demonstrate the same probing depth (Fig 206). Because of gingival recession and limited inflammation (edema) in the gingival margin, smokers in particular may have advanced periodontal attachment loss but limited probing depth.

On the other hand, some drugs, systemic diseases, and hormonal changes may result in extremely hyperplastic gingiva, with formation of pseudopockets and relatively limited probing attachment loss. The absence of deep pockets is usually a good indicator of periodontal stability, while deepened pockets indicate periodontal instability.

The size and shape of the periodontal probe, the force with which the probe is applied, and the health of the attachment apparatus can affect the measurement. For example, inflamed connective tissue exhibits reduced resistance and will result in a 0.5- to 1.0-mm overestimation of probing attachment loss, while the more resistant healthy connective tissue may result in a 0.5- to 1.0-mm underestimation of probing attachment loss.

Radiographs

Conventional radiographs

For detailed analyses of the alveolar bone, it is usual practice to take intraoral complete-mouth radiographs, supplemented with four vertical bitewing radiographs. A standardized technique is used, eg, film holders are attached to the long cone. The radiographs provide information about the height and configuration of the interproximal alveolar bone and disclose the presence of calculus and defects on the approximal root surfaces.

In experimental studies, measurement of interproximal alveolar bone loss is facilitated by the use of special radiographic film equipped with a millimeter grid and a viewer with ×10 magnification. The normal threshold for concluding that there is no loss of alveolar bone is a distance of 1.5 to 2.0 mm from the cementoenamel junction to the most coronal level of intact supporting bone.

Compared with individual periapical radiographs, vertical bitewing radiographs require a smaller radiation dose because several maxillary and mandibular posterior teeth are included on one piece of film. The bone height is generally imaged very accurately along the root surface because of the ease of directing the x-ray beam perpendicular to the tooth, either by eye or with a specially designed vertical bitewing positioning device.

For detailed analysis of infrabony pockets, special millimeter-graded probes can be inserted in the pockets during radiography, and the aforementioned film with a millimeter grid can be used.

A particularly useful technique for monitoring the clinical outcome of regenerative therapy is placement of a periodontal probe to indicate CAL as pretreatment and posttreatment radiographs are exposed (Figs 207a and 207b).

To arrive at a correct diagnosis with respect to the alveolar bone level, the presence of angular bony defects and interdental osseous craters, and so on, an additional method, called *sounding*, may be used. While the site is under local anes-

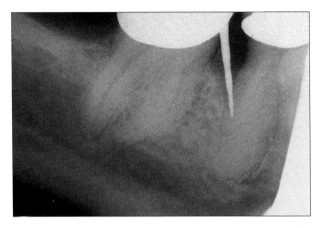

Fig 207a Periodontal probe inserted to the bottom of a three-wall intrabony defect at the distal aspect of the mandibular right first molar before regenerative treatment.

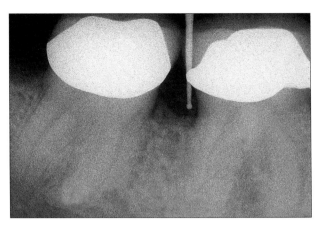

Fig 207b Radiograph at reexamination about 2.5 years after treatment.

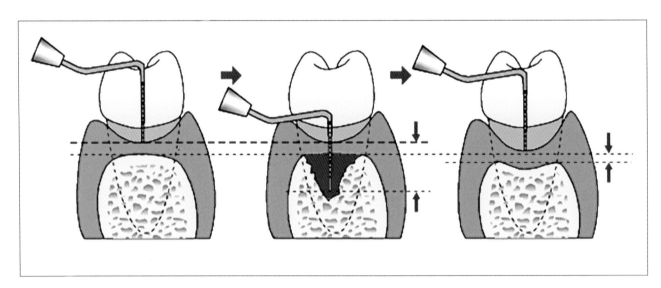

Fig 208 Relationship of probing attachment levels to radiographic change. (Modified from Goodson et al, 1984. Reprinted with permission.)

thesia, the periodontal probe is inserted in the pocket, the tip is forced through the supra-alveolar connective tissue to contact the bone, and the distance from the cementoenamel junction to the bone is assessed in millimeters.

Conventional radiographic evaluation of periodontal status also has some important limitations, for example, the fact that there must be major loss of mineral mass (more than 50%) before it can be detected on a radiograph by the naked eye. In a study by Goodson et al (1984), standardized radiographs and repeated periodontal probing measurements were made for untreated subjects with destructive periodontal disease who were monitored for 1 year. Radiographs of selected sites were taken at 6 and 12 months and attachment levels were measured monthly. Significant PAL generally preceded radiographically detectable bone loss by 6 to 8 months.

Figure 208 from the study illustrates possible attachment level and alveolar bone changes during a period of actively destructive periodontal disease. The earliest phase results in medullary bone loss and an accompanying increase in PAL. During this phase, radiographic evidence of bone loss is not apparent because the cortical bone height remains unchanged. At the end of the acute burst of active destructive disease, the probing attachment depth resumes a stable level, and the underlying bone undergoes remodeling. At that time, radiographic evidence of bone loss is detected because the level of crestal alveolar bone has decreased, even though there has been repair of the approximal bone defect. This decrease occurs because the bone mass of the cortical bone was greater than that of the total spongiform bone, and the natural shape of the alveolar bone is being reestablished.

Subtraction radiographs

Over the past 20 years, subtraction radiography has been applied with increasing frequency for detailed longitudinal evaluation of the outcome of periodontal therapy in experimental studies (Gröndahl, 1997; Gröndahl and Gröndahl, 1983; Gröndahl et al, 1987). The technique is especially useful for studies of regeneration and for evaluation of therapy in furcation involvement in mandibular molars.

Computer programs are able to analyze the information in the source radiographs and present it in a form that can be more readily interpreted by the clinician or may provide a quantitative measure of the amount of bone loss or gain. Such methods are termed *image-processing techniques.* Computer image processing of high-quality images makes it possible to detect bone change of less than 5% with better than 90% sensitivity, specificity, and overall accuracy (Jeffcoat, 1992; Jeffcoat and Reddy, 1993; Jeffcoat et al, 1995).

Image-processing techniques have been developed to enhance the detection of small osseous changes over short periods of time. These include digital subtraction radiography and computer-assisted densitometric image analysis. Digital subtraction radiography is especially useful for detecting small changes in hard tissues between examinations. All unchanged structures are subtracted from a set of two radiographs, leaving only the area of change. This image-processing technique subtracts unchanging teeth, cortical bone, and trabecular pattern, leaving only the bone gain or loss standing out against a neutral gray background on the subtraction image. By convention, bone gain is shown as a light area and bone loss as a dark area.

In computer-assisted densitometric image analysis, the images are not always displayed, but the numeric values after subtraction in areas of interest are analyzed to detect osseous changes. Additional software can localize the area of bone change and superimpose it on the original radiograph to facilitate interpretation by a clinician.

The first step in subtraction is digitization, which simplifies the information in the radiograph to a form that can be understood by a computer that analyzes and displays the information. The use of subtraction radiography requires that radiographs be taken with similar contrast, density, and angulation. Meticulous attention to detail is critical when radiographs are exposed for use in digital radiographic techniques.

Color coding of subtraction images improves the ability of clinicians inexperienced in reading subtraction images to detect bone loss or gain. In the color-coded images, bone gain may appear as shades of green and bone loss as shades of red. Among the systems available are the Digora image plate system (Soredex) for digital intraoral radiography (Fig 209), which reduces radiation exposure by as much as 90%; the CDR system (Schick; Fig 210); Sivision (Sirona); the Everest RVG system (Trophy Radiologie); DSR (Electro Medical Systems); VistaRay (Dürr); and the Sens-A-Ray system (Regam Medical Systems).

The subtraction image itself can be used to make direct measurements, in millimeters, of bone change along the root surface. In addition, the mass of the region of bone change can be calculated by incorporating a reference wedge in the original radiographic image. Software permits the actual bone loss or gain to be quantified in milligrams.

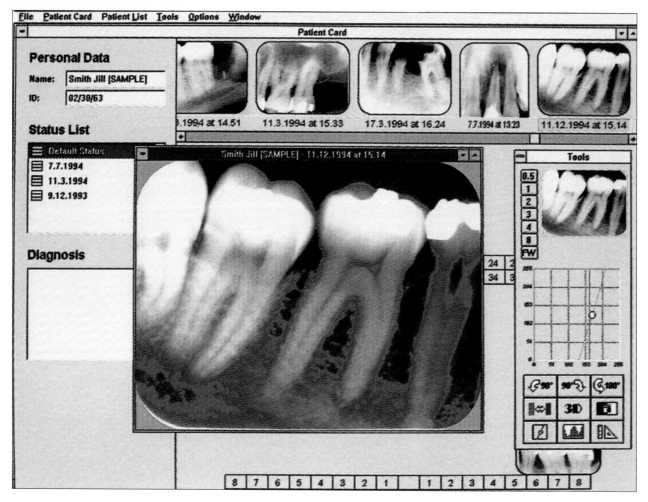

Fig 209 Digital intraoral radiography using the Digora image plate system. With computer-aided digital subtraction radiography, bone loss or bone regeneration can be measured and visualized with color within 2 to 4 months.

WOUND HEALING RELATED TO REPAIR AND REGENERATION

Nonsurgical periodontal treatment, alone or in combination with periodontal surgery and supplemented by excellent gingival plaque control, can successfully heal infectious inflamed periodontal tissues and arrest the progression of periodontitis. Such treatments may regenerate bone (bone fill) and occasionally some other tooth-supporting structures. These healing effects are regarded as repair, with a combination of connective tissue adhesions and attachment or formation of a long junctional epithelium, as discussed earlier.

Regeneration of the complete periodontal support, on the other hand, includes the formation of new cementum with inserting collagen

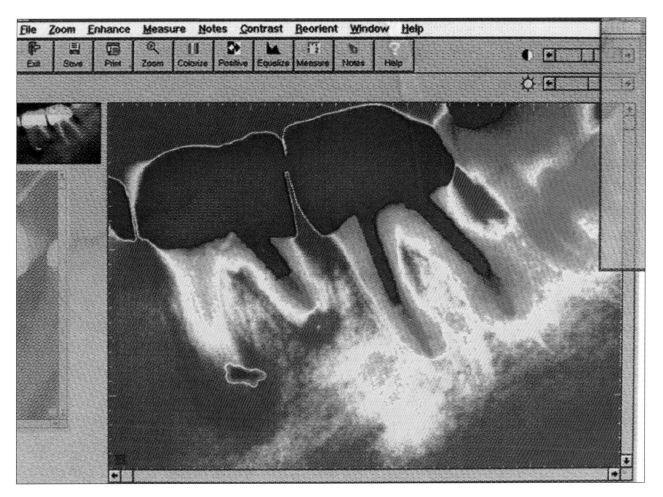

Fig 210 Color coding of subtraction radiographic images using the CDR system.

fibers on the previously periodontitis-affected and instrumented root surfaces and regrowth of alveolar bone, particularly in bone defects (vertical intrabony and furcation-involved defects).

However, regeneration of root cementum with inserting collagen fibers may also be achieved as an effect of regenerative therapy without formation of new alveolar bone, for example,

at sites with well-mineralized horizontal alveolar margins on iatrogenically exposed buccal root surfaces. That means a fibrous reattachment can be achieved without apposition of bone.

Although many of the cellular and molecular events in the healing of periodontal wounds are similar to those seen elsewhere in the body, differences complicating the periodontal healing process do exist. Animal research (Araújo et al, 2003; Cardaropoli et al, 2005; Caton and Nyman, 1980; Caton et al, 1980) has confirmed that periodontal surgical wounds go through the same sequence of healing events as all incisional wounds: formation of a fibrin clot between the flap margin and the root surface followed by replacement of this fibrin clot with a connective tissue matrix attached to the root surface. When this fibrin linkage is maintained, a new connective tissue attachment to the root surface develops. If the fibrin linkage is disrupted, an attachment of the long junctional epithelium type results.

It has been suggested that these regenerative failures may result when the tensile strength of the fibrin clot is exceeded, resulting in a tear (Araújo et al, 1998). Mobility of the flap (wound margin) positioned directly adjacent to the potential regenerative site may be a potential cause of this tear. On the other hand, healing of periodontal surgical wounds has been suggested to differ from other wounds in several features; factors such as the presence of multiple specialized cell types and attachment complexes, the stromal-cellular interactions, the diverse microbial flora, and the avascular tooth surfaces complicate the process of periodontal regeneration. Better understanding of these special factors involved in the periodontal wound-healing process should allow more predictable treatment outcomes following periodontal regenerative therapy.

After flap surgery, the instrumented root surfaces may be repopulated by four different types of cells:

1. Epithelial cells
2. Cells derived from the gingival connective tissue
3. Cells derived from the alveolar bone
4. Cells derived from the periodontal ligament

Animal experiments by Nyman et al (1980) and Karring et al (1980) have shown that neither bone nor connective tissue cells can induce new attachment with collagen fibers that insert into newly formed cementum on instrumented, periodontitis-affected, transplanted roots. Instead, healing resulted in root resorption and ankylosis.

On the other hand, other animal experiments by Nyman et al (1982a) have shown that new alveolar bone may be formed without ankylosis and root resorption along transplanted roots with remaining intact periodontal ligament. Thus the researchers concluded that only periodontal ligament cells have the potential to induce regeneration of a complete new periodontal attachment. However, it has been suggested that bone and connective tissue cells may also contribute to regeneration of lost periodontal support (Giannobile and Somerman, 2003; Hughes et al, 2006).

The periodontal ligament cells are a heterogenous group of cells that may have the capacity to function as osteoblasts or cementoblasts during the regenerative process. The cells may also function as regulators or inhibitors of mineral formation and thus prevent ankylosis during regeneration. Some subpopulations of the cells may either inhibit or promote formation of mineralized tissues (bone and cementum). However, the factors and cells involved in the regeneration of the periodontium and the function and the relative contributions of periodontal ligament cells, osteoblasts, root surface cells, and paravascular cells in the regenerative environment are still not entirely understood, in spite of the progress and extensive ongoing research in this field (for review, see Polimeni et al, 2006).

METHODS AND MATERIALS FOR REPAIR AND REGENERATION OF LOST PERIODONTAL TISSUES

Clinical studies have shown that flap surgery procedures followed by maintenance care and excellent gingival plaque control may result in repair (bone fill) of two- and three-wall intrabony defects (Polson and Heijl, 1978; Prichard 1957a, 1957b; Rosling et al, 1976a). Bone replacement grafts, barrier membranes (GTR), biomaterials, and growth factors have been used in conjunction with coronally placed flaps to promote regeneration.

Bone replacement grafts

Bone replacement grafts represent the first attempts at regenerative therapy of intraosseous defects. Bone replacement grafts have been widely used in two- and three-wall intrabony defects, mostly in the United States.

Graft material has also been used in grade II furcation defects. Four different graft materials have been used for bone replacement in regenerative or repair therapy.

1. *Autogenous graft:* Harvested from an intraoral or extraoral donor site in the same individual. The graft may consist of cortical, cancellous, or marrow bone.
2. *Allogeneic graft:* Harvested from a genetically dissimilar donor of the same species as the recipient. The graft material can be either frozen cancellous bone and marrow or freeze-dried bone.
3. *Xenogeneic graft:* Harvested from a donor of another species.
4. *Alloplastic material:* Synthetic or inorganic implant material.

The following concepts are behind the use of graft materials in regenerative or repair therapy:

- Autogenous bone grafts contain vital bone-forming cells (osteogenesis effect).
- Bone grafts may serve as a scaffold for bone formation (osteoconductive effect).
- Bone grafts may contain bone-inducing substances (osteoinductive effect).

However, the use of autogenous bone grafts or other graft materials cannot result in complete regeneration of the connective attachment because only periodontal ligament cells are able to form new collagen fibers that insert into new cementum, as discussed earlier. Thus, only repair of the alveolar bone defect may be expected with the use of graft materials. Gain of probing attachment and bone fill has been confirmed by reentry and radiographs in several case report studies (for review, see Brunsvold and Mellonig, 1993), but histologic evidence for true new attachment is lacking or very limited.

Autogenous bone grafts

Narrow grafts of intraoral autogenous cancellous bone are usually obtained from the maxillary tuberosity, mandibular retromolar area, healing extraction sites, or edentulous areas of the jaws. Extraoral autogenous grafts are usually obtained from iliac cancellous bone with marrow. However, because of the morbidity associated with the donor site and the risk of root resorption (Ellegaard et al, 1973, 1974), iliac crest marrow grafts are not used in regenerative therapy today. Intraoral as well as extraoral bone grafts may, on average, result in 3 to 4 mm of bone fill in intraosseous bone defects, according to several case report studies (Nabers and O'Leary, 1965; Robinson, 1969).

Allogeneic bone grafts

Three main types of allogeneic bone grafts are commercially available: frozen iliac cancellous bone and marrow, freeze-dried bone allograft (FDBA), and demineralized freeze-dried bone allograft (DFDBA). Of these, DFDBA has been most frequently used and evaluated in regenerative therapy for intraosseous defects.

In controlled clinical trials, FDBA and DFDBA have resulted in 1.3 to 2.6 mm and 1.7 to 2.9 mm of bone fill, respectively. In randomized clinical trials, DFDBA has resulted in significantly more gain of bone fill than open flap debridement (OFD). However, controlled human histologic studies have also shown that DFDBA may result in limited periodontal regeneration compared to OFD (for reviews, see Reynolds et al, 2003; Trombelli et al, 2002).

The controversial results regarding the effect of DFDBA on the regeneration of periodontal intraosseous defects, along with great differences in the osteoinductive potential (ranging from high to no osteoinductive effect) of commercially available DFDBA and the risk for disease transmission (although minute), have raised concern about the clinical applicability of DFDBA. In countries of the European Union, commercially available DFDBA is not granted CE marking, which would permit distribution of the material within the union.

Alloplasts

Six basic types of alloplastic materials are commercially available: bioactive glass, nonporous hydroxyapatite, hydroxyapatite cement, porous hydroxyapatite (replamine form), β-tricalcium phosphate, and a calcium-layered polymer of polymethyl methacrylate and hydroxyethyl methacrylate. It has been reported that porous and nonporous hydroxyapatite materials and polymethyl methacrylate–hydroxyethyl methacrylate polymer are nonresorbable, while tricalcium phosphate and bioactive glass are bioresorbable (Dragoo and Kaldahl, 1983; Froum et al, 1982; Froum and Stahl, 1987; Moskow and Lubarr, 1983).

In controlled clinical studies, both nonporous and porous alloplasts have resulted in 1.6- to 3.5-mm defect closure compared to the 0.5- to 0.7-mm closure obtained with OFD (for review, see Trombelli et al, 2002). However, histologic evaluation shows that the graft material tends to be encapsulated by connective tissue with minimal or no bone formation (Ganeles et al, 1986). Thus, alloplasts seem to act as a nonirritating filler of intraosseous defects.

Xenografts

A xenograft (heterograft) is a graft taken from a donor of another species. These grafting materials are also referred to as *anorganic bone* because proprietary processes are suggested to remove all cells and proteinaceous material, leaving behind an inert absorbable bone scaffolding on which revascularization, osteoblast migration, and woven bone formation supposedly occur. There are very few human clinical data supporting the use of these materials for management of periodontal defects. In addition, concerns over the risk of transmission of prion-mediated diseases have arisen.

Outcomes

In a systematic review, Reynolds et al (2003) analyzed the efficacy of bone replacement grafts in the treatment of periodontal osseous defects. The review included 49 controlled studies on the clinical outcome of intrabony defects and 17 studies of furcation defects following grafting procedures. The authors developed the following conclusions:

- Bone replacement grafts generally increase bone level, reduce crestal bone loss, increase CAL, and reduce probing depth more effectively than do OFD procedures in the treatment of intrabony defects.
- Hydroxyapatite and bone allograft provide similar improvements in clinical measures in the treatment of intrabony defects.
- The combination of bone grafts and barrier membranes may provide superior clinical outcomes to grafts alone in the treatment of intrabony defects.
- Insufficient studies of comparable design are available for meta-analysis of treatment results for furcation defects.
- Histologic evidence indicates that autogenous bone and DFDBA support the formation of a new attachment apparatus.
- Histologic evidence indicates that alloplastic grafts support periodontal repair rather than regeneration.

Guided tissue regeneration

According to the previously discussed animal experiments by Nyman et al (1980) and Karring et al (1980), only cells derived from the periodontal ligament have the capacity to form new root cementum with inserting new principal fibers, resulting in new attachment. Based on these results, the same research team developed the so-called guided tissue regeneration technique. To prevent the root surface from repopulating with cells derived from epithelium, bone, and connective tissue, a tailored barrier was placed between the flap and the root surface after OFD. In this way, periodontal ligament cells could repopulate the debrided and cleaned root surface without competition from other cells in the space between the barrier and the root cementum.

Nyman et al (1982b) presented the pioneering report of a human root treated according to the principles of GTR. Because of severely advanced periodontal breakdown, the tooth was scheduled for extraction, allowing histologic documentation of the treatment result. A periodontal defect measuring 11 mm from the cementoenamel junction to the bottom of the defect was diagnosed during periodontal surgery. A tailored, nonresorbable micropore filter was placed as a barrier between the flap and the root surface and coronally fixed to the tooth before the flap was tightly resutured, creating a space between the barrier membrane and the root surface. Three months after GTR treatment, the tooth was removed with the buccal periodontium still attached. Histologic analysis demonstrated 7 mm of new connective tissue attachment extending coronally from the base of the original defect.

The outcome from this pioneering human GTR case was later confirmed in a controlled experimental split-mouth study in monkeys (Gottlow et al, 1984) as well as in case reports in humans (Gottlow et al, 1986). Variations in the amount of new attachment achieved in these studies can be explained by differences in amounts of remaining periodontal ligament tissue (ie, differences in the availability of progenitor cells and in defect morphology) as well as by technical problems, for example, difficulty in achieving proper flap coverage of the membranes.

The amount of regeneration possible seems to be limited by the position of the membrane: The coronal extent of the newly formed periodontal ligament does not exceed the level of the coronal margin of the membrane. Thus, the more coronal the membrane, the more extensive the regeneration (Gottlow et al, 1986).

Over the past two decades, GTR therapy has evolved in both surgical technique and membrane technology. Both factors must be considered critically. In 1982, investigation began of materials that would limit the migration of epithelium around dental implants and teeth. It had been speculated that specific porosities ingrown with connective tissue would stop or slow the migration and pocketing of epidermal and epithelial tissues. This phenomenon was called *contact inhibition*. Around natural teeth, the ingrowth or attachment of Sharpey fibers and surrounding fiber bundles occurs at the base of a sulcus, where epithelial downgrowth ends. Accordingly, the first design criterion evolved: Membranes needed an organized open microstructure to encourage tissue in-

tegration and thereby limit epithelial migration while creating a stable site for wound healing.

In addition, it was determined that membrane materials should also be easy to cut and shape, tolerate suturing, and be easy to remove in case of complications. It also became apparent that membranes placed completely subgingivally were easier for the clinician to manage and more comfortable for the patient than those that extended into the mouth.

Thus, the evolution of membrane development suggests five essential design criteria: *(1)* tissue integration; *(2)* cell occlusivity; *(3)* clinical manageability; *(4)* space-making capacity; and *(5)* biocompatibility. These criteria may be applied to select the appropriate materials and designs for specific GTR applications. Nonresorbable as well as bioresorbable membranes (barriers) are commercially available. Special titanium-reinforced nonresorbable barriers are also available.

Nonresorbable membranes

In the first GTR studies by Nyman et al (1982b) and Gottlow et al (1984), the tailored micropore filter membranes were placed so that they extended coronally and were glued to the crown to exclude epithelium from the healing site. These membranes did not meet the first design criterion (facilitating ingrowth to limit the epithelium and to stabilize wound healing), and consequently, the epithelium was able to migrate around the membranes. This migration led to secondary pocketing, recession, and gross membrane exposure.

Experiments were conducted to investigate whether wrapping porous e-PTFE structures around teeth would help to stabilize the gingival flaps and exclude epithelium from healing periodontal defects. The results showed that e-PTFE membranes limited the migration of epithelium, stabilized the wound, and kept epithelium (and associated pocketing) out of the healing periodontal defect (Gottlow et al, 1986).

Original e-PTFE membranes. With the aforementioned design criteria established, WL Gore began working on a two-part material: *(1)* an open microstructure collar that could be implanted sub-

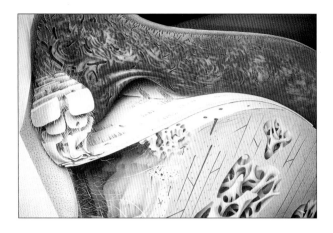

Fig 211 Nonresorbable e-PTFE barrier membrane in situ. (Courtesy of WL Gore.)

gingivally, ingrow with connective tissue, and limit epithelial migration; and *(2)* an occlusive portion that would still attach to stabilize the wound area, separate cell types for GTR, have a structure strong enough to retain sutures snugly around the tooth, be easy to cut and shape without leaving sharp edges to perforate tissue, and in the event of complication, be easily removable (Fig 211). By 1988, clinical testing of e-PTFE membranes had been in progress for more than 3 years. Researchers reported clinically significant gains in attachment level, reduction in probing depths, and improvement of prognosis for grade II furcations and two- and three-wall intrabony defects (Becker et al, 1987, 1988; Gottlow et al, 1986; Nyman et al, 1987). Figures 212a to 212d illustrate GTR with a nonresorbable membrane in an intraosseous periodontal defect.

An assortment of transgingival configurations of nonresorbable barrier membranes have been designed to fit different types of periodontal defects. The configuration most suitable for covering the defect is selected, and additional shaping is performed so that the defect is covered completely and the membrane extends at least 3 mm on the bone beyond the defect margin. This assures stability and protects the underlying blood clot during healing. It is essential to ensure good adaptation of the barrier material to the alveolar bone surrounding the defect and to avoid overlapping or folding of the material.

Although exceptions exist, most barrier materials are fixed to the tooth with a sling suturing technique. For optimal performance, the barrier should be placed with its margin apical to the flap margin. To maximize coverage of the barrier, a horizontal releasing incision in the periosteum may assist in the coronal displacement of the flap during the suturing of the wound. However, the blood supply to the flap must not be compromised. The interproximal space near the barrier should be closed first. A vertical mattress suturing technique is advocated to ensure adequate closure.

Case 1. A 45-year-old nonsmoking woman exhibited grade II to III furcation involvement on the buccal aspect of the mandibular left first molar (Fig 213a). The pretreatment radiograph revealed more than 50% loss of alveolar bone in the furcation area (Fig 213b). The initial buccal probing depth was 12 mm.

Before surgery, the patient received oral hygiene education, PMTC, and nonsurgical periodontal treatment including scaling, debridement, and root planing. In response to treatment, the buccal probing depth decreased by 3 mm, and the gingival margin healed.

The furcation area was exposed by open full-thickness flap surgery with marginal incisions placed buccally and lingually and two vertical releasing incisions placed buccally. The buccal pocket epithelium and the granulation tissue in the furcation defect were carefully removed. The narrow dome of the deep furcation area was briefly scaled with a universal curette; this was followed by final minimally invasive scaling, debridement, and root planing (Fig 213c). The root surfaces were cleaned of debris and washed with

Figs 212a to 212d GTR treatment of an intraosseous defect with a nonresorbable membrane. (Courtesy of Guidor.)

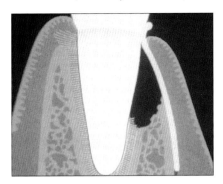

Fig 212a The membrane has been placed to create a space favorable to migration of periodontal ligament cells.

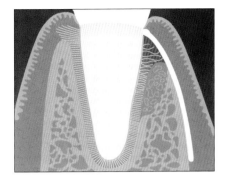

Fig 212b The intrabony defect heals gradually with formation of new bone and periodontal ligament.

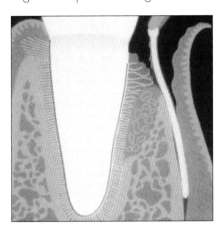

Fig 212c After about 6 weeks, a flap is surgically raised and the membrane is removed.

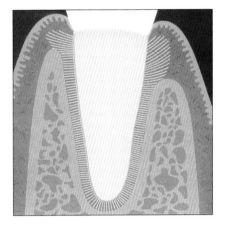

Fig 212d Successful regeneration has been achieved, resulting in complete bone fill in the defect as well as new periodontal ligament and supra-alveolar fibers.

sterile saline. After debridement and root planing were completed, only a partial, paper-thin lingual bone wall remained (Fig 213d). At surgery, vertical probing attachment loss was 12 mm, and horizontal attachment loss was 9 mm.

For regenerative therapy by GTR, a single-tooth nonresorbable Gore-Tex e-PTFE membrane (WL Gore) was applied to the buccal surface. After fixation of the barrier membrane to the tooth (Fig 213e), the flap was replaced and sutured so that it completely covered the membrane (Fig 213f). From 1 week before to 6 weeks after surgery, chemical plaque control was established through twice-daily rinses with 0.2% chlorhexidine (CHX) solution.

Depending on the outcome of presurgical subgingival microbiology and sensitivity analysis and the patient's general health status, antibiotics may be used as a supplement to regenerative therapy. However, in this case no antibiotics were used. An extrasoft toothbrush was used twice daily in the treated area from day 2 after surgery. The sutures were removed after 3 weeks. Six weeks after treatment, a second flap surgery had to be performed to remove the nonresorbable barrier membrane (Figs 213g and 213h). The advanced furcation defect was already filled with noninflammatory, nonmineralized osteogenic tissue (Fig 213i).

Figs 213a to 213n Case 1.

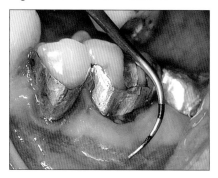

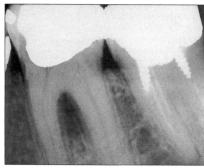

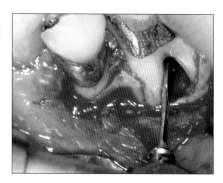

Fig 213a The furcation probe shows the clinically diagnosed vertical depth of a very advanced furcation defect located at the buccal surface of the mandibular left first molar.

Fig 213b There is advanced loss of alveolar bone in the furcation area of the mandibular left first molar (May 1990).

Fig 213c An extremely advanced furcation defect is visible during debridement and root planing with a PER-IO-TOR 4 reciprocating instrument (Dentatus).

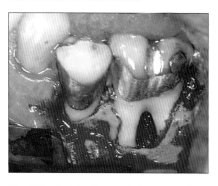

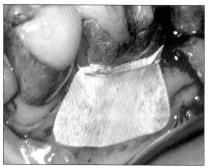

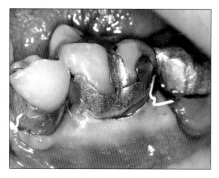

Fig 213d Mechanical cleaning of the advanced defect has been completed.

Fig 213e An e-PTFE membrane is fixed over the defect.

Fig 213f The replaced and sutured flap completely covers the barrier membrane.

For the first month after removal of the membrane, the patient was included in a weekly maintenance program including self-care education and PMTC; thereafter, the patient returned once a month for the following 6 months. At the 1-year reexamination, the buccal probing depth was only 1 mm (Fig 213j). The patient then consented to direct inspection of the healing tissue by reentry surgery. Figure 213k shows complete bone regeneration of the initially very advanced furcation defect. New periodontal ligament tissues were present on the buccal surfaces, which were not covered by bone. A radiograph taken at the same examination revealed total arrest of the extremely advanced furcation bone defect and the formation of a new periodontal ligament space all around the furcation area (Fig 213l).

Because of the maintenance program based on excellent gingival plaque control, at the 8-year follow-up there was no deterioration in the initial healing. There was still complete arrest of the bone level in the furcation area (Fig 213m), and the probing depth was still only 1 mm. After 1 and 8 years, the vertical and horizontal probing attachment gain was more than 9 mm. In addition, the health of the marginal gingiva was excellent (Fig 213n; Heden G and Axelsson P, unpublished data, 1990 and 1998).

Titanium-reinforced e-PTFE membranes. When the anatomy of the residual bone does not permit creation and maintenance of space at the defect site, it becomes necessary to use adjunctive materials such as bone replacement grafts. However, a commercially available membrane that achieved

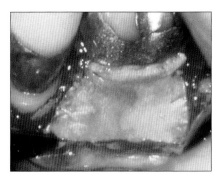
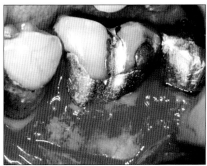
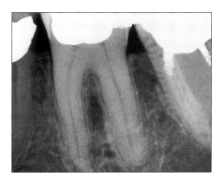

Figs 213g and 213h The barrier is removed 6 weeks after treatment.

Fig 213i The furcation defect is filled with noninflammatory, nonmineralized osteogenic tissue at the time of membrane removal.

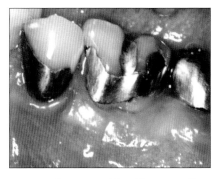
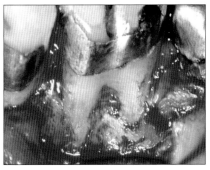
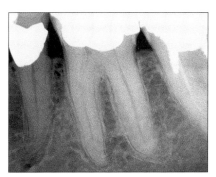

Fig 213j Gingival health is excellent 1 year after treatment, and only a 1-mm probing depth is measured buccally.

Fig 213k Complete bone regeneration is found in the furcation defect 1 year after treatment. The results are confirmed by reentry as well as by the presence of periodontal ligament on the buccal root surfaces.

Fig 213l The advanced furcation defect has totally regenerated, and a new periodontal ligament space has formed around the furcation area (May 1991).

Fig 213m The bone level is stable 8 years after regenerative therapy.

Fig 213n The probing depth is 1 mm at the 8-year follow-up. There has been no deterioration of the initial healing. Healthy gingiva and vertical and horizontal attachment gains of more than 9 mm have been maintained for 8 years.

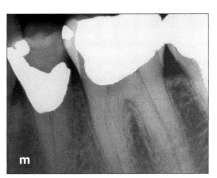
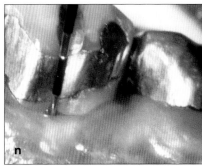

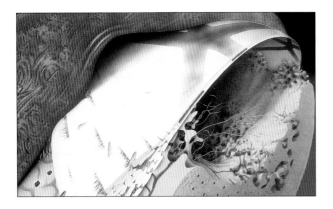

Fig 214 Titanium-reinforced e-PTFE barrier membrane in situ over an intrabony osseous defect. (Courtesy of WL Gore.)

the same goal could contribute greatly to regenerative treatment in non–space-making defects.

The stiff yet flexible e-PTFE membranes are efficient for the treatment of defects where the anatomy of the remaining bone permits creation of an adequate space. However, in periodontal and bony defects that do not allow natural creation of space, additional membrane support becomes necessary to ensure good results. Collapse of the membrane from occlusive pressure on the soft tissue flap and concomitant loss of the regenerative space can compromise the result, especially in applications where the material is left in place for 2 to 6 months, such as wide two-wall interproximal defects and wide advanced furcation defects.

In an effort to improve the space creation and maintenance in non–space-making defects, a titanium-reinforced e-PTFE membrane has been designed (titanium-reinforced Gore-Tex). A titanium frame is completely enclosed within nonresorbable e-PTFE regenerative material; the surface characteristics are equivalent to those of standard configurations (Fig 214). Four precut transgingival configurations have been designed to fit three different types of defects: mucogingival recession, intrabony, and furcation defects.

The advantages of titanium-reinforced configurations of Gore-Tex regenerative material are improved shapability and adaptability, providing for enhanced space-making in transgingival and submerged applications. The titanium-reinforced configurations maintain their shape in bone applications as well as anterior and posterior interproximal applications. Furthermore, when titanium-reinforced configurations are used, bone-grafting supplements may be less critical to space maintenance for a regenerative result.

Although the handling of the titanium-reinforced configurations is similar to that of the standard configuration of Gore-Tex membranes, there are some variations in manipulation and placement. Because of the rigidity of the titanium frame, the titanium-reinforced configurations must conform properly to the underlying structures. Proper trimming and adaptation of the material can prevent perforations of the underlying soft tissue flap.

The modified papilla preservation technique was designed for self-supporting barrier membranes to obtain primary closure of the interdental space over the membrane (Fig 215), resulting in better protection of the membrane from the oral environment (Cortellini et al, 1995). The technique involves the elevation of a full-thickness palatal flap that includes the entire interdental papilla. The buccal flap is mobilized with vertical and periosteal incisions and coronally positioned to cover the membrane. A first suture (horizontal internal crossed mattress suture) is placed beneath the mucoperiosteal flaps between the base of the palatal papilla and the buccal flap. The interproximal portion of this suture hangs on top of the membrane, allowing the coronal displacement of the buccal flap. To ensure passive primary closure of the interdental tissues over the membrane, a second suture (a vertical internal mattress suture) is placed between the buccal aspect of the interproximal papilla (that is, the most coronal portion of the palatal flap that includes the interdental papilla) and the most coronal portion of the buccal flap. This suture is free of tension.

The modified papilla preservation technique can successfully be applied in sites where the in-

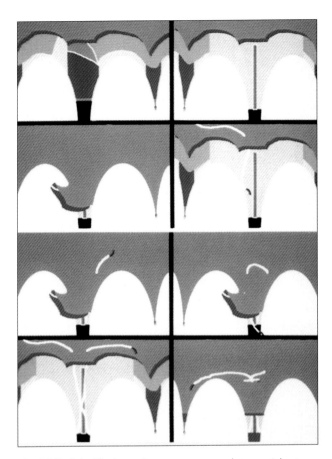

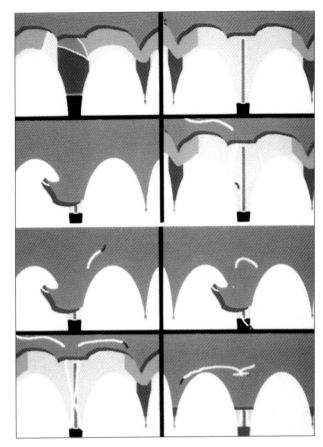

Fig 215 Modified papilla preservation technique. A horizontal incision is made in the buccal keratinized gingiva at the base of the papilla and connected with mesiodistal intrasulcular incisions; then, a full-thickness buccal flap is raised. The residual papilla is dissected from the neighboring teeth and bone. Thereafter, a full-thickness palatal flap, including the interdental papilla, is raised. Vertical and periosteal incisions are used to mobilize the buccal flap if necessary for accessibility during debridement of the defect. After placement of the membrane barrier, a horizontal internal crossed mattress suture is placed beneath the mucoperiosteal flaps between the base of the palatal papilla and the buccal flap. The interdental position of this suture hangs on top of the membrane, thus allowing the coronal displacement of the buccal flap. A second vertical internal mattress suture is placed between the most coronal position of the palatal papilla and the buccal flap for complete closure without tension. (From Cortellini et al, 1995. Reprinted with permission.)

Fig 216 The simplified papilla preservation method begins with an incision across the defect-associated papilla. It starts from the gingival margin at the buccolingual angle of the involved tooth and continues to the midinterdental portion of the papilla under the contact point of the adjacent tooth. The scalpel blade is held parallel to the long axis of the teeth. After elevation of the full-thickness buccal flap, the dissected papilla tissue, together with the palatal or lingual flap tissues, is elevated. After defect debridement and placement of the barrier, primary closure of the flaps is achieved with a horizontal internal mattress suture running from the base of the keratinized tissue at the midbuccal aspect of the uninvolved tooth to the same location at the base of the oral flaps. The suture contacts the approximal root surface, hangs on the residual bone crest, and is fixed to the oral flap. The interdental tissues above the membrane barriers are finally sutured for complete closure with one or two interrupted sutures, depending on the width and thickness of the tissues. (From Cortellini et al, 1999. Reprinted with permission.)

terdental space width is at least 2 mm at the most coronal portion of the papilla. When interdental spaces are narrower, the technique is difficult to apply. The simplified papilla preservation flap has been proposed for narrow interdental spaces

(Cortellini et al, 1999). An offset mattress suture runs along the root surface of the tooth approximal to the defect and runs over the residual bone crest, preventing apical displacement of the resorbable barrier membrane (Fig 216).

Figs 217a to 217j Case 2. (Courtesy of Dr P. Cortellini.)

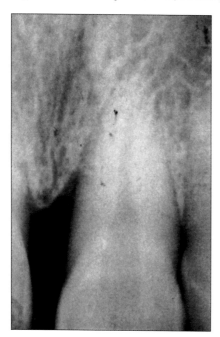

Fig 217a The pretreatment radiograph reveals a mesial intraosseous defect at the maxillary left central incisor.

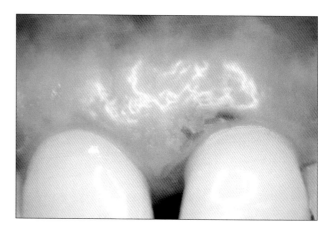

Fig 217b The gingival status at baseline is shown.

Case 2. A bone defect was present mesial to the maxillary left central incisor (Figs 217a and 217b). The wide interproximal defect was mainly a non-supportive one-wall defect with a suprabony component and a wide palatal bone dehiscence (Fig 217c). The membrane of choice was a titanium-reinforced e-PTFE barrier to provide proper support of the interdental soft tissue (Fig 217d). Primary closure of the interdental space was obtained with a double-layer suturing technique, including a crossed internal mattress suture and a vertical internal mattress suture, according to the previously described modified papilla preservation technique (Fig 217e).

Primary closure was maintained up to 6 weeks, when the barrier membrane was removed (Fig 217f). After membrane removal, the defect appeared to be completely filled with regenerated tissue (Fig 217g). The flap was resutured to protect the regenerated tissue (Fig 217h). The clinical appearance after 6 years showed optimal preservation of the interdental tissues (Fig 217i), and the 6-year radiograph confirmed resolution of the defect (Fig 217j).

Case 3. An advanced iatrogenic recession defect was present on the buccal surface of a maxillary right canine (Fig 218a). A flap with vertical releasing incisions was raised, and the root surface was mechanically and chemically cleaned. A single-tooth narrow transgingival titanium-reinforced e-PTFE barrier membrane was placed (Fig 218b). The excellent result after 1 year is shown in Fig 218c.

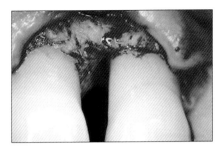

Fig 217c The nonsupportive one-wall defect is exposed.

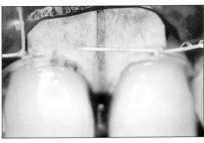

Fig 217d A titanium-reinforced e-PTFE barrier is placed over the defect.

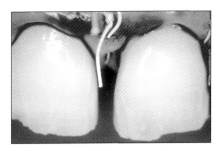

Fig 217e The modified papilla preservation flap is sutured.

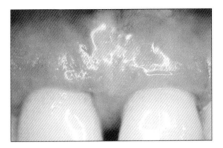

Fig 217f The gingiva appears healthy before removal of the barrier, 6 weeks after treatment.

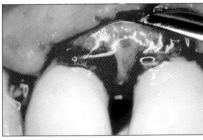

Fig 217g The defect is completely filled with regenerated tissue after removal of the barrier.

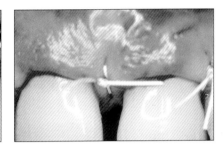

Fig 217h The flap is resutured after barrier removal.

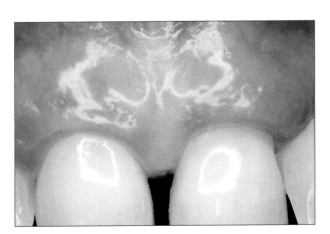

Fig 217i The clinical status 6 years after treatment is excellent.

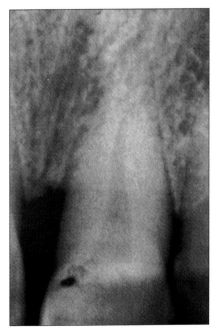

Fig 217j A radiograph taken 6 years after treatment reveals complete resolution of the defect.

Figs 218a to 218c Case 3.

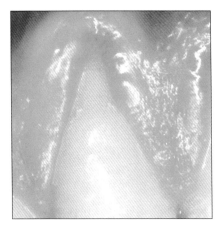 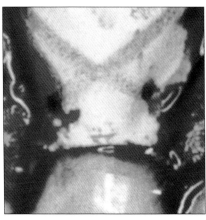 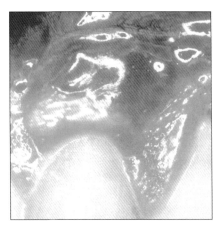

Fig 218a An advanced iatrogenic recession defect is present on the buccal surface of a maxillary right canine.

Fig 218b An e-PTFE membrane is placed during regenerative therapy.

Fig 218c The result after 1 year is excellent.

Bioresorbable membranes

Although successful treatment results have been reported for nonresorbable barrier membranes (Cortellini and Bowers, 1995; Gottlow, 1994; Karring et al, 1993; Machtei and Schallhorn, 1995), these barriers have some definite disadvantages. They have to be surgically removed, usually about 6 weeks after implantation. A second surgical intervention may traumatize and infect the newly formed immature periodontal tissues, jeopardizing the intended new attachment formation. Other negative factors are inconvenience and extra costs for the patient. Such problems would be overcome if the GTR device were bioresorbable.

Another drawback of GTR barriers is the frequent incidence of apical downgrowth of the dentogingival epithelium along the surface of the connective tissue flap facing the barrier (Cortellini et al, 1990, 1993; Machtei et al, 1994). This is especially likely to occur if the nonresorbable e-PTFE membrane is not fully covered by the resutured full-thickness flap. Apical downgrowth will lead to pocket formation and/or gingival recession with exposure of the barrier, which in turn will result in infection and gingival inflammation. This may seriously disturb the healing process, markedly reducing or even preventing regenera-

tion. The nonresorbable barrier, commercially available since 1988, had a cervical collar with large pores intended to prevent epithelial downgrowth along the barrier by encouraging ingrowth of connective tissue into the pores (see Fig 211). However, this collar was often exposed to the oral cavity and did not fulfill its intended function; instead of being filled with ingrowing connective tissue, it harbored large amounts of oral microorganisms (Machtei et al, 1994).

It was therefore necessary to design a barrier that would minimize gingival flap recession and epithelial downgrowth from the gingival margin. In addition, the optimal goal would include development of a bioresorbable membrane to eliminate the need for a second flap surgery. Based on the knowledge gained from GTR research and studies of implant–soft tissue integration, the following design criteria were considered requirements for a successful bioresorbable barrier for periodontal regeneration:

- Rapid integration with the adjacent connective tissue
- Maintenance of space for selective tissue ingrowth
- Effective anchorage to the tooth
- Bioresorbability

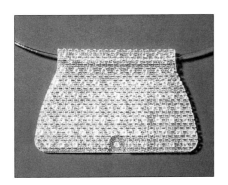

Fig 219a Outer side of a Guidor resorbable barrier membrane.

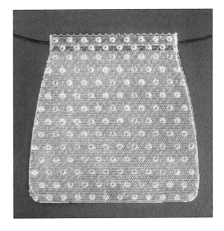

Fig 219b Inner side of a Guidor resorbable barrier membrane.

- Biocompatibility
- Tailored and controlled resorption pattern
- Initial dimensional stability
- Suitable malleability

A double-layered barrier was designed to fulfill these requirements (Guidor Matrix Barrier, Guidor); the outer layer that faces the gingiva has large perforations to promote rapid ingrowth of gingival connective tissue through the perforations (Fig 219a), while the inner layer has smaller perforations (Fig 219b). The outer and inner layers are separated by spacers to form an interspace for the ingrowth of the gingival tissue. In addition, spacers maintain a gap between the root surface and the barrier to facilitate stabilization of the blood clot and coronal regrowth of the periodontal ligament with inserting fibers in newly formed root cementum.

There are eight configurations designed to fit various kinds of defects, and a resorbable suture is fixed to each configuration. The bioresorbable barrier is made of a special combination of polylactic acids blended with citric acid ester in such a way that the resorption does not start until after 6 weeks and then proceeds slowly. Figures 220a to 220d illustrate successful treatment of a periodontal defect with a Guidor resorbable barrier. Guidor barriers were the first

bioresorbable barriers cleared by the US Food and Drug Administration.

Resolut bioresorbable barriers (WL Gore) are made from essentially pure polyglycolic acid and polylactic acid polymers and trimethylene carbonate. The barriers are designed to maintain integrity and separate the periodontal tissues for about 6 weeks, which allows regeneration of the periodontal ligament–bone complex along the root. The material is resorbed through hydrolysis into lactic acid and glycolic acid and is completely eliminated as carbon dioxide and water during the subsequent few months.

Resolut barrier membranes are designed to encourage rapid tissue incorporation of the matrix portion of the material. This incorporation helps stabilize the material and wound. The ingrowth of connective tissue also prevents formation of pseudopockets by inhibiting epithelial migration between the flap and the barrier membrane. Six transgingival configurations are available to fit various types of periodontal defects; the barriers are fixed to the tooth by individual placement of an included resorbable suture.

Vicryl periodontal mesh (Ethicon) is another synthetic resorbable barrier membrane. The material is woven from the same copolymer of glycolide and lactide used to produce Vicryl synthetic absorbable sutures, which have a long

189

Figs 220a to 220d Guided tissue regeneration with a Guidor bioresorbable barrier membrane. (Courtesy of Guidor.)

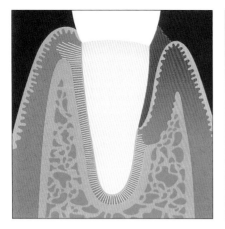 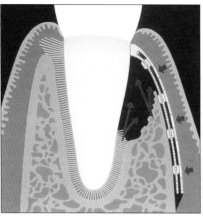 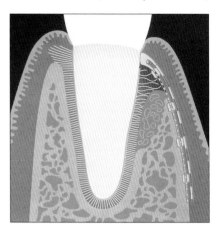

Fig 220a Periodontal intraosseous defect.

Fig 220b The double-layered Guidor bioresorbable barrier has been placed and tightly covered *(short red arrows)* by the mucogingival flap. The *long red arrows* indicate expected regeneration of the alveolar bone and periodontal ligament.

Fig 220c The barrier has partially resorbed, and the periodontal tissues have almost completely regenerated.

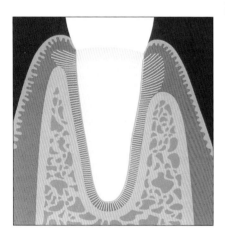

Fig 220d Successful regeneration.

history of safe and successful use by dentists and physicians internationally. For periodontal application, the tightly woven mesh is preferable to the knitted version. The pore size allows the passage of critical fluids while providing a barrier to larger cells.

Vicryl periodontal mesh is available in four shapes and sizes, each with an appropriate length of preattached Vicryl ligature. The mesh maintains its integrity during the period of most active tissue regeneration and is completely absorbed within 90 days of insertion.

Bioresorbable collagen barrier membranes are also available for GTR therapy. Collagen is an extracellular macromolecule of the periodontal connective tissue and alveolar bone and is physiologically metabolized; it is chemotactic for fibroblasts, hemostatic, a weak immunogen, and a scaffold for migrating cells. The hemostatic effect is achieved by aggregating the platelets, which may facilitate early clot formation and wound stabilization. These effects are considered to be essential for successful regeneration. The chemotactic effect on fibroblasts results in promotion of primary wound closure.

Bio-Gide (Osteohealth) and BioMend (Zimmer Dental) are two commercially available collagen barriers. Both are made of xenogeneic collagen and maintain their barrier function for about 6 weeks before resorption.

Figs 221a to 221d Case 4.

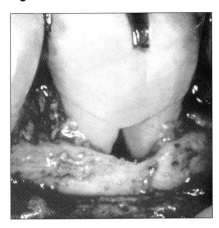

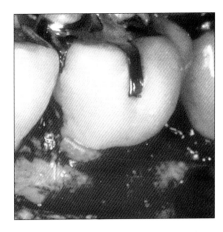

Fig 221a A grade II furcation defect is present on the buccal aspect of a mandibular molar.

Fig 221b A Guidor straight matrix barrier is placed and fixed over the defect.

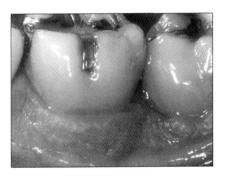

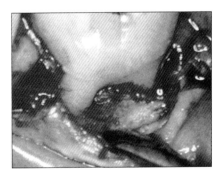

Fig 221c One year after GTR treatment, the defect is completely closed.

Fig 221d Reentry after 1 year reveals complete bone fill of the defect.

Case 4. A 39-year-old man had a grade II buccal furcation defect with a horizontal depth of 7 mm on a mandibular molar (Fig 221a). Following flap elevation, careful debridement, scaling, and root planing, a Guidor barrier was placed over the defect (Fig 221b), and the flap was sutured to cover the matrix completely. One year later, the defect was found to be completely closed (Fig 221c). Reentry at that time revealed complete bone fill of the furcation defect (Fig 221d).

Case 5. A 45-year-old man presented with a grade II furcation defect on the maxillary first molar; the defect was 8 mm deep in a horizontal direction (at the top of the furcation) and had a 1-mm intrabony component (Fig 222a). Full-thickness flaps were elevated, and the defect was carefully debrided (Fig 222b). The restricted entrance to the defect, the presence of an intrabony defect component, and the coronal level of interproximal bone crest were all morphologic characteristics of a defect with a favorable prognosis for regeneration. In such cases, however, small apertures make proper debridement difficult, and enlargement of the entrance is sometimes necessary.

A straight matrix barrier configuration was selected and tightly attached to the tooth with the preattached ligature. The barrier covered the defect and 3 mm of the surroundings (Fig 222c). The flap was repositioned coronal to its presurgical

Figs 222a to 222f Case 5.

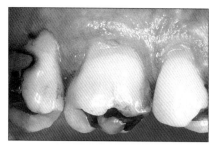

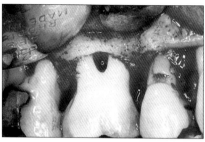

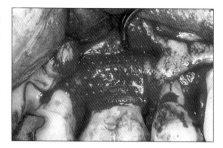

Fig 222a A grade II furcation defect is present on the buccal aspect of a maxillary first molar.

Fig 222b The defect is exposed during OFD.

Fig 222c A straight matrix bioresorbable barrier is placed.

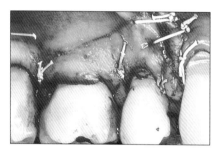

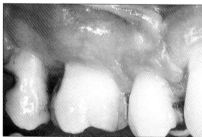

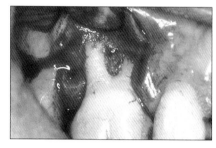

Fig 222d The flap is replaced and sutured.

Fig 222e The gingiva appears healthy 6 months after treatment.

Fig 222f Complete closure of the defect with alveolar bone is confirmed by reentry 1 year after treatment.

level and secured with interproximal mattress sutures (Fig 222d).

One month postsurgery the tissues appeared healthy, without signs of inflammation or an adverse response to the device. Although some material was exposed, it was left untrimmed and had completely disappeared 8 weeks after surgery, at which time the patient resumed mechanical toothcleaning, including the use of interproximal brushes. At the 6-month evaluation, some gingival recession had occurred (Fig 222e), but probing indicated that the furcation was closed. At the 1-year examination, a reentry procedure confirmed complete closure of the defect with bone (Fig 222f).

Case 6. A 71-year-old woman presented with a defect distal to the mandibular right canine, involving attachment loss of 15 mm from the cementoenamel junction, and an intrabony defect 11 mm deep (Figs 223a and 223b). Although deep, the intrabony defect was narrow and confined to only one root surface, that is, a three-wall intrabony defect, offering favorable conditions for regeneration of both the periodontal ligament and the bone.

Buccal and lingual mucoperiosteal flaps that extended one tooth mesial and one tooth distal to the defect area were raised. The defect was carefully debrided (Fig 223c), and the root surface was scaled and planed. A curved bioresorbable matrix barrier was selected and trimmed to cover the defect (Fig 223d). The flap was repositioned, with tight interproximal suturing, resulting in complete coverage of the defect as well as the membrane (Fig 223e).

The sutures were maintained for 1 month. At 6 months, the probing attachment gain was 8 mm, or about 75% of the initial defect depth (Fig 223f). A radiograph taken 1 year after surgery revealed extensive bone fill (Fig 223g).

Figs 223a to 223g Case 6. (From Gottlow et al, 1994. Reprinted with permission.)

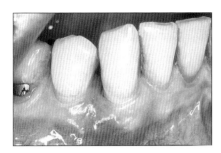

Fig 223a An interproximal three-wall intrabony defect is present at the mandibular right canine.

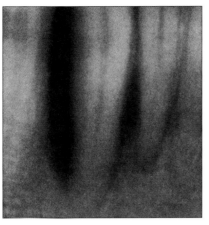

Fig 223b The initial presurgical radiograph reveals the extent of the defect.

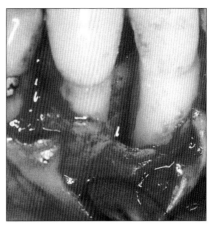

Fig 223c The intrabony defect is exposed after open flap debridement.

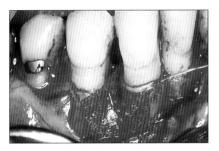

Fig 223d A curved bioresorbable matrix barrier is trimmed to cover the defect and is attached to the tooth by the preattached ligature.

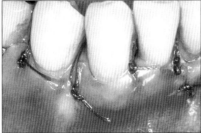

Fig 223e The flap is sutured with close adaptation between buccal and lingual flaps and complete coverage of the defect and device. Healing at 1 month is shown.

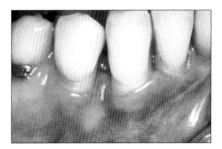

Fig 223f At 6 months, probing reveals an 8-mm gain in attachment (75% of attainable attachment).

Fig 223g A radiograph taken 1 year postsurgery reveals the extensive bone fill of the defect.

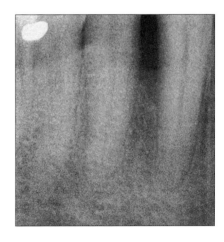

Figs 224a to 224e Case 7. (From Gottlow et al, 1994. Reprinted with permission.)

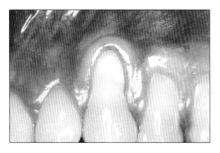

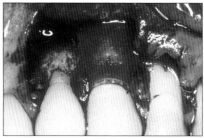

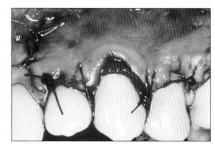

Fig 224a A 5-mm buccal gingival recession defect is present on the maxillary left canine.

Fig 224b A bioresorbable matrix barrier is attached, covering the defect and a 2-mm-wide surrounding zone.

Fig 224c Some of the matrix barrier is exposed following suturing of the flap.

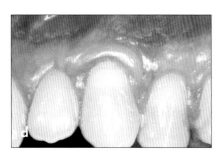

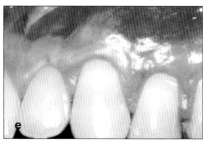

Fig 224d The gingival status 2 months after treatment is shown.

Fig 224e The gingival margin is healthy and located 3.5 mm coronal to the presurgical level after 6 months.

Case 7. A young man had a 5-mm gingival recession on the buccal aspect of the maxillary left canine (Fig 224a). The probing depth was 1 mm. A full-thickness flap and a split-thickness flap were raised without involving the papillae. The full-thickness flap was extended approximately 3 to 4 mm apical and lateral to the bone crest so that the peripheral part of the barrier was on the bone. A bioresorbable straight barrier configuration was placed over the defect and a 2-mm-wide zone of the surrounding bone (Fig 224b). The coronal portion of the matrix barrier extended slightly coronal to the buccal cementoenamel junction, resulting in some barrier exposure following coronal repositioning and suturing of the flap (Fig 224c).

One month after surgery, barrier exposure persisted, but without further gingival recession, and the soft tissues were not inflamed. Two months after surgery, the exposed part of the barrier membrane had disappeared (Fig 224d). At 3 months and 6 months postsurgery, the gingival margin was 3.5 mm coronal to the presurgical level, and the buccal probing depth was 1.0 mm (Fig 224e).

Case 8. After initial nonsurgical treatment and improved plaque control, a 7-mm mesial probing depth remained on the mesial surface of a mandibular left first molar (Fig 225a). The baseline radiograph revealed a narrow, deep intrabony defect mesial to the molar (Fig 225b).

The interdental space was accessed with a modified papilla preservation technique for GTR therapy (Fig 225c). After removal of granulation tissue and final cleaning of the root surface, a narrow, 6-mm-deep three-wall intrabony defect was exposed (Fig 225d). The membrane of choice was a bioresorbable barrier, well supported by bony walls (Fig 225e). Primary closure was obtained with a double-layer suturing technique, including an offset internal mattress suture and a modified internal mattress suture (Fig 225f). At 5 years, the defect was completely resolved (Fig 225g); the site exhibited healthy gingival conditions and only a 2-mm probing depth (Fig 225h).

Figs 225a to 225h Case 8. (Courtesy of Dr P. Cortellini.)

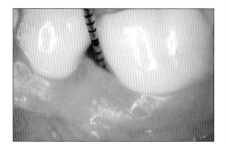

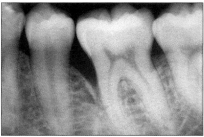

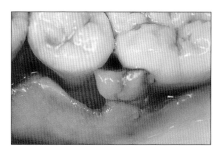

Fig 225a An intrabony osseous defect is present mesial to the mandibular left first molar.

Fig 225b A narrow intrabony defect is visible on the pretreatment radiograph.

Fig 225c The papilla is elevated according to the modified papilla preservation flap technique.

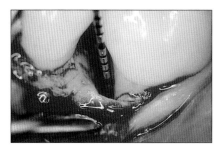

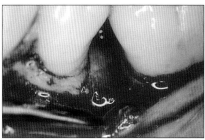

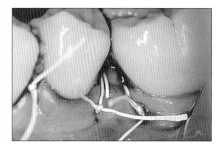

Fig 225d The narrow intrabony three-wall osseous defect is exposed after removal of granulation tissue and debridement.

Fig 225e A bioresorbable barrier (Resolut) is placed and attached over the defect.

Fig 225f The flaps are resutured with resorbable mattress sutures.

Fig 225g A radiograph taken 5 years after the GTR treatment reveals that the defect is completely resolved.

Fig 225h After 5 years, a 2-mm probing depth is measured mesially.

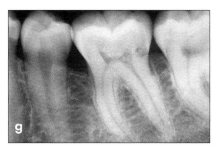

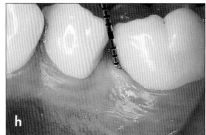

Figs 226a to 226f Case 9. (Courtesy of Dr P. Cortellini.)

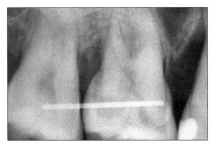

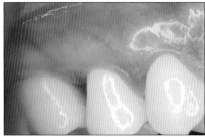

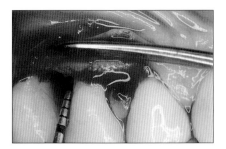

Fig 226a A deep intrabony osseous defect is located distal to the maxillary right second premolar.

Fig 226b The clinical status at baseline is shown.

Fig 226c The narrow, two- and three-wall intrabony osseous defect is 9 mm deep.

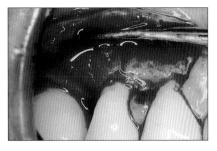

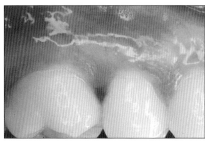

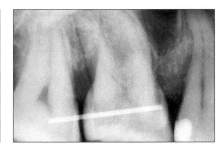

Fig 226d The regenerative strategy of choice is a combination of a bovine-derived bone xenoograft and a bioresorbable collagen barrier.

Fig 226e The gingiva is healthy, and there is no interdental recession 3 years after treatment.

Fig 226f A radiograph taken 3 years after treatment reveals that the deep defect is completely resolved.

Case 9. A deep intrabony defect was located distal to the maxillary right second premolar (Fig 226a). There was slight recession of the interdental papilla in the interproximal space between the second premolar and first molar (Fig 226b). The defect was a narrow 9-mm-deep two- and three-wall intrabony defect (Fig 226c).

The interdental space was accessed with a simplified papilla preservation technique (see Fig 216). The regenerative strategy of choice was a combination of a bovine-derived bone xenograft and a bioresorbable collagen barrier (Fig 226d). Primary closure was obtained with a double-layer suturing technique, including a crossed internal mattress suture and a modified internal mattress suture. The 1-year probing depth was only 3 mm. After 3 years, the site showed healthy gingival conditions and no interdental recession (Fig 226e). The radiograph taken 3 years after GTR therapy revealed that the deep defect was completely resolved (Fig 226f).

Outcomes

Histologic evaluation of wound healing following GTR therapy. Graziani et al (2005) performed a histologic evaluation of wound healing following GTR therapy for experimentally created dehiscence-type defects in monkeys. After debridement and root planing, a flap was raised, and a bioresorbable barrier (Guidor) was placed on one side of the jaw and a nonresorbable e-PTFE barrier (Gore-Tex) was placed on the contralateral segment. Wound healing was evaluated histologically at 6 weeks, 6 months, and 2 years after GTR. A new attachment apparatus was developed after only 6 weeks of healing. A 10- to 20-μm-thick layer of acellular extrinsic fiber cementum had formed along the instrumented root surface. At 6 months, the thickness of the supracrestal cementum was comparable to that at 6 weeks, while the thickness of the cementum at the bone crest had increased from 40 to 60 μm. In this zone, the cementum consisted of an inner layer of acellular extrinsic fiber cementum attached to the root dentin and an outer layer of cellular mixed fiber cementum. At 2 years, the periodontal tissues resembled the pristine periodontal apparatus.

In an earlier experimental study in dogs, Araújo et al (1997) evaluated the dynamics of periodontal tissue formation in grade III furcation defects. Histologic analyses were performed 2, 4, 8, and 20 weeks after GTR therapy with bioresorbable barriers.

At 2 weeks of healing, the furcation was occupied by granulation tissue in the coronal portion and by connective tissue in the remaining area. In some areas, the collagen fibers in the connective tissue lateral to the root ran parallel to the root surface. In other areas, however, this connective tissue contained strands of fine collagen-like fibers extending in a perpendicular direction from the dentinal surface (phase I in cementum formation).

At 4 weeks of healing, the tissues in the furcation comprised a small area of granulation tissue, frequently at the most coronal portion of the defect; a large area of connective tissue; and a limited area of newly formed bone. The connective tissue in direct contact with the root presented the previously described features, but in some areas the fibers extending from the root were embedded in a matrix substance (phase II in cementum formation).

At 8 weeks, the furcation was occupied by a large area of woven bone and to a lesser extent by connective tissue, bone marrow, lamellar-like bone (including primary and secondary osteons), and periodontal ligament. The root surface was covered by new cementum in different phases of formation. In some areas, the new cementum contained intrinsic fibers and cells (phase III in cementum formation).

At 20 weeks of healing, the furcation defect was occupied by lamellar bone, bone marrow, periodontal ligament, and some residual connective tissue. The lamellar bone, along with a layer of bundle bone, was found mainly at the periphery of the bone tissue, while in the center a large bone marrow space was present. Lamellar bone frequently failed to form in the fornix region of the furcation, however. The entire root surface was covered by new cementum that contained cells and extrinsic and intrinsic fibers.

These results indicate that tissue formation and differentiation in a furcation defect after GTR follow an orderly sequence of events. The granulation tissue that occupies a large area of the furcation defect at 2 weeks of healing is gradually replaced by connective tissue. In later stages of healing and depending on its location, this connective tissue is replaced by cementum, periodontal ligament, or bone tissue.

Clinical effects of GTR therapy. The clinical effects of GTR therapy on intrabony defects, furcation defects, and gingival recession have been evaluated in meta-analyses as well as systematic reviews.

Intrabony defects. Needleman et al (2005) presented a systematic review on the effect of GTR for intrabony defects. The inclusion criteria for this review were:

- Randomized controlled trials (RCTs) of at least 12 months' duration
- Chronic periodontitis or periodontitis (aggressive periodontitis was excluded) in subjects aged 21 years or older
- GTR versus OFD
- GTR plus bone substitutes versus OFD

Of 626 published articles, only 17 RCTs fit the above inclusion criteria. Of these, three were multicenter studies, and eight were split-mouth studies. Changes in attachment levels, probing depth, gingival recession, and alveolar bone levels were the most important clinical variables in this systematic review.

The GTR test groups achieved significantly greater attachment gains than did the OFD control groups. The mean difference between test and control sites was 1.20 mm. However, there was substantial variation between the results of different studies, ranging from 0.02 to 3.60 mm. The possible reasons for this large range will be discussed later. There was no significant difference between the use of nonresorbable and resorbable barriers.

In another systematic review (Murphy and Gunsolley, 2003) that included 19 studies (broader inclusion criteria required a minimum of 6 months after treatment), GTR provided a significantly greater mean gain (1.15 mm) in clinical attachment level than OFD. However, the range was 0.20 to 2.90 mm.

Two meta-analyses have reported greater benefits to GTR than found in the aforementioned systematic reviews. One meta-analysis found a 2.7-mm difference in attachment gain between GTR and OFD (Laurell et al, 1998). The authors compared OFD, bone replacement grafts, and GTR for surgical treatment of intrabony defects in studies over a 20-year period. For OFD, grafts, and GTR, the mean gains in CAL were 1.5, 2.1, and 4.2 mm, respectively, and the mean gains in bone fill were 1.1, 2.2, and 4.2 mm, respectively. In a meta-analysis by Cortellini and Tonetti (2000), the weighted mean of the reported results was a gain of 3.8±1.7 mm in CAL after GTR treatment, a value that was 1.6 mm more than that attained after OFD alone.

Furcation defects. Two systematic reviews have been published on the effect of GTR compared with OFD for furcation defects. Jepsen et al (2002) analyzed 16 RCTs of at least 6 months' duration and concluded:

- The placement of barrier membranes (GTR surgery) could improve the clinical condition of mandibular and maxillary grade II furcation defects.
- There were no or very limited improvements in clinical conditions of mandibular or maxillary grade II furcations following open flap debridement.
- A significantly greater reduction in horizontal furcation depth of mandibular and maxillary grade II furcation defects (as measured during a surgical reentry procedure) was accomplished by GTR when compared with OFD.
- A complete closure of grade II molar furcation defects following placement of barrier membranes appears to be an unpredictable outcome.
- Significantly greater improvements in vertical probing attachment were observed following GTR compared with OFD in mandibular and maxillary grade II furcations.

- There are only limited data on the effects of GTR in grade III furcations. A complete closure (as evaluated during reentry) was never reported.

In another systematic review, Murphy and Gunsolley (2003) analyzed 28 relevant RCTs, systematic reviews of RCTs, cohort studies, and case-control studies of GTR in furcation defects. In 11 studies, GTR with e-PTFE barriers resulted in 1.39 ± 0.36 mm greater gain in weighted mean vertical PAL than did OFD (*P* < .0001). In a single study, use of a polymeric resorbable barrier resulted in a 2.50-mm greater gain in vertical periodontal attachment than did OFD. A meta-analysis evaluating the effect on vertical probing depth revealed that GTR resulted in a significantly greater reduction than did OFD (*P* < .0001). A meta-analysis also demonstrated that GTR resulted in significantly greater gain of horizontal open probing attachment than did OFD (*P* < .01).

No significant difference was observed between nonresorbable and resorbable barriers, but the combination of barrier and augmentation material (bone replacement grafts) significantly enhanced the gain in vertical periodontal attachment level (PAL) compared with a barrier alone (*P* = .039).

Long-term patient-centered outcomes, such as tooth loss and ease of maintenance, were not reported in the studies selected for inclusion in the aforementioned systematic reviews. However, Eickholz et al (2006) presented the 10-year results of a split-mouth study comparing the effect of nonresorbable or bioresorbable barrier membranes on grade II furcation defects. The mean gains in horizontal PAL at 1 and 10 years, respectively, were 1.9 and 1.1 mm with the nonresorbable membranes and 1.9 and 1.7 mm with the bioresorbable membranes. The mean gain in bone at 10 years was 0.8 mm with the nonresorbable membrane and 1.1 mm with the bioresorbable membrane. At 10 years, 15 of 18 treated defects were stable (83%). One patient lost two teeth during the 10-year period.

Gingival recession. Roccuzzo et al (2002) presented a systematic review of different plastic surgical methods for treatment of localized gingival recessions. The following periodontal plastic surgery procedures were compared: GTR (with either resorbable or nonresorbable barrier membranes), free gingival graft, connective tissue graft, coronally advanced flap, and laterally positioned flap.

The authors found 30 studies that fit the inclusion criteria they had set forth. Their review of the results demonstrated the following weighted mean values for reduction of gingival recession: GTR with resorbable barrier membranes, 2.85 mm; GTR with nonresorbable barrier membranes, 3.70 mm; connective tissue graft, 3.10 mm; coronally advanced flap, 2.68 mm. Only limited data existed for the free gingival graft and laterally positioned flap, and the predictability appeared to be low for both methods. However, all the other treatment procedures reduced gingival recession, increased attachment level, and enhanced root coverage, but the heterogeneity was marked both between and within the different treatment groups.

In a meta-analysis, Al-Hamdan et al (2003) compared the effect of GTR with conventional mucogingival surgery on treatment of gingival recessions. Both procedures produced statistically significant decreases in recession depth ($P < .05$). Conventional mucogingival surgery achieved 81.0% ± 6.7% root coverage. With GTR, the posttreatment values corresponded to 72.0% ± 9.1% root coverage.

The long-term effect of GTR on gingival recession was presented in a 10-year study by Trombelli et al (2005). At 6 months postsurgery, recession depth was 0.9 ± 0.6 mm. The recession depth increased to 1.0 ± 1.3 mm at 4 years and 1.3 ± 1.5 mm at 10 years. The 10-year recession depth was not significantly different from the 6-month and 4-year recordings.

Long-term outcomes. In the systematic reviews and meta-analyses of studies performed 6 or 12 months after treatment, the total gain of vertical and horizontal attachment for GTR represents the difference between GTR and OFD plus the gain of vertical and horizontal CAL for OFD. How-ever, gain of vertical and horizontal CAL mostly means repair (bone fill of the defects) for OFD and "true" regeneration for GTR, as discussed earlier. These facts may be of great importance for the long-term outcomes of the two different therapies. In a recent meta-analysis of RCTs, Tu et al (2008) showed that the initial gain in CAL after regenerative therapy was maintained after several years, in contrast to the temporary effects of OFD.

Gottlow et al (1992) showed that the results of GTR treatment could be maintained over periods of up to 5 years if good maintenance (supportive) care is established. In a split-mouth study, Eickholz et al (2004) randomly compared the long-term outcomes of two bioresorbable barriers. The gain in CAL achieved after GTR therapy was still stable in more than 80% of the treated defects after 5 years.

In another long-term study, Cortellini and Tonetti (2004) evaluated the effect of GTR therapy on CAL and tooth survival in 175 patients with one deep intrabony defect. Ten years after treatment, the survival of these initial severely diseased teeth was 96%. The percentages of positive outcomes were smaller in smokers and in the 33% of patients who did not follow a periodontal maintenance program.

The long-term stability of mandibular furcation defects regenerated following GTR alone or in combination with citric acid root conditioning and bone grafting was evaluated by McClain and Schallhorn (1993). Of the 57% of the furcation defects that were assessed as completely filled at 6 and 12 months, only 29% were completely filled after 4 to 6 years. However, 74% of the furcations treated with a combination of GTR and DFDBA were completely filled at both the short- and long-term evaluations, suggesting that the results obtained with the combined procedure were more stable over time (for further review, see Cury et al, 2003; Machtei et al, 1996; Stavropoulos and Karring, 2004).

Factors that influence short- and long-term outcomes. Even if the GTR studies analyzed in systematic reviews and meta-analyses represent fewer than 5% of all the published studies because of strict inclusion criteria (mainly RCTs with 12 months' or at least 6 months' duration), the heterogeneity of the outcome among the previously cited studies is surprising. Furthermore, the differences in the outcomes of GTR among the hundreds of excluded case reports, uncontrolled and nonrandomized studies with different sample sizes, study durations, operators, materials, and methods must be striking.

Several factors, separately and in combination, may positively or negatively influence the short- and long-term outcomes of GTR therapy at the site, subject, and group levels. These factors may explain the great heterogeneity of the results reported for GTR therapy at site and subject levels and between different studies. The following groups of factors may influence the outcome of GTR therapy:

- Patient factors:
  - Internal modifying factors (eg, genetics, diabetes)
  - External modifying factors (eg, smoking, self-care, compliance)
- Defect factors:
  - Morphology of intraosseous defects
  - Morphology of furcation defects
  - Morphology of recession defects
- Professional presurgical treatment:
  - Detailed diagnosis and history taking
  - Patient education (self-care and self-diagnosis)
  - Scaling, root planing, and debridement
  - PMTC
  - Antimicrobial treatment (chemical plaque control and use of antibiotics)
- GTR treatment:
  - Surgical technique
  - Mechanical cleaning
  - Root surface conditioning
  - Barrier selection and trimming
  - Skill of the operator
- Professional postsurgical treatment:
  - Antimicrobial treatment (chemical plaque control and use of antibiotics)
  - Maintenance (supportive) care (intervals, methods, and materials)
  - Reexaminations (variables)
- Study design:
  - Study duration and sample size
  - Consecutive case series
  - Controlled studies

- RCTs
- Parallel groups
- Split-mouth design

Patient factors. Internal modifying factors such as genetics may increase or reduce the individual's susceptibility to chronic infectious diseases such as the periodontal diseases. For example, reduced function of the phagocytizing polymorphonuclear cells and genetic polymorphism of proinflammatory interleukins such as interleukin 1 may significantly increase the susceptibility to periodontitis. Some chronic diseases, such as poorly controlled diabetes, are also regarded as internal modifying prognostic risk factors for periodontal disease (for details, see chapter 5 and volume 3 of this series [Axelsson, 2002]).

Among external modifying factors, cigarette smoking is well documented as an extremely powerful external prognostic risk factor for periodontal disease progression (Axelsson, 2002). Only one RCT included in a systematic review of GTR conducted by Needleman et al (2005) evaluated the role of smoking on the outcome of GTR therapy (Mayfield et al, 1998a). In this study, nonsmokers exhibited significantly more gain in CAL 12 months after GTR therapy than did smokers (1.9 mm versus 0.8 mm, respectively). In addition, nonsmokers showed a significant, 1.1-mm mean gain in bone level while smokers had a nonsignificant, 0.1-mm gain.

In a retrospective study, Tonetti et al (1995) examined the effect of cigarette smoking on the healing response following GTR in deep intrabony defects. The oral hygiene of both groups was good, but smokers had significantly higher complete-mouth plaque scores. At membrane removal, no significant differences between smokers and nonsmokers were observed in terms of percentage of tissue gained. At the 1-year follow-up, however, smokers had gained significantly less probing attachment level than nonsmokers. A multivariate model, correcting for the oral hygiene level of the patients and the depth of the intrabony component, indicated that smoking was in itself a significant factor in determining the clinical outcome. It was concluded that cigarette smoking is associated with reduced healing response after GTR treatment.

In a retrospective analysis of 47 deep intrabony defects 1 year after treatment, Stavropoulos et al (2004) also reported that smoking affects the outcome of GTR therapy negatively. Smokers gained approximately 1.1 mm less in CAL than nonsmokers (3.2 ± 1.4 mm versus 4.3 ± 1.3 mm, respectively) and had approximately seven times less chance of gaining 4 mm in CAL than patients who did not smoke.

The precise mechanism by which smoking interferes with the outcome of GTR is not yet understood, but nicotine and smoking by-products adversely affect the proliferation, attachment, and chemotaxis of periodontal ligament cells and enhance the effect of periopathogenic toxins. In addition, nicotine is known to induce vasoconstriction, thereby reducing peripheral blood supply, and carbon monoxide is known to reduce oxygen transport and metabolism. Thus, smoking may interfere with several stages of the reparatory and regenerative process in the periodontal wound and thereby compromise healing in general. This in turn may explain the impaired flap survival, characterized by the increased frequency of membrane exposure observed in smokers as compared with nonsmokers (for details on local and systemic negative effects of smoking, see Axelsson, 2002).

Other external prognostic risk factors for progression of periodontal disease are acquired systemic diseases and infectious diseases (human immunodeficiency virus and AIDS), psychosocial stress, low educational level, low compliance, and poor self-care habits. Among these factors, meticulous gingival plaque control by the patient, preoperatively and particularly postoperatively, is the most important determinant of successful GTR therapy (Cortellini et al, 1994; Tonetti et al, 1995, 1996).

In published studies, the standard of oral hygiene is usually based on plaque recording. However, differences in the way plaque scores are reported between studies prevent sensible comparison. For instance, some studies present complete-mouth plaque scores, others measure plaque at the experimental sites only, and still others present Plaque Index values. Most studies, however, do not present any plaque data at all. Therefore, meta-analyses and systematic reviews on the role of oral hygiene are still lacking. However, based on the limited available reported data, the role of excellent presurgical and postsurgical gingival plaque control by the patient in the successful outcome of GTR should not be underestimated.

For 1 or 2 weeks before surgery, mechanical gingival plaque control by self-care should be supplemented by chemical plaque control with a 0.1% or 0.2% CHX rinse immediately after every mechanical toothcleaning procedure. Because CHX is a cation, toothpastes without anions, such as lauryl sulfate and monofluorophosphate, must be used. Postoperatively, the patient is given special instruction in hygiene for the surgically treated areas. For the success of the procedure, it is essential that the area be kept free of gingival plaque. Care should be taken to avoid disturbing the wound mechanically.

After surgery, the patient should refrain from flossing or other interdental cleaning techniques in the treated area for up to 6 weeks. However, an extrasoft toothbrush can be used without pressure beginning day 3 postsurgery. During this period, the patient should be instructed to rinse with an antimicrobial agent such as CHX after every toothcleaning procedure.

Patients should be scheduled for postsurgical follow-up at least every second week during the initial healing period of 6 weeks for evaluation of the self-care procedures and needs-related supplementary PMTC. After this healing period, efficient mechanical toothcleaning, including toothbrushing, flossing, and other interdental cleaning techniques, can be resumed, even in the treated area.

It is obvious that patient selection is of great importance for the outcome of GTR therapy. The most favorable outcome of GTR therapy may be predicted in unstressed, nonsmoking patients with excellent general health, excellent levels of gingival plaque control by self-care, and good compliance.

Defect factors. The width, depth, and number of bony walls may influence the outcome of GTR therapy in intrabony defects. The most successful results may be predicted in deep, narrow two- and three-wall defects, while the outcome in wide, shallow one-wall defects seems to be unpredictable (Tonetti et al, 1993, 1996).

Treatment of approximal maxillary grade II furcation defects and maxillary and mandibular grade III furcation defects with GTR therapy is unpredictable. On the other hand, mandibular grade II furcation defects in the first and second molars, either buccal or lingual, with deep pockets at baseline and a gingival thickness of more than 1 mm may achieve predictable benefits of GTR therapy (Jepsen et al, 2002.)

A meta-analysis (Al-Hamdan et al, 2003) showed no difference in posttreatment recession reduction between 363 defects with a mean pretreatment recession depth of less than 4.0 mm and 330 recession defects with a mean pretreatment recession depth of 4.0 mm or greater. However, gain of CAL was significantly greater for deep recession defects than for shallow recession defects. On the other hand, shallow recession defects exhibited a higher percentage of complete root coverage than deep defects.

In another systematic review, Hwang and Wang (2006) evaluated the role of gingival thickness in the outcome of different recession treatment methods. The mean initial thickness ranged from 1.0 to 1.5 mm in 7 of 15 studies and from 0.7 to 1.0 mm in 8 studies. A critical threshold thickness of more than 1.0 mm existed for weighted mean and complete root coverage. Further simple linear regression revealed that there was a high correlation between weighted thickness and weighted root coverage when GTR therapy and connective tissue grafting were employed but not when coronally advanced flap therapy was utilized. The follow-up time did not affect the percentage of root coverage.

Professional presurgical treatment. Detailed clinical diagnosis and history taking are key to successful outcomes of GTR therapy because of the importance of selecting suitable patients and defects for the procedures.

In addition, before GTR therapy, it is important that the total amount of the oral microflora and particularly the number of periopathogens be reduced as much as possible. With the stringent application of the so-called complete-mouth disinfection principle, all infectious inflamed sites in the oral cavity should be healed before the GTR surgery. In this way the surgical procedure is facilitated because probing depths and bleeding are decreased, improving visibility and accessibility and reducing surgery time and postsurgical gingival recession. In addition, infectious contamination from other infected sites is prevented.

Heitz-Mayfield et al (2006) reported that the presence of high bacterial load and specific periopathogen complexes in deep periodontal pockets associated with intrabony defects had a significant negative impact on the 1-year outcome of surgical regenerative treatment. Rüdiger et al (2003) assessed the dynamics of bacterial colonization in intraosseous defects following GTR therapy with bioresorbable barriers. At the 12-month reexamination, the colonization of periodontal pathogens at sites treated by GTR was correlated with the intraoral presence of these pathogens before surgery, in spite of supportive care every 3 months postsurgery.

If colonization of GTR sites by periopathogens is to be prevented, intraoral suppression or eradication of these pathogens is required before surgery. Therefore, it is important to carry out oral microbiology analyses and sensitivity tests at least in the sites that are selected for regenerative therapy. Based on these analyses and the general health status of the patient, supplementary use of antibiotics and other intensified antimicrobial treatment may be indicated. Presurgically, local antimicrobial treatment may be performed with the use of controlled slow-release CHX chips, slow-release metronidazole gel, controlled slow-release doxycycline gel, slow-release minocycline gel, or controlled slow-release tetracycline fibers.

Systemic antibiotics are usually administered for 10 days, starting 2 days before GTR surgery. The most common systemic antibiotic prescription is 250 to 400 mg of metronidazole three times daily as monotherapy or in combination with 375 mg of amoxicillin three times daily, depending on the results of microbiologic analyses. In smokers, a higher dose of metronidazole (400 mg three times daily) is recommended.

In an RCT, Reddy et al (2003) evaluated the supplementary effect of a CHX chip placed in the pockets 1 week before GTR treatment and compared the results to those of a placebo chip. Nine months after therapy, the sites treated with CHX exhibited significantly greater gains than the placebo group in mean bone height (3.5 ± 0.45 mm compared to 2.6 ± 0.34 mm, respectively) and bone mass (5.6 ± 0.7 mg compared to 2.6 ± 0.3 mg, respectively).

Very limited data have been reported on the supplementary effect of antibiotics to GTR therapy, despite the fact that antibiotics are frequently included in GTR therapy. Sander et al (1994) evaluated the effect of slow-release metronidazole dental gel (Elyzol, Colgate) as a supplement to GTR therapy. Six months after removal of the membrane, the median gain in probing attachment level as a percentage of the initial defect depth was 92% for Elyzol-treated defects and 50% for control defects (*P* = .001), indicating that local application of metronidazole gel has a beneficial effect on healing of periodontal vertical defects treated by GTR.

Demolon et al (1993) reported that systemic administration of amoxicillin and clavulanate for 10 days, as a supplement to GTR therapy on grade II furcation defects, had positive short-term clinical effects and effects on the incidence of periopathogens such as *Tannerella forsythia*, *Porphyromonas gingivalis*, *Prevotella intermedia*, and *Aggregatibacter actinomycetemcomitans* (*Aa*). However, at follow-up 1 year later, this initial effect did not result in significant differences in bone regeneration and probing attachment level compared to the results of GTR therapy without systemic use of antibiotics (Demolon et al, 1994).

The most successful systemic use of antibiotics in periodontal therapy to date is the combination of amoxicillin and metronidazole as a supplement to scaling, root planing, and debridement. In *Aa*-associated periodontal diseases, *Aa* was eliminated from the oral cavity for 2 years after such therapy (Pavicić et al, 1994). To date, no meta-analyses or systematic reviews of RCTs have evaluated the supplementary effect of the aforementioned combination of systemic antibiotics with GTR therapy. For details on the use of antibiotic therapy, see chapter 3.

GTR treatment. The special techniques and flap designs for GTR in different periodontal defects were described earlier. The outcome of the GTR therapy is influenced by how closely the recommended technique is followed and the skill of the operator.

The first step after raising of the flap is careful removal of all granulation tissue in the defect to reduce bleeding and optimize visibility and accessibility. Afterward, supplementary minimally invasive mechanical cleaning (debridement) is performed. It is critical not to expose the root dentin and dentinal tubules during scaling and root planing (for details, see chapter 1). A clean root cementum surface is most important for the outcome of periodontal tissue regeneration (Blomlöf et al, 1987, 1989). Care should therefore have been taken during presurgical scaling, root planing, and debridement to preserve as much root cementum as possible.

After mechanical cleaning, the root surface is chemically cleaned and conditioned. These procedures reduce the risk for infectious contamination and healing disturbance and enhance healing potential. Conditioning of the root surface has been shown to alter the diseased root surface, creating a surface that can favorably influence wound healing. In addition, scaling, root planing, and debridement leave a smear layer, with remnants of contaminated cementum and calculus on the root surface. In vivo and in vitro studies indicate a greater potential for cell and fiber attachment to conditioned root surfaces (Blomlöf and Lindskog, 1995; Blomlöf et al, 1996).

Other factors, such as spatial relationships and wound stabilization, may also influence the extent and predictability of periodontal wound healing following root surface demineralization. A critical event in periodontal wound healing is the establishment and maintenance of a fibrin clot that adheres to the root surface. Appropriate root surface conditioning may therefore regulate the adsorption of plasma proteins, enhance adhesion of the blood clot, and stimulate deposition of collagen against the root surface. An understanding of the early events in wound healing, therefore, appears critical to the selection of appropriate agents and their potential to promote regeneration (Polimeni et al, 2006).

As an adjunct to scaling, root planing, and debridement, agents used to date for root surface conditioning include citric acid, ethylenediaminetetraacetic acid (EDTA), phosphoric acid, and tetracycline hydrochloride. Apart from dissolving the smear layer, some etching agents, depending on application time, also seem able to dissolve parts of the mineralized root surface, exposing collagenous fibers. Although there are conflicting results regarding the etching effect (Mariotti, 2003), depending on the mode of application, an etched root surface generally appears to promote better healing than an unconditioned root surface (Blomlöf and Lindskog, 1995). To ensure the efficacy of the etchant, various modes of application have been suggested, such as rubbing, burnishing, and continuous dripping from a syringe. Impregnating the surface by burnishing or rubbing with a cotton pellet may be more efficient than passive application of the etchant (Blomlöf et al, 1996).

Blomlöf and Lindskog (1995) studied the texture of dentinal surfaces after citric acid, phosphoric acid, or EDTA etching. The possible effects on early cell and tissue colonization were also assessed. EDTA, active at neutral pH, selectively removed mineral from a dentin surface, exposing a collagenous matrix. By contrast, etching with citric or phosphoric acid, both of which are active at low pH, appeared to remove not only the mineral component but also the collagenous matrix. The EDTA-treated dentinal surfaces appeared to be more receptive to cellular colonization and subsequent connective tissue formation than surfaces etched at low pH.

Mayfield et al (1998b) evaluated the supplementary effect of EDTA root surface conditioning on GTR. After 12 months, subjects treated with EDTA showed greater mean gains in CAL and probing bone levels than did subjects treated without EDTA, regardless of whether they were smokers or nonsmokers.

In contrast a meta-analysis and systematic review (Mariotti, 2003) stated that the use of citric acid, tetracycline, or EDTA to modify the root surface provides no benefit of clinical significance to regeneration in patients with chronic periodontitis. However, histologic evidence seems to suggest that new connective tissue attachment and limited regeneration may result from root surface demineralization (Blomlöf et al, 1996). However, this histologic healing pattern does not result in significant improvement in clinical conditions beyond nondemineralized control sites (Mariotti, 2003). Appropriate conditioning of root surfaces is likely to be important for enhancing pre-

dictability of regenerative therapies. Research focused on identifying factors that can detoxify roots and influence appropriate cell attachment is needed to identify the best root conditioning therapies.

Selection of membrane type, whether nonresorbable or bioresorbable, as well as membrane configuration and shaping might be important to outcomes. However, in their systematic review, Needleman et al (2005) found no significant differences between nonresorbable and resorbable barriers. At least for the patient's comfort, a bioresorbable barrier should be preferred because nonresorbable barriers need a second flap surgery for removal, which also could increase the risk of infection in the newly regenerated tissues. On the other hand, titanium-reinforced barriers are more efficient space holders than are bioresorbable barriers for wide defects.

Instability of the barrier membrane and premature exposure may also impair the outcome of GTR therapy (Machtei, 2001). Although the membrane material used for GTR therapy is submerged following application, the coronal part often becomes exposed to the oral cavity at the margin of the covering gingiva. The membrane often is further exposed by a gradual recession of the gingival tissue during the period of insertion, probably because the epithelium migrates apically along the inner surface of the covering tissue, thereby forming a pocket that allows further bacterial contamination of the membrane.

Exposure of the membrane material to the oral cavity results in bacterial contamination of both the outer and inner surfaces of the membrane. The presence of these microorganisms in the membrane material and the healing wound may negatively interfere with the formation of both new connective tissue attachment and alveolar bone following the GTR procedure (Gottlow et al, 1984; Magnusson et al, 1985). Thus, it is reasonable to assume that prevention of bacterial contamination following the GTR procedure may favor the regeneration of lost periodontal tissue (Karring, 2000).

Special surgical techniques intended to retain the interdental soft tissues have been proposed to achieve and maintain primary closure during wound healing, thereby preventing exposure of the barrier. It has been suggested that such methods could produce greater clinical improvements.

One of these techniques is the modified papilla preservation technique, described earlier (Cortellini et al, 1995; see Fig 215). The modified papilla preservation technique allows primary closure of the interdental space, resulting in better protection of the membrane from the oral environment (Cortellini et al, 1995). The simplified papilla preservation flap has been proposed for narrow interdental spaces (Cortellini et al, 1999; see Fig 216).

In an RCT, Cortellini et al (1995) showed that the modified papilla preservation technique and GTR resulted in a significantly greater mean gain in CAL than either conventional GTR therapy alone or OFD (5.3 ± 2.2 mm, 4.1 ± 1.9 mm, and 2.5 ± 0.8 mm, respectively).

Meta-analysis of six RCTs involving the modified papilla preservation technique (Needleman et al, 2005) did not show a statistically significant difference compared with the overall estimate, despite the apparent greater attachment gain (0.75 mm; 95% confidence interval (CI) = –0.10, 1.59; $P = .09$). However, the 95% CI only just included a value of "no difference," suggesting that papilla preservation might be important and should be examined in future studies.

Professional postsurgical treatment. Machtei et al (2003) evaluated the supplementary effect of aggressive anti-infective therapy to GTR treatment on grade II furcation defects in smokers. Thirty-eight smokers were randomly assigned to a test or a control group. In the test group, 25% metronidazole gel was applied to the outer surface of the nonresorbable barrier during GTR surgery. The test group rinsed with 0.2% CHX solution twice daily and had an intake of 100 mg of doxycycline daily for 6 to 8 weeks until the barrier was removed. The control group rinsed with 0.2% CHX solution twice daily and received 100 mg of doxycycline daily for only 1 week after the GTR surgery. During the first 6 to 8 weeks, the test group received PMTC once per week and the control group, biweekly. Thereafter supportive preventive treatment was performed once a month until the 1-year reexamination. At 1 year, the mean gain in vertical CAL was significantly greater in the test group than in the control group. At reentry, the mean distance from the cemento-

enamel junction to the new tissue crest was 5.2 ± 0.4 mm in the test group and 6.3 ± 0.3 mm in the control group ($P < .05$). The authors concluded:

> While smoking prevented tissue maturation and mineralization, the anti-infective protocol enhanced these processes, resulting in a more favorable outcome. It is therefore suggested that when GTR is performed for [grade II] furcation defects in smokers, anti-infective therapy should be incorporated into the treatment protocol to enhance the regenerative outcome in these patients.

The role of an excellent maintenance program on the long-term effects of GTR therapy on deep human intrabony defects was evaluated by Cortellini et al (1994). Following GTR treatment, 40 deep intrabony defects in 23 patients gained a mean 4.1 mm of CAL after 1 year of stringent plaque control. In the subsequent 3 years, 15 patients (22 sites; group A) were recalled every 3 months. In this group, the attachment level remained stable. Conversely, at the 4-year follow-up, 8 patients (18 sites; group B) who received only sporadic care had lost 2.8 ± 2.7 mm of the CAL gained at 1 year. Patients in group A had significantly lower mandibular complete-mouth plaque and bleeding scores than did patients in group B at 4 years. Furthermore, bleeding on probing, plaque, *P gingivalis*, and *P intermedia* were detected significantly more frequently in group B. Risk assessment analysis indicated that compared to patients undergoing regular recall, in patients receiving only sporadic care, there was a 50-fold greater risk of probing attachment loss at GTR sites 1 to 4 years postoperatively. It was concluded that the stability of gained clinical attachment was dependent on stringent plaque control.

Gottlow et al (1992) also evaluated whether new attachment achieved by GTR can be maintained over longer periods of maintenance therapy. In 39 patients, 88 sites in 52 teeth with various types of periodontal defects were treated by GTR. The effect of treatment was evaluated by assessing CAL preoperatively and 6 months postoperatively. Only sites that had gained 2 mm or more CAL at the 6-month examination (baseline) were regarded as successful and scheduled for further monitoring. At baseline, 80 such sites were identified: All sites were monitored for 1 year, 65 for 2 years, 40 for 3 years, 17 for 4 years, and 9 for 5 years (71 sites lost to follow-up after 5 years). The results demonstrated that the attachment gain achieved by GTR treatment could be maintained over periods up to 5 years in a maintenance program based on high-quality gingival plaque control.

The results shown in case 1 and described in other studies (Cortellini and Tonetti, 2004; Cury et al, 2003; Eickholz et al, 2004, 2006, 2007; Gottlow et al, 1992; Machtei et al, 1996; Stavropoulos and Karring, 2004; Trombelli et al, 2005) have shown that the gains in CAL achieved through GTR therapy in intrabony defects, furcation defects, and recession defects can be maintained for several years if patients participate in a good supportive care program.

Study design. Of the hundreds of published GTR studies during the last two decades, the vast majority are case series reports and consecutive uncontrolled longitudinal studies followed by controlled longitudinal studies. The number of patients and treated sites in the different studies varies from a few to several hundreds, and the duration of observation ranges from 6 months up to 10 years. Details about history taking and methods and materials used during presurgical and postsurgical treatment are often insufficient, and those aspects that are reported are diverse.

Even if important information and knowledge can be received from many of these studies, it is always necessary to compare apples and oranges because of the great heterogeneity. Very few studies are so-called RCTs. In the previously discussed systematic review comparing the effect of GTR therapy on intrabony defects with that of OFD (Needleman et al, 2005), only 17 of 626 studies matched the inclusion criteria (RCTs with a minimum of 12 months' duration). In the included studies, the differences in mean gain in CAL for GTR compared with OFD ranged from 0.0 to 3.6 mm. Because of insufficient information about history taking (smoking, self-care, and dental care habits as well as general health status) and material and methods of presurgical and

postsurgical treatment, it was impossible to evaluate the influence of such factors.

However, split-mouth studies may overcome some of these problems, because the influence of genetics; systemic diseases; smoking, self-care, dental care, and dietary habits; and the operator's skill and experience will be the same for the test and control sites. In addition, protection from bias might be more straightforward in split-mouth studies. For instance, selection bias might be less of a risk because the patient represents both experimental groups. Furthermore, it might be more successful to maintain masking for patient, examiner, and therapist if the patient represents both groups.

In fact, the variation in the results in six split-mouth RCTs in the systematic review by Needleman et al (2005) was significantly less than the variation among seven parallel-group RCTs included in the same review. Thus, to reduce the variation among clinical GTR trials, they should be split-mouth RCTs. In addition, strict and standardized research protocols have to be followed regarding patient selection, variables included in history taking and diagnosis, methods and materials for presurgical treatment, GTR treatment, and postsurgical treatment (maintenance care).

Multicenter studies carried out at university clinics should follow the same research protocols. Even when the same protocols were used, there was a great range in the gains in mean CAL (1.6 to 5.0 mm) among 10 studies in 7 different countries (Tonetti et al, 2004). Therefore, the influence of the operator's skill and experience should not be underestimated.

Biomaterials

In the early study by Nyman et al (1982b), histologic specimens from some sites regenerated with the GTR technique revealed that there is often an artifactual defect between regenerated cementum and root dentin. Araújo et al (1997) observed that cementum resulting from GTR therapy apparently is different from cementum formed during tooth development (acellular cementum). Therefore, application of the term *regeneration* has been questioned in relation to GTR therapy. The term *true periodontal regeneration* has been defined as "healing after periodontal treatment that results in the regain of lost supporting tissues including new acellular cementum attached to the underlying dentin surface, a new periodontal ligament with functionally oriented collagen fibers inserting into the new cementum and new alveolar bone attached to the periodontal ligament" (Araújo et al, 1998; Wang et al, 2005).

Thus the optimal aim for regenerative therapy should be to develop methods and materials that can simulate the original development of the periodontal tissues. The development of the periodontal ligament and the alveolar bone is associated with the development of the teeth. Experimental studies indicate that the maintenance of the periodontal ligament and the alveolar bone is also regulated by cells close to the root surface (Araújo et al, 1997). Therefore, if the ambition is to regenerate the periodontal ligament and the alveolar bone that have been lost to periodontitis, regenerative techniques should aim at establishing new cementum and adjacent cells. If this can be accomplished, the periodontal ligament and alveolar bone are regenerated as a result of the cells at a healthy root surface.

During natural tooth development, the root formation is initiated by the downgrowth of the Hertwig epithelial root sheath. The epithelial root sheath constitutes an apical extension of the enamel organ. The root sheath cells form and secrete enamel matrix proteins during root formation. Enamel matrix proteins secreted on the newly formed root dentin attract and stimulate mesenchymal cells to differentiate, and cementoblasts are induced on the root dentin surface, resulting in the formation of root cementum. The root cementum produced in the initial stage contains no cells and is called *acellular cementum.* Principal fibers are embedded in this acellular cementum, and the cementum functions to maintain attachment to the tooth.

Following the production of root cementum, a series of cell inductions occur, and the periodontal ligament and alveolar bone proper are formed. Thus, enamel matrix proteins secreted by the Hertwig epithelial sheath play an important role not only in cementogenesis on roots but also in the development of the periodontal attachment apparatus.

The enamel matrix is composed of a number of proteins, such as amelogenin, amelin, enamelin, tuft protein, proteases, and albumen. Amelogenin exists in several different sizes and is by far the most abundant component, constituting more than 90% of the organic fraction. Amelogenin has been stable for millions of years of evolution, and several laboratory studies (Gestrelius et al, 1997a, 1997b, 2000; Hammarström, 1997) have proven that it is well accepted in human tissues without any immunologic reactions. Therefore, enamel matrix proteins are an attractive possibility for simulating nature in periodontal regenerative therapy.

Emdogain (Straumann), based on purified acid extract of porcine enamel matrix derivatives (EMDs) mixed with propylene glycol alginate in gel form, was introduced in Sweden in 1995 (Figs 227a to 227e). Some years later it was accepted in other European countries, the United States, and Japan.

In a pioneering experimental study, Hammarström et al (1997) showed that regeneration of acellular root cement and periodontal ligament with principal fibers attaching into the cementum can be achieved with EMDs (Figs 228a and 228b).

In a split-mouth experimental study, Araújo et al (1998) investigated the effect on periodontal tissue healing when GTR was followed by application of Emdogain to the root surface. Grade III furcation defects were created, and GTR was performed in dogs. In the experimental site, after phosphoric acid gel was applied to the exposed root surfaces, Emdogain was applied to all the instrumented parts of the root before a Resolut barrier was placed. The contralateral premolar received the same treatment, but acid etching was not performed and EMD gel was not applied before barrier installation.

Histologic analyses of the sites after 4 months showed the furcation defects of both the test and control groups to be occupied with similar amounts of mineralized bone, bone marrow, periodontal ligament tissue, and residual connective tissue. In the apical half of the furcation in the test group, however, the new cementum was found to be acellular and thin (12 μm) and to contain extrinsic and intrinsic fibers. In addition,

Figs 227a to 227e Effect of surgical application of Emdogain to a periodontal defect. (Courtesy of Biora.)

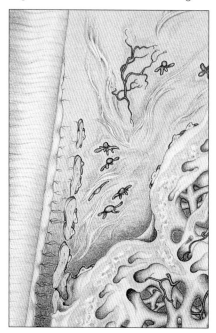

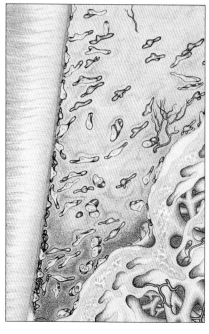

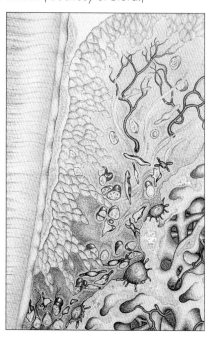

Fig 227a Periodontal defect showing inflammation, attachment loss, and epithelial downgrowth.

Fig 227b After surgical application, Emdogain proteins aggregate and form an insoluble matrix on the root surface. A coagulum fills the defect, and mesenchymal cells migrate to the lesion and attach to the protein matrix.

Fig 227c A new attachment with cementum and ligament is formed along the root surface treated with Emdogain. The restrictive effect of Emdogain on epithelial cells prevents oral epithelium from growing into the lesion.

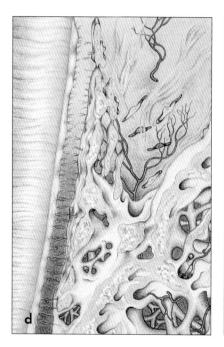

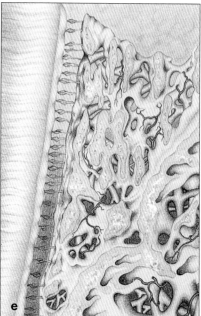

Fig 227d Bone formation starts as the Emdogain proteins aggregate and form an insoluble matrix on the root surface, not just at the periphery of the defect. Subsequently, new alveolar bone will fill the defect.

Fig 227e A new functional attachment is achieved with time.

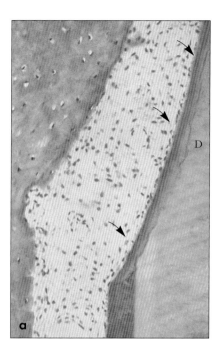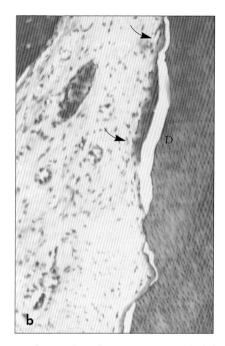

Figs 228a and 228b Histologic evaluation of periodontal regeneration with *(a)* and without *(b)* EMDs in monkeys. *(a)* A layer of acellular cementum firmly attached to the dentin (D) has formed in the cavity *(arrows)*, where enamel matrix had been placed before reimplantation. *(b)* Fragments of a cellular, poorly attached hard tissue *(arrows)* have formed in the cavity. (H&E, original magnification ×1,500.) (From Hammarström, 1997. Reprinted with permission.)

this new acellular cementum contained more inserting collagen fibers (extrinsic fibers) than did the new thick (32-µm) cellular cementum in the coronal part of the defect in the test group and the entire instrumented surface of the root in the control group. These observations seemed to confirm that EMD, when applied onto an instrumented and acid-etched dentinal surface, may create an environment conducive to the formation of acellular cementum (for review, see Araújo et al, 1998; McGuire and Cochran, 2003).

Not all the effects of EMD on regenerative therapy are known, but some important factors have been shown. Results from cell culture experiments strongly support the hypothesis that EMD facilitates periodontal ligament cell attachment and growth (Gestrelius et al, 1997b; Rodrigues et al, 2007). Moreover, attachment of periodontal ligament cells to EMD seems to generate an intracellular cyclic adenosine monophosphate signal to increase their proliferation and general metabolism as well as their production and secretion of vari-

ous autocrine growth factors. Acting in concert, these growth factors hold a potential for triggering dormant regenerative processes in surrounding cells and tissues. Also, the restrictive effect of EMD on epithelial cell growth could be beneficial by hindering growth of epithelium in a periodontal lesion during the wound-healing phase and the early regenerative process (Lyngstadaas et al, 2001; Van der Pauw et al, 2000). EMD also enhances the differentiation of periodontal ligament mesenchymal cells to cementoblasts, fibroblasts, and osteoblasts. In addition, EMD has been shown to have a positive effect on the composition of bacterial species in the postsurgical periodontal wound by selectively restricting growth of periopathogens that could hamper wound healing and negatively affect the outcome of regenerative procedures (Spahr et al, 2002). Topically applied Emdogain has been shown to enhance the early healing of soft tissue wounds after nonsurgical instrumentation (Wennström and Lindhe, 2002; for a review of the biologic effects of EMD, see Bosshardt, 2008).

Clinical use

Emdogain is available as a gel in a syringe with a cannula ready to be used, but it must be refrigerated until some minutes before use. Three different syringe packages are available: Emdogain gel 0.3 mL, Emdogain gel 0.7 mL, and Emdogain gel TS. Emdogain gel 0.3 mL should be used at one or a maximum of two sites. Emdogain gel 0.7 mL should be used at three to four individual sites.

Emdogain gel TS consists of two components, the enamel matrix protein (Emdogain gel) and synthetic alloplastic bone graft particulate (PerioGlas, NovaBone), which are mixed together just before application. The resulting formulation is easy to handle, does not migrate from the surgical site, and adapts readily to the defect. Treatment with Emdogain gel TS ensures that the soft tissues of the periodontium are well supported while the unique properties of Emdogain gel initiate the regenerative process. Emdogain gel TS is preferable in any defect where additional tissue support is desired, for example, wide two-wall intrabony defects and furcation defects.

The main indications for use of Emdogain gel are one-, two-, and three-wall intrabony defects and grade II furcation involvement in mandibular molars and buccal sites of maxillary molars. However, recessions and grade II furcation defects at free and accessible approximal surfaces of maxillary molars and first premolars may also be successfully treated with Emdogain during regenerative therapy. Combinations of Emdogain gel and bioresorbable barriers or titanium-reinforced nonresorbable barriers may sometimes be more useful and efficient than Emdogain gel alone (Araújo and Lindhe, 1998).

Preoperative preparation. As with GTR therapy, the protocol includes comprehensive history taking and clinical diagnosis, followed by education and training of the patient in self-diagnosis and self-care to optimize daily gingival plaque control. To reduce the microbial challenge as much as possible, comprehensive minimally invasive scaling, root planing, and debridement, combined with bactericidal antimicrobial pocket irrigation (0.1% iodine solution), are followed by

PMTC to eliminate the subgingival biofilm, nonattaching microflora, and calculus. So-called complete-mouth disinfection is performed, including not only toothcleaning but also tongue scraping and chemical plaque control (Axelsson et al, 1987b; Quirynen et al, 1995).

The effect of this initial hygiene phase is evaluated by DNA probe analysis of the subgingival microflora in all sites scheduled for regenerative therapy. Antibiotics are not usually necessary but may be used restrictively in the most highly susceptible patients, patients with cardiovascular disease or diabetes, and when there are persistently high counts of the most virulent pathogens: *P gingivalis*, *T forsythia*, and *Aa*. For patients with high counts of all three pathogens, amoxicillin (375 mg) with metronidazole (400 mg) is used 3 times per day for 10 days, starting 2 days preoperatively. If the sites to be treated are not infected with *Aa*, only metronidazole should be used. Alternatively, the sites could be treated topically with tetracycline fibers, metronidazole gel, or doxycycline gel during the week before treatment.

For self-care, the patient should supplement mechanical plaque control and tongue scraping with a CHX mouthrinse (0.12%) used twice a day during the week before treatment. However, a toothpaste without anions, such as sodium lauryl sulfate or monofluorophosphate, must be used to avoid inactivation of the cationic CHX.

A final subgingival debridement combined with antimicrobial irrigation is carried out to remove remaining biofilms and to increase the accessibility of the antibiotics 2 days before surgery. The aim is to achieve an oral cavity and, particularly, preoperative lesions that are as free of infection as possible. As an effect of this intensive presurgical treatment, even the sites that will receive regenerative therapy are healed. Therefore, bleeding during surgery is significantly reduced, which optimizes both the accessibility for the Emdogain gel and the outcome of therapy.

Surgical protocol. An intracrevicular incision is combined with a vertical releasing incision, and a mucoperiosteal (full-thickness) flap is elevated (Figs 229a and 229b). After removal of granulation tissue to optimize accessibility and reduce

Figs 229a to 229h Surgical protocol for use of Emdogain in an intraosseous defect. (Courtesy of Biora.)

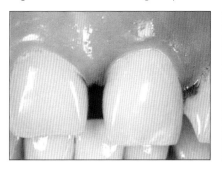 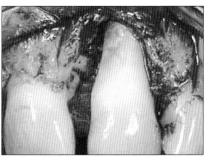 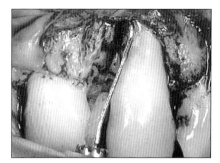

Fig 229a Presurgical view. A deep intraosseous defect exists mesiobuccal to the maxillary left central incisor.

Fig 229b An intracrevicular incision is combined with vertical releasing incisions, then a full-thickness flap is elevated.

Fig 229c After removal of granulation tissues, the root surface is cleaned by minimally invasive debridement.

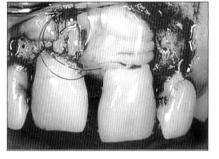 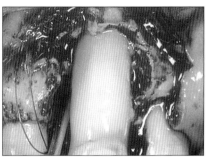 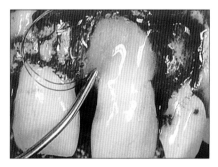

Fig 229d The root is chemically conditioned, and debris is removed with an EDTA gel.

Fig 229e The area is rinsed with saline solution and dried with cotton pellets.

Fig 229f Emdogain gel is applied to the entire root surface to the bottom of the defect. The absence of blood contamination ensures optimal accessibility.

Fig 229g A modified mattress suture is placed.

Fig 229h The flap is replaced to its preoperative position and sutured.

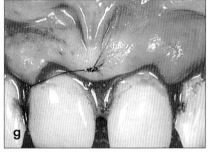 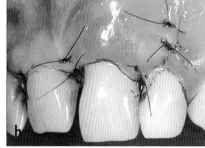

bleeding, supplementary mechanical cleaning of the root surface is completed with minimally invasive instrumentation (Fig 229c). Thereafter, the root surface is chemically cleaned and conditioned (for removal of smear layer and limited demineralization of the surface) with an EDTA gel for 2 minutes (Fig 229d). The root surface and the bone defect are carefully irrigated with saline solution and dried (Fig 229e). These steps, along with presurgical healing of the infectious inflamed periodontal tissue, ensure optimal accessibility for application of Emdogain gel with the syringe (Fig 229f). The entire exposed root surface is generously covered with Emdogain gel. To allow rapid flap closure, it is recommended that the sutures be attached before application of the Emdogain gel (see Fig 229e). The tailored flap is sutured tightly with a modified mattress suture to cover the entire defect, enclose the gel, and stabilize the blood clot during early healing (Figs 229g and 229h). After the suturing is completed, some of the remaining gel should be applied to cover the incision wounds, particularly in the sulcus. Normally, the sutures are removed after 2 weeks.

The solubility of the enamel proteins is both pH and temperature dependent. Because the pH will reach body temperature soon after the flaps have been replaced and sutured, the enamel proteins will start precipitating almost immediately. Thus, aggregates of enamel proteins will adsorb to the root surface and form an insoluble surface matrix that can interact with cells originating in the periodontal ligament and, maybe, endosteal surfaces in marrow spaces, periosteum, and vasculature.

Detectable amounts of enamel proteins are present at the site of application for up to 2 to 3 weeks before being enzymatically degraded. Although this appears to be a sufficiently long period of time to permit colonization of cells with the potential to initiate cementum formation and periodontal regeneration, it is important not to delay wound healing unnecessarily; the surgeon should avoid overuse of adrenaline-containing local anesthetics in the immediate area of the periodontal defect, use a skillful surgical technique, and strive for optimal wound stability.

The viscosity of the vehicle will change rapidly following flap closure and become very watery. The vehicle will leave the surgical area rapidly and no traces will be left after 12 to 24 hours. The vehicle will therefore neither interfere with the formation of the coagulum or cellular ingrowth nor act as a barrier or space maintainer.

Postsurgical protocol. The patient should take ibuprofen tablets (400 mg), which have analgesic and anti-inflammatory effects, four times during the first 36 hours postsurgery. The patient must refrain from interdental mechanical toothcleaning near the wound for the first 4 weeks of healing. However, a special extra-extrasoft toothbrush may be used with caution around the treated teeth beginning 2 to 3 days after surgery. All other tooth surfaces as well as the dorsum of the tongue should be comprehensively cleaned to prevent reinfection of the treated sites. Use of a CHX mouthrinse (0.12%) twice a day should continue for 6 weeks after treatment.

Needs-related PMTC is carried out every 2 weeks during the first 6 weeks and once a month during the following 5 to 6 months. However, during the first 2 weeks postsurgery, cleaning at the treated sites is restricted to the use of cotton pellets soaked in a bactericidal iodine solution to avoid mechanical disruption of wound healing. Beginning 7 months postsurgery, supportive care at needs-related intervals of every 2 to 4 months is recommended (see chapter 5).

Measurement of probing depth and attachment level is not recommended until 6 months postsurgery. The first radiographic evaluation is recommended after 6 to 12 months.

Case 10. A 63-year-old man with cardiovascular disease who was a former smoker (10 cigarettes per day for 45 years = 23 pack years) had chronic periodontitis. Several teeth exhibited deep pockets, in particular the maxillary left lateral incisor (11 mm distally) and the maxillary left first premolar (14 mm mesially, 10 mm distally, and 12 mm lingually). Because it was extremely mobile, the maxillary left first premolar was temporarily fixed to the canine and second premolar. A radiograph taken with a probe in situ revealed a very deep intrabony defect mesial to the maxillary left first premolar (Fig 230a). Oral microbiologic analyses showed this defect to have the highest checkerboard DNA-DNA hybridization score (5) for *P gingivalis* and *Treponema denticola* and a score 2 for *T forsythia* in this particular defect. As a supplement to the usual presurgical treatment, systemic antibiotics (amoxicillin, 350 mg, and metronidazole, 400 mg, three times per day) were prescribed for 10 days (starting 2 days before surgical treatment).

In this case, a full-thickness flap was raised from the distal aspect of the left central incisor to the buccal aspect of the left second premolar because Emdogain gel was to be used on the root surfaces of the lateral incisor, canine, and first premolar. After removal of the granulation tissue, supplementary minimally invasive mechanical cleaning and planing of the roots, and irrigation with saline solution, the very deep two- and three-wall defect on the mesial aspect of the first premolar was exposed (Fig 230b).

Because of the tailored intensive presurgical treatment and the removal of the granulation tissue, the root surface was free of blood, which optimized the accessibility for chemical conditioning of the root surface with EDTA gel (Fig 230c), irrigation with saline solution, drying, and sub-

Figs 230a to 230g Case 10.

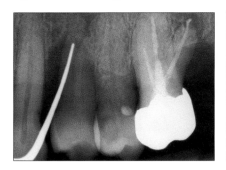

Fig 230a A periodontal probe reveals advanced loss of periodontal support on the mesial of the maxillary left first premolar in a heavy smoker positive for genetic polymorphism of interleukin 1.

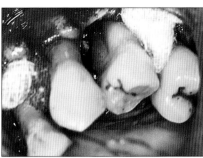

Fig 230b The intrabony defect is visible mesial to the maxillary left first premolar after removal of granulation tissue.

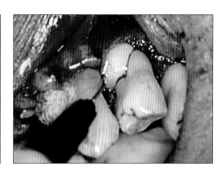

Fig 230c After minimally invasive mechanical cleaning of the root surface, the EDTA gel is applied. After 2 minutes, the gel is removed by irrigation with saline solution, and the root surface is dried.

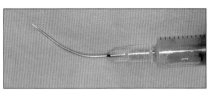

Fig 230d Emdogain gel in the syringe, ready to use.

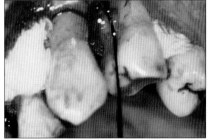

Fig 230e The Emdogain gel is applied to the intrabony defect. It also will be applied to the roots of the central incisor, canine, and second premolar.

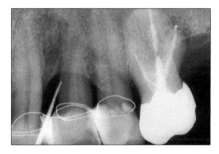

Fig 230f A probe inserted to the bottom of the defect 5 to 6 months after treatment reveals 5 to 6 mm of bone gain compared to the baseline radiograph (see Fig 230a).

Fig 230g A radiograph taken 6 years after treatment reveals that the gain of alveolar bone observed after 5 to 6 months has been maintained.

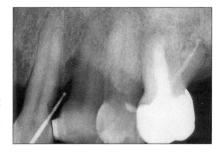

sequent application of the Emdogain gel (Figs 230d and 230e). The flap was sutured with the modified mattress suture, and the interproximal space was tightly closed.

Ibuprofen (400 mg) was administered during the following 36 hours. The sutures were removed after 2 weeks. Good wound healing and no postsurgical complications were observed.

The patient was scheduled for a personalized supportive care program at needs-related intervals. At the first reexamination after almost 6 months, a radiograph taken with a probe in situ showed a 5- to 6-mm bone gain (Fig 230f). The gain in CAL was 7 mm. At the most recent reexamination, after 6 years, the gains in alveolar bone and CAL observed after 6 months were still maintained (Fig 230g). The patient exhibited excellent plaque control and gingival health. The probing depths were 3 mm mesially, 1 mm buccally, 2 mm distally, and 1 mm lingually.

Figs 231a to 231f Case 11. (Courtesy of Dr P. Cortellini.)

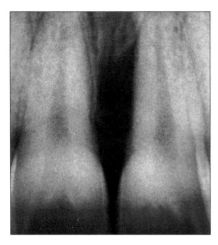

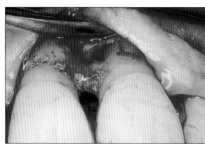

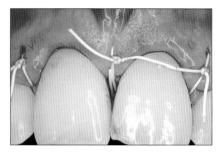

Fig 231a A deep intraosseous defect is located mesial to the maxillary left central incisor.

Fig 231b The narrow interdental space is accessed with simplified papilla preservation flap surgery. The exposed 9-mm-deep, two- and three-wall defect is complex, with a palatal bone dehiscence and a small bone bridge coronally between the central incisors.

Fig 231c After regenerative therapy with Emdogain, the flaps are replaced with a single modified interdental suture.

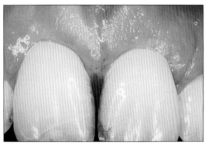

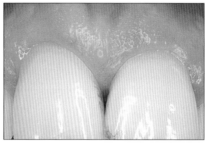

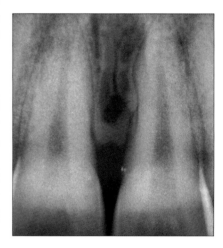

Fig 231d Primary closure is obtained after 1 week.

Fig 231e After 3 years, there is no interdental recession.

Fig 231f A radiograph taken 3 years after treatment reveals that the deep defect is completely resolved, with a well-mineralized bone margin.

Case 11. A radiograph revealed a deep defect mesial to the maxillary left central incisor (Fig 231a). The narrow interdental space was accessed with a simplified papilla preservation technique (Fig 231b). The defect was a 9-mm, complex two- and three-wall intrabony defect with a palatal bone dehiscence. A bone bridge was still present between the central incisors. After regenerative treatment with Emdogain, primary closure of the involved interdental space was obtained with a single modified interdental suture (Fig 231c). Primary closure was obtained after 1 week, and the interdental soft tissues were well-supported by the bone bridge (Fig 231d). After 3 years, no interdental recession had occurred (Fig 231e). A radiograph taken 3 years after treatment revealed that the deep defect was completely resolved (Fig 231f).

Figs 232a to 232f Case 12. (Courtesy of Dr G. Heden.)

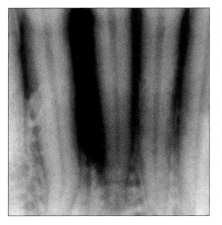

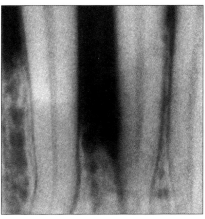

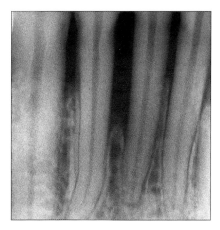

Fig 232a A deep periodontal defect, extending almost to the apex, is present at the distal surface of the mandibular right central incisor.

Fig 232b Initial nonsurgical treatment and systemic antibiotics have resulted in no gain of alveolar bone.

Fig 232c Regenerative treatment with Emdogain has resulted in substantial gain of alveolar bone only 1 year after application.

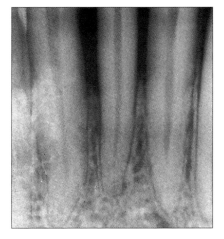

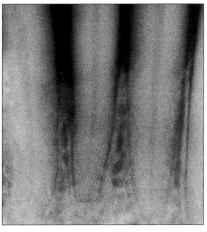

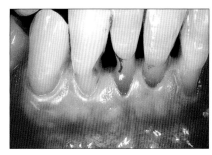

Fig 232d The bone gain has continued at the 5-year reexamination.

Fig 232e The bone level is stable after 14 years.

Fig 232f The clinical appearance is healthy 14 years after treatment.

Case 12. A 38-year-old woman who was a light smoker with hormonal problems had a deep periodontal defect distal to the mandibular right central incisor, according to clinical probing and a radiograph (Fig 232a). Initial nonsurgical treatment and systemic administration of doxycycline because of a very high *Aa* level resulted in minimal healing (Fig 232b). Subsequently, regenerative therapy with flap surgery and Emdogain gel was performed. After 1 year, substantial gain of alveolar bone was observed (Fig 232c). The gains continued after 5 years (Fig 232d), and the bone level

and clinical status were stable after 14 years (Figs 232e and 232f).

Case 13. An 18-year-old nonsmoking, healthy woman had localized aggressive periodontitis. Retrospective bitewing radiographs had revealed localized loss of alveolar bone mesially at the maxillary and mandibular right first molars (Figs 233a and 233b). No special periodontal treatment had been performed until the patient had reached the age of 17 years.

Figs 233a to 233e Case 13. (Courtesy of Dr G. Heden.)

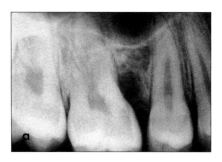 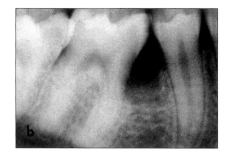

Figs 233a and 233b Deep intraosseous defects are present mesial to the maxillary and mandibular right first molars in a young adult with localized aggressive periodontitis.

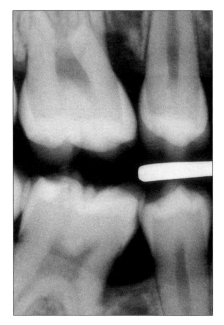 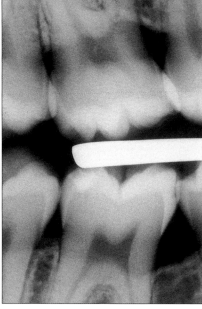 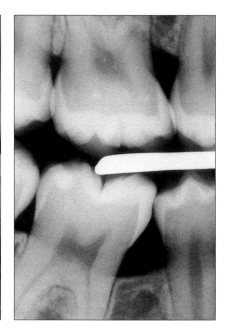

Fig 233c A bitewing radiograph before regenerative treatment with Emdogain reveals the extent of the defects.

Fig 233d A bitewing radiograph reveals substantial gain of alveolar bone at the mesial surfaces of both first molars 1 year after treatment.

Fig 233e The gain achieved by regenerative treatment has been maintained, with a well-mineralized bone margin, 3 years after treatment.

Initial education in self-care, PMTC, nonsurgical debridement, and topical use of doxycycline to treat the high levels of *Aa* were followed 6 months later with Emdogain regenerative therapy.

Figure 233c shows a bitewing radiograph taken before regenerative therapy. A bitewing radiograph after 1 year revealed an obvious gain of alveolar bone mesial to the maxillary and mandibular first molars (Fig 233d). This gain was maintained and stable, with a well-mineralized alveolar bone margin, after 3 years (Fig 233e).

Case 14. A 45-year-old nonsmoking man presented with a combined one- and two-wall periodontal defect on the distal surface of the maxillary left first premolar. An inserted probe revealed the most apical part of the defect on the baseline radiograph (Fig 234a). The probing depth was 9 mm distally and lingually. The maxillary left first molar exhibited through-and-through grade III furcation involvement between the mesiobuccal and palatal roots. The distobuccal root had been hemisectioned several years previously. After hemisection of the mesiobuccal root, regenera-

Figs 234a to 234d Case 14.

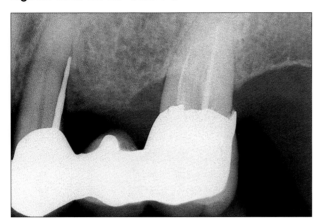

Fig 234a A one- and two-wall alveolar bony defect is present at the distal surface of the maxillary left first premolar, and a mesial defect is present at the left first molar.

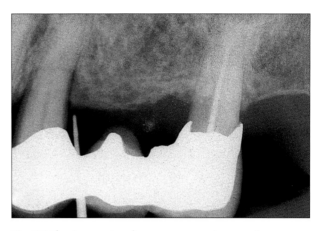

Fig 234b Six months after regenerative therapy, there is considerable gain in probing attachment, and new bone has formed up to the horizontal crest distal to the first premolar.

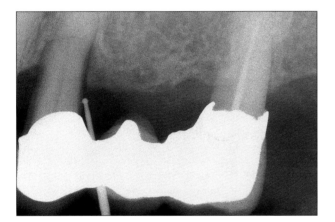

Fig 234c The result is well maintained 6 years after treatment.

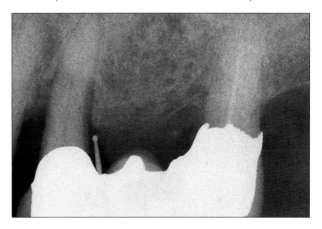

Fig 234d The site remains healthy 10 years after treatment.

tive therapy with flap surgery and Emdogain gel was carried out distolingually at the first premolar and mesiobuccally at the first molar. After only 6 months, the inserted probe clearly revealed considerable gain in probing attachment, and new bone had formed up to the horizontal crest distal to the first premolar (Fig 234b).

As an effect of the personalized supportive care program, this result was well maintained after 6 years (Fig 234c) and at the most recent re-examination, 10 years after treatment (Fig 234d). The probing depths were 3 mm mesially, 1 mm buccally, 2 mm distally, and 1 mm lingually at the first premolar, and 2 mm mesially, 2 mm buccally, 2 mm distally, and 1 mm lingually at the first molar. The gingival condition and the plaque control were excellent.

Case 15. A 70-year-old male former smoker (32 pack years) testing positive for genetic polymorphism of the proinflammatory cytokine Il-1 presented with a medical history of regular use of five drugs related to cardiovascular disease. A baseline full-mouth radiograph (Fig 235a) and clinical examination revealed severe untreated periodontal disease involving most of his remaining teeth.

The maxillary first premolars and right first molar were extracted because of furcation involvement. The extremely mobile mandibular incisors were provisionally stabilized with bonded composites. The prognoses for the left maxillary and right mandibular canines seemed to be hopeless. Baseline radiographs showed an extremely deep intrabony defect mesially at the left maxil-

Figs 235a to 235h Case 15.

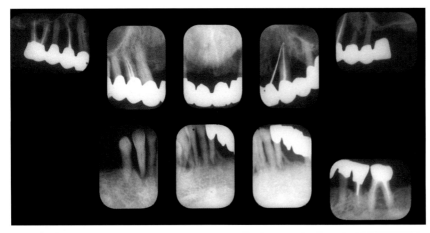

Fig 235a Baseline complete-mouth radiographs and clinical examinations show severe untreated periodontal disease involving most of the remaining teeth. The maxillary first premolars and right first molar were untreatable and therefore were extracted.

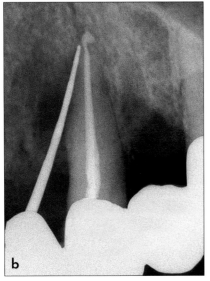

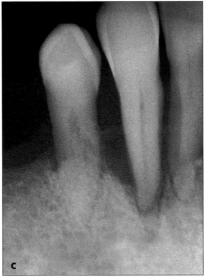

Figs 235b and 235c Baseline radiographs with a probe inserted show a very deep intrabony defect mesial to the maxillary left canine (b) and almost around the apex distal to the mandibular right canine (c).

lary canine (Fig 235b) and almost apical marginal communication distally at the right mandibular canine (Fig 235c). The pocket depths at the left maxillary and right mandibular canines, respectively, were 12 and 10 mm mesially, 3 and 3 mm buccally, 10 and 14 mm distally, and 10 and 3 mm lingually. The mesial site of the left maxillary canine exhibited the highest level (score 5) of *P gingivalis*, *T forsythia*, and *T denticola*, while the distal site of the right mandibular canine showed somewhat lower levels.

After comprehensive presurgical treatment, regenerative therapy with flap surgery plus Emdogain gel was carried out in the right mandibular quadrant at the first premolar mesially, the canine mesially and distally, and the lateral incisor

mesially, and at the left maxillary canine mesially, distally, and palatally. In addition, systemic administration of amoxicillin and metronidazole was supplemented.

Radiographs 1 year later showed about 14 mm of bone level gain at the mesial surface of the left maxillary canine (Fig 235d) and about 5 to 6 mm at the distal surface of the right mandibular canine (Fig 235e). This gain was well maintained at the 5-year (Fig 235f) and 7-year reexaminations (Figs 235g and 235h). The patient also exhibited excellent gingival health and very shallow pockets (7 years after treatment, left maxillary and right mandibular canines, respectively: 2 and 3 mm mesially, 1 and 1 mm buccally, 2 and 3 mm distally, and 2 and 2 mm lingually).

Figs 235d and 235e Radiographs 1 year after regenerative treatment with Emdogain show about 14 mm of alveolar bone gain mesial to the maxillary left canine *(d)* and 5 to 6 mm distal to the mandibular right canine *(e)* compared to baseline (see Figs 235b and 235c).

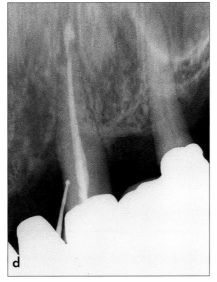
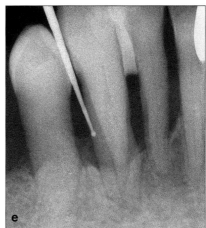

Fig 235f Complete-mouth radiographs 5 years after treatment.

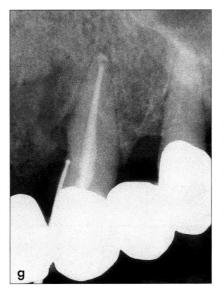
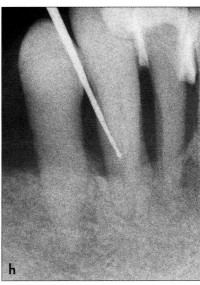

Figs 235g and 235h Radiographs 7 years after treatment show that the bone gain achieved after 1 year was well maintained.

Figs 236a to 236f Case 16.

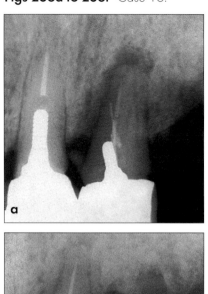

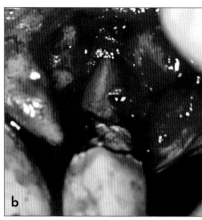

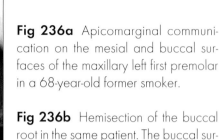

Fig 236a Apicomarginal communication on the mesial and buccal surfaces of the maxillary left first premolar in a 68-year-old former smoker.

Fig 236b Hemisection of the buccal root in the same patient. The buccal surface of the palatal root is visible to the apex. Gutta-percha filling is visible through the thin buccal root wall.

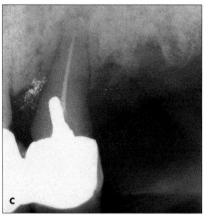

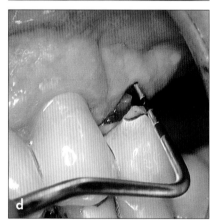

Fig 236c Radiograph 4 months after hemisection of the buccal root and regenerative therapy with Emdogain shows considerable bone gain around the apex and mesially along the remaining palatal root.

Fig 236d Gingival condition 1 year after treatment. The buccal pocket depth was only 1 mm.

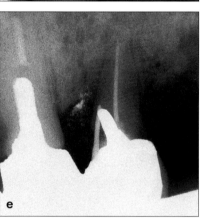

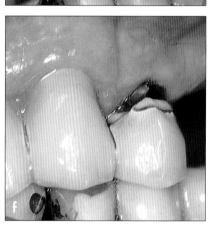

Fig 236e Radiograph 7 years after treatment with a probe inserted mesially shows that the remaining root was still well maintained.

Fig 236f Gingival condition 7 years after treatment.

Case 16. A 68-year-old male former smoker (more than 20 cigarettes per day for more than 40 years = 50 pack years) had an apical-marginal communication on the mesial and buccal surfaces of his maxillary left first premolar (Fig 236a). Because the tooth was the posterior abutment of a 4-unit fixed partial denture, hemisection of the buccal root was planned after explorative flap surgery. However, after hemisection, the entire buccal surface of the lingual root was visible up to the apex

(Fig 236b). The gutta-percha root filling material was visible through the thin buccal root wall. As a last resort, the buccal root surface was nonaggressively mechanically and then chemically cleaned and surface conditioned with EDTA gel, after which Emdogain gel was applied, and the flap was sutured.

Considerable regeneration of alveolar bone around the apex and the mesial aspect of the lingual root was found only 4 months postsurgery

Figs 237a to 237d Case 17.

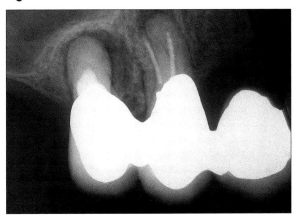

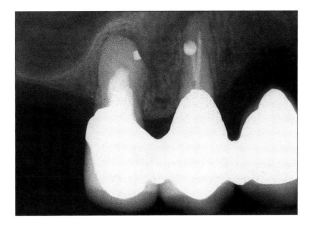

Fig 237a An apicomarginal communication is present along the mesiobuccal root surface of the maxillary right second premolar, and an apical lesion is present on the first premolar.

Fig 237b There is complete regeneration of alveolar bone at both premolars 3 months after retrograde root filling of the buccal root of the first premolar and a mesioapical perforation at the second premolar, followed by regenerative therapy with Emdogain apically at the first premolar and mesioapically at the second premolar.

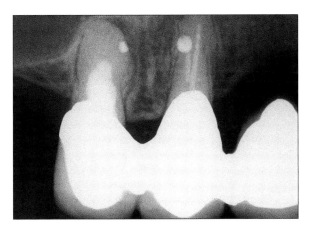

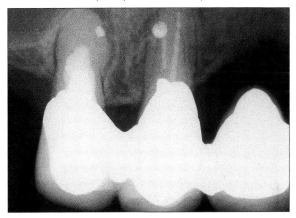

Fig 237c The initial result has been maintained after 3 years.

Fig 237d Complete regeneration of alveolar bone has been maintained after 5 years.

(Fig 236c). On the buccal surface, the probing depth was only 1 mm, and the margin of the gingiva was located at the exposed tip of the post 1 year after treatment (Fig 236d). More than 7 years after treatment, the tooth and gingival health were still well maintained (Figs 236e and 236f).

Case 17. A 63-year-old nonsmoking woman had a marginal-apical communication along the mesiobuccal surfaces of the maxillary right second premolar and an apical periodontal lesion on the first premolar (Fig 237a). During open flap surgery, a perforation or accessory root canal less than 1 mm in diameter mesioapically was dis-

covered at the maxillary right second premolar. After preparation of this hole and the apex of the buccal root of the first premolar, retrograde root filling with silver–glass-ionomer material, comprehensive mechanical cleaning and chemical conditioning of the exposed root surfaces, and regenerative treatment with Emdogain gel was performed at the mesiobuccal surfaces and around the apex of the second premolar and apical to the first premolar. Only 3 months after treatment, complete regeneration of alveolar bone was achieved at both the first and second premolars (Fig 237b). This result was maintained after 3 years (Fig 237c) and 5 years (Fig 237d).

Figs 238a to 238g Case 18.

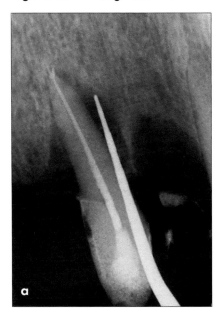 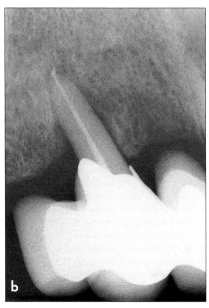

Fig 238a Baseline radiograph with a probe inserted to the bottom of a deep intrabony defect mesial to the right maxillary canine.

Fig 238b Radiograph 6 months after regenerative therapy with Emdogain and 1 month after a fixed prosthesis was placed shows a dramatic regeneration of alveolar bone mesial to the maxillary right canine and pocket depth reduction from 14 to 2 mm.

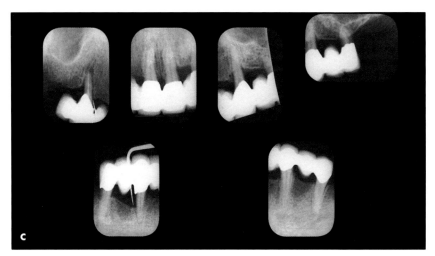

Fig 238c The complete-mouth radiographs more than 2 years after treatment.

Case 18. A 58-year-old male smoker (one pack per day for more than 40 years = more than 40 pack years) had very advanced, untreated aggressive periodontitis but was otherwise healthy according to his medical history. Only 20 teeth remained, of which 11 were untreatable and had to be extracted. In the maxilla, only the canines, central incisors, and the left second premolar could be retained; in the mandible, only the two canines and the second premolars could be saved.

After initial diagnosis, history taking, education in self-care, scaling, root planing, debridement, and extraction of untreatable teeth, provisional prostheses were constructed.

The prognosis for the maxillary right canine was highly questionable, as disclosed on the radiograph, which was taken with a periodontal probe inserted mesiolingually almost to the apex (Fig 238a). The probing depths were 14 mm mesially, 8 mm lingually, 8 mm distally, and 4 mm buccally. Checkerboard DNA probe analyses from the examined sites showed the maximum score of 5 for *P gingivalis*, *T forsythia*, *T denticola*, and somewhat lower levels for *Aa*. Because the canine was the most posterior tooth on the maxillary right side, it was a key tooth for construction of a fixed prosthesis; therefore, every effort was made to save this tooth.

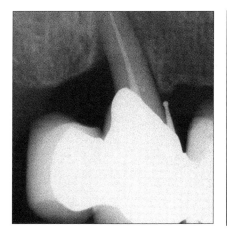

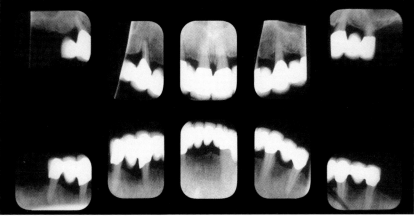

Fig 238d Close-up radiograph 5 years after treatment.

Fig 238e Complete-mouth radiographs 6.5 years after treatment.

Fig 238f Close-up radiograph more than 9 years after treatment shows that the alveolar bone gain that had been achieved at 6 months was still maintained.

Fig 238g Clinical view 9 years after treatment shows healthy gingiva and excellent plaque control. Pocket depths were only 2 mm mesiodistally and 1 mm buccolingually.

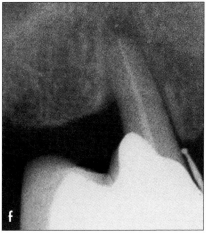

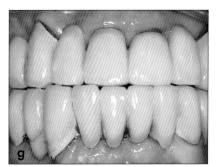

After optimal plaque control, including full-mouth disinfection and repeated debridement to eliminate all subgingival biofilms, regenerative therapy was carried out. The technique involved flap surgery, debridement, chemical conditioning of the root surface, and the use of Emdogain gel. To optimize the healing potential, the patient stopped smoking, and systemic metronidazole plus amoxicillin were administered starting 2 days before therapy (400 mg metronidazole and 375 mg amoxicillin, 3 times per day for 10 days) on the basis of the checkerboard DNA probe analyses.

Because dramatic healing was achieved after only 5 months, a fixed prosthesis was constructed.

Figure 238b shows a control radiograph taken after placement of the prosthesis (6 months after treatment). Probing depth had decreased from 14 to 2 mm mesially, and the above-mentioned aggressive periopathogens either had disappeared entirely or were found at the lowest level (score 1). This alveolar bone gain was shown to be maintained at re-examinations 2, 5, 6, and 9 years after treatment (Figs 238c to 238f). The pocket depths at the 9-year reexamination were only 2 mm mesially, 1 mm buccally, 2 mm distally, and 1 mm palatally. In addition, the gingival condition and plaque control were excellent (Fig 238g).

Figs 239a and 239b Case 19.

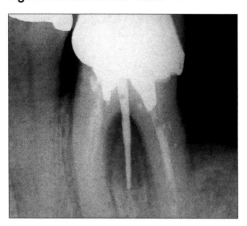 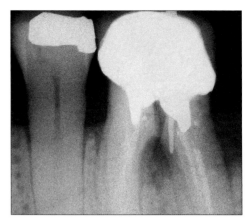

Fig 239a A probe inserted in the pretreatment radiograph reveals a very deep grade II to III furcation defect buccal to the mandibular left first molar.

Fig 239b A radiograph taken 6 months after advanced odontoplasty and regenerative therapy with Emdogain reveals about 5-mm vertical regeneration of the furcation defect. The vertical probing depth has been reduced from 11 to 3 mm and the horizontal depth from 7 to 2 mm.

Figs 240a and 240b Case 20.

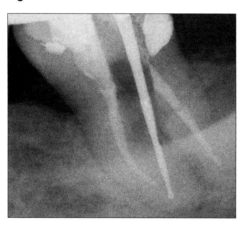 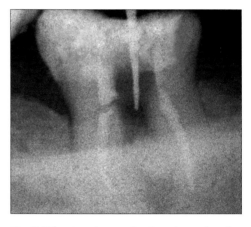

Fig 240a An inserted probe reveals a very deep furcation defect, extending almost to the apex, at the buccal aspect of the mandibular left second molar.

Fig 240b A radiograph taken 6 months after regenerative therapy with Emdogain reveals a dramatic 10-mm vertical gain of alveolar bone in the defect.

Case 19. A 54-year-old woman who was a smoker (36 pack years) had advanced chronic periodontitis. The mandibular left first molar had a very advanced grade II to III furcation defect buccally (Fig 239a). The vertical pocket depth was 11 mm, and the horizontal pocket depth was 7 mm. After a deep buccal odontoplasty was performed on the nonvital tooth, regenerative therapy with flap surgery and Emdogain gel was performed. The surgical procedures were supplemented with systemic administration of antibiotics (amoxicillin plus metronidazole) for 10 days.

At the 6-month reexamination, considerable gain of bone had been achieved in the furcation defect, and the vertical probing depth was reduced to 3 mm (Fig 239b).

Figs 241a and 241b Case 21.

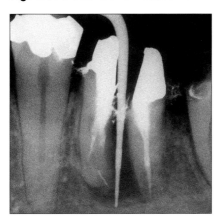

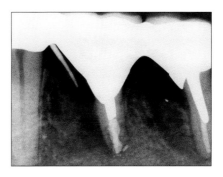

Fig 241a Baseline radiograph shows advanced grade III furcation (through and through) defects at the mandibular left first and second molars. The roots of first molar were already separated because of apicomarginal communication at the mesial root.

Fig 241b Radiograph 1 year after hemisection and extraction of the mesial roots and regenerative therapy with Emdogain, followed by placement of a fixed prosthesis. About 8 to 10 mm of alveolar bone had been regenerated mesial to the distal roots of the mandibular left first and second molars.

Case 20. A 69-year-old man exhibited an extremely advanced vertical grade II buccal furcation defect, almost reaching the apex, at the mandibular left second molar (Fig 240a). The vertical probing depth was 14 mm. The two roots were located tightly together, and the curved apex of the mesial root seemed to be fixed to the distal root. Hemisection did not seem to be a feasible treatment option. Therefore, an advanced odontoplasty was performed on the crown, and the groove between the two roots of the nonvital tooth was recontoured. Regenerative therapy with flap surgery and application of Emdogain gel was performed.

At the reexamination after 5 to 6 months, an extremely rapid gain of alveolar bone level, about 10 mm, was observed (Fig 240b). The vertical probing depth was reduced to 2 mm.

Case 21. A 58-year-old nonsmoking man with generalized aggressive periodontitis had several severely diseased teeth, including mandibular left first and second molars with grade III ("through-and-through") furcation involvement (Fig 241a). After hemisection and extraction of the mesial roots, regenerative therapy with Emdogain gel was carried out around the distal roots. Because of the aggressive periodontitis and very high levels of *P gingivalis*, *T forsythia*, and *T denticola* as well as *Aa*, systemic administration of amoxicillin and metronidazole for 10 days was provided. A dramatic gain of periodontal support was achieved at the 6-month reexamination, allowing the distal roots of the two molars to be used as abutments for a fixed prosthodontic reconstruction. Figure 241b shows the result 1 year after regenerative therapy.

Figs 242a to 242f Case 22.

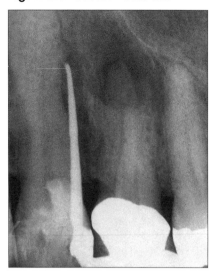

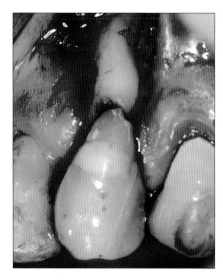

Fig 242a Baseline radiograph with a probe inserted to the bottom of a deep periodontal defect distal to the maxillary left canine. In addition, an apical periodontal lesion is shown at the adjacent first premolar.

Fig 242b A raised mini-flap shows loss of alveolar bone buccally and distally almost to the apex.

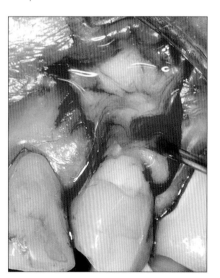

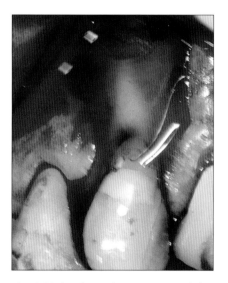

Fig 242c After nonaggressive mechanical debridement, the exposed root surface was conditioned with EDTA gel.

Fig 242d After saline rinsing and drying, Emdogain gel was applied, covering the entire exposed root surface.

Case 22. A 65-year-old nonsmoking woman with general good health exhibited a severe localized periodontal defect close to a marginal apical communication at the buccal and distal surface of the maxillary left canine. The pocket depths were 12 mm buccally and 14 mm distally. A radiograph showed advanced loss of alveolar bone distally and a pea-sized apical lesion on the adjacent first premolar (Fig 242a).

A full-thickness mini-flap was raised. After removal of granulation tissue distally, the root surface was exposed almost to the apex, particularly

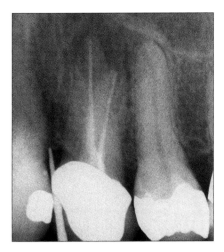

Fig 242e Radiograph 1 year after treatment with a probe inserted to the bottom of the pocket showed that alveolar bone had been regenerated to only 3 mm from the cementoenamel junction. In addition, the apical destruction at the maxillary left first premolar was almost completely remineralized after endodontic treatment.

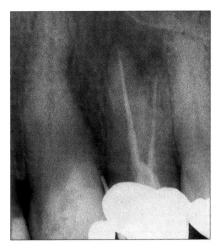

Fig 242f Radiograph 6 years after treatment shows that the result achieved at 1 year was maintained.

at the distal surface, which exhibited a concavity apically (Fig 242b). After nonagressive mechanical debridement, root surface conditioning with EDTA gel (Fig 242c), rinsing with saline solution, drying, and application of Emdogain gel (Fig 242d), the flap was sutured. The maxillary left first premolar was endodontically treated.

At the 1-year reexamination, radiographs showed that a gain in alveolar bone had been achieved up to only 3 mm from the cementoenamel junction at the distal surface of the left maxillary canine and that the pocket depth was only 1 mm buccally and 2 mm distally (Fig 242e). In addition, the apical lesion on the first premolar was almost completely healed following endodontic treatment. As a result of the customized supportive care program, the effect achieved at the 1-year reexamination was well maintained after 6 years (Fig 242f).

Combination of EMD and other materials. In deep two- and three-wall intrabony defects, EMD alone will result in successful regeneration of lost periodontal tissues with good predictability. However, in wide one- and two-wall intrabony defects and furcation defects, the outcome of EMD alone has been less predictable. The viscous Emdogain gel alone cannot maintain the space and height for the intended amount of regenerated bone fill. Particularly in wide one- and two-wall intrabony defects, the flap will collapse into the defect.

If Emdogain gel and a synthetic alloplastic bone graft particulate (PerioGlas) are mixed (Emdogain gel TS), such defects will be filled, and the soft tissue flap will be supported in the expected position. An alternative to the synthetic alloplastic bone graft could be an autogenous bone graft (for review, see Trombelli and Farina, 2008).

The combination of Emdogain gel TS and resorbable barriers could be even more successful in the treatment of wide one- and two-wall intrabony defects and furcation defects (Araújo and Lindhe, 1998). Under special conditions in extrawide and shallow one- and two-wall intrabony defects, the combination of Emdogain gel and titanium-reinforced nonresorbable barrier tailored as a valve could be the method of choice.

Factors for success

The short- and long-term gains in periodontal support that were achieved in this case series represent the effect of a series of important steps:

- Comprehensive history taking and diagnosis, intensive elimination of the subgingival biofilm and infection, and establishment of excellent gingival plaque control and complete-mouth disinfection before surgery.
- Tailored mini-flap surgery; minimally invasive supplementary mechanical cleaning of the visible exposed root surfaces; chemical cleaning and conditioning of the root surface with EDTA gel; and the application of Emdogain gel.
- Excellent gingival plaque control during the healing phase and the subsequent maintenance program. This is the key to long-term success.
- Cessation of smoking in smokers.
- Supplementary treatment with antibiotics based on analyses of the subgingival microflora, periodontal susceptibility, and general health conditions.

Surgeons who neglect to complete all these steps and just open a flap at infectious sites and apply Emdogain gel to root surfaces that are covered with blood and remaining microbial biofilms will always fail, even if surgery is supplemented with antibiotics.

For the author, routine use of Emdogain, beginning in 1995, represented a paradigm shift in treatment of periodontal intraosseous and furcation defects. Some of the reasons the author prefers Emdogain to the use of barrier membranes are:

- Emdogain is much more user friendly.
- It is more cost effective because four to six sites can be treated with one 0.7-mL syringe at one appointment.
- When the previously discussed presurgical and postsurgical treatment protocols are used in combination with Emdogain gel, at least some gain of periodontal support can always be expected. This has been the author's experience in hundreds of patients treated since 1995.

Therefore, Emdogain gel has been used routinely in every flap surgery for treatment of periodontal defects. So far, no postsurgical complications, such as abscesses, have occurred. Even postsurgical pain has been very limited.

This case series has shown that successful periodontal regeneration can be achieved within 6 months and maintained for many years in teeth with very advanced loss of periodontal support with intraosseous as well as furcation defects. On the other hand, extraction of teeth and subsequent replacement with implants has mushroomed worldwide during the last decade, although patients susceptible to periodontal diseases are at least as susceptible to peri-implantitis. Even if it will take 2 to 10 years for implants to be completely lost because of peri-implantitis, it will take about 10 times more years before natural teeth are lost because of periodontal disease in periodontitis-susceptible patients. Thus, only the top of the peri-implantitis iceberg is visible so far because more than 90% of the implants worldwide have been placed during the last decade.

It must also be observed that several cross sectional, retrospective, and prospective analytical studies have shown a close relationship between periodontal diseases (chronic infectious inflammatory diseases), cardiovascular diseases, and diabetes. Ongoing intervention studies also indicate a causative relationship. Infectious inflamed periodontal tissues around the remaining natural teeth have to be healed before placement of the implant to prevent infection around the implant (peri-implantitis). In addition, patients have to be kept in a maintenance program based on excellent plaque control for optimal long-term outcome of implant treatment. Thus, it seems fair to raise the following provocative question: Should replacement of treatable natural teeth with implants, resulting in peri-implantitis, lost alveolar bone, and possible impaired general health, be regarded as at least maltreatment and possibly a crime?

Outcomes

Intraosseous defects. A systematic review by Trombelli et al (2002) that compared the effect of Emdogain EMD combined with OFD to OFD alone in the treatment of periodontal intraosseous defects was based on RCTs of at least 6 to 8 months' duration. Five studies were selected for review. The weighted mean differences between EMD and OFD were 1.3 mm (95% CI = 0.8, 1.9; $P < .005$) in clinical attachment gain and 1.6 mm (95% CI = 0.6, 2.6; $P < .002$) in probing depth reduction.

A systematic review by Giannobile and Somerman (2003) was based on quasi-randomized clinical trials of at least 6 months' duration. Among the eight studies they reviewed was the pioneer split-mouth multicenter RCT by Heijl et al (1997) in which 33 subjects with paired one- and two-wall osseous defects were treated randomly with either OFD (modified Widman flap) plus EMD or OFD plus a placebo gel. The mean gains in CAL after 36 months were 2.2 mm for OFD plus EMD and 1.7 mm for OFD plus placebo. There was a 2.7-mm gain in the bone level at EMD sites, while the bone level was unchanged at the placebo sites.

A systematic review by Esposito et al (2003) was based on RCTs of 12 months' duration. Ten studies could be evaluated according to their inclusion criteria. The combination of EMD and OFD resulted in a 1.3-mm greater weighted mean gain in CAL (95% CI = 0.8, 1.8) than did OFD alone ($P < .001$) and a 1.0-mm greater reduction in probing depth (95% CI = 0.5, 1.4; $P < .002$).

In a meta-analysis, Heijl and Gestrelius (2001) evaluated the effect of EMD plus OFD in intrabony defects in a total of 10 studies. At the 12- to 14-month reexaminations, a mean 4.4- mm probing depth reduction and a mean 3.5-mm CAL gain had been achieved. A mean gain of 3.5 mm in bone level was confirmed from radiographs or reentry (five studies).

Sanz et al (2004) compared the effect of EMD plus OFD with GTR plus OFD in a multicenter RCT study at 7 centers in 3 countries involving 75 patients. Results at the 1-year follow-up demonstrated mean CAL gains of 3.1 mm for the EMD-treated defects and 2.5 mm for GTR-treated defects ($P < .05$). A statistically significant difference was found also in the incidence of complications (6% for EMD versus 10% for GTR). Furthermore, the multivariate analysis confirmed that there was a significant center effect (2.6 mm) between best and worst treatment outcomes.

Recently Heden and Wennström (2006) showed that the effect of EMD plus OFD achieved after 1 year was not only maintained but improved after 5 years. One year following regenerative surgery, a mean CAL gain of 4.3 mm ($P < .001$), a mean probing depth reduction of 4.9 mm ($P < .001$), and a mean recession reduction of 0.6 mm ($P < .001$) were recorded. At the 5-year follow-up, a further CAL gain of 1.1 mm ($P < .01$), probing depth reduction of 0.3 mm ($P > .05$), and recession reduction of 0.8 mm ($P < .01$) had taken place. Radiographs revealed that the bone defects had been reduced in depth by an average of 2.9 mm at 1 year ($P < .001$). No statistically significant alteration in defect depth was observed between the 1- and 5-year follow-up examinations. The stepwise regression analysis identified the degree of recession and residual probing depth at 1 year as significant predictors of CAL change between 1 and 5 years.

In a split-mouth RCT, Sculean et al (2006) compared the long-term effects of EMD with GTR with bioresorbable barriers in a limited number of patients. Both treatments resulted in gains in CAL at 1 year, and no statistically significant differences in CAL were found between the 1- and 8-year results for either group. Thus it could be concluded that the results achieved after 1 year were maintained in both treatment categories for 8 years.

In a 4-year prospective controlled clinical study, Sculean et al (2007) showed that EMD treatment of intrabony defects resulted in almost 4 mm of CAL gain after 1 year, which was maintained over the 4-year period.

Furcation defects. So far, no RCTs comparing the effect of EMD plus OFD with OFD alone on furcation defects have been published. However, Jepsen et al (2004), Meyle et al (2004), and Hoffman et al (2006) presented the results of a multicenter split-mouth RCT comparing the effect of EMD plus OFD with the effect of GTR (Resolut bioresorbable barrier) plus OFD on grade II buccal mandibular defects.

Both treatment modalities led to significant clinical improvements. The median reduction of open horizontal furcation depth was 2.8 mm with the corresponding interquartile interval (1.5 mm, 3.5 mm) at EMD sites and 1.8 mm (1.0 mm, 2.8 mm) at GTR sites. In patients with poor oral hygiene, EMD resulted in significantly greater reduction in the horizontal defect than GTR. In nonsmokers, EMD treatment also resulted in greater reduction of the horizontal defect than GTR treatment (2.75 mm versus 1.75 mm, respectively [Hoffman et al, 2006]).

Recession defects. In a split-mouth RCT by McGuire and Nunn (2003), the effect of coronally advanced flap in combination with either EMD or connective tissue graft on recession defects was evaluated. The results after 12 months showed that a coronally advanced flap with EMD was superior to the subepithelial connective tissue graft with regard to early healing and patient-reported discomfort. No significant difference in the amount of root coverage was found between the EMD and connective tissue graft sites. On average, a gain of 4.5 mm of tissue coverage on the previously exposed root surfaces was achieved with both treatment groups.

In a more recent RCT, Castellanos et al (2006) compared the effect of a coronally advanced flap plus EMD with a coronally advanced flap alone in class II recessions larger than 2 mm. After 12 months, vertical recession was reduced from 2.68 ± 1.63 mm to 0.36 ± 0.60 mm in the EMD group and from 2.31 ± 1.52 mm to 0.90 ± 0.95 mm in the coronally advanced flap group.

Spahr et al (2005) compared the long-term effect of coronally advanced flaps used in conjunction with EMD to that of coronally advanced flaps alone on Miller class I and II recession defects. Complete root coverage was maintained over 2 years in 53% of the EMD sites but in only 23% of the coronally advanced flap sites. A total of 47% of treated recessions in the flap-only group deteriorated again in the second year after therapy, compared to 22% in the EMD group.

Thus, coronally advanced flaps used in combination with EMD seemed to result in better long-term stability than coronally advanced flaps

alone. The reason may be that coronally advanced flaps never will result in regeneration with new cementum and inserting principle fibers covering the entire defect. At best, such coverage will take place in the most apical part of the defect, while the majority of the defect will be covered via connective tissue adhesion and epithelial downgrowth. In contrast, McGuire and Cochran (2003) demonstrated histologic evidence in humans of new cementum formation with inserting periodontal ligament fibers and some bone formation after treatment with coronally advanced flaps and EMD (for review, see Cairo et al, 2008).

Heterogeneity of outcomes. Similar to outcomes of GTR treatment, the outcomes of EMD regenerative therapy reported in different controlled studies also exhibit a large range. In a systematic review by Giannobile and Somerman (2003), the mean gain in CAL ranged from 2.2 to 4.8 mm among 8 RCTs. In a meta-analysis of multicenter RCTs, Tonetti et al (2002) reported that the mean gain in CAL achieved at 10 specialist centers in 7 different countries was 3.1 mm. However, the difference in gain between the best-performing center and the worst-performing center was more than fourfold higher than the effect achieved by application of EMD. In a meta-analysis of 12 controlled studies, the mean gain in CAL was 3.2 mm, but the results ranged from 1.7 to 4.5 mm (Kalpidis and Ruben, 2002).

These variations are influenced by the same factors that affect the outcomes of GTR therapy: patients factors, defect factors, professional presurgical treatment, EMD plus surgical procedures, professional postsurgical treatment, and study design. For example, a recent meta-analysis of RCTs showed that the initial gain of CAL after EMD treatment is not temporary, as it is in randomized controls receiving OFD (Tu et al, 2008). Therefore, only the long-term effect in RCT studies should be considered relevant. However, there are some important differences between the surgical procedures for GTR and EMD.

GTR-specific considerations.

- Selection and trimming of barrier membranes are time consuming. As a consequence, only one or two barriers are usually placed during an appointment. Patients with several sites selected for regenerative therapy need more appointments.

- Because of postsurgical pain and discomfort, the total treatment time for the patients with several treated sites has to be expanded to some weeks, which also may limit systemic use of antibiotics during all the surgeries.
- Nonresorbable barriers require two surgical procedures, increasing the risk of bacterial contamination of the barrier and the newly regenerating tissues.
- The barrier may be exposed because of gingival recession, which may allow epithelial downgrowth, pocket formation, and bacterial disturbance of the wound healing.
- The trimmed barrier will not only cover the defect completely but also extend at least 3 mm on the bone beyond the defect margins after placement. Therefore, a flap larger than the barrier has to be raised for a complete coverage.
- The titanium-reinforced nonresorbable barrier is an excellent space holder for wide defects.
- Correctly selected and trimmed barriers in combination with tailored flap surgery will favor blood clot and wound stabilization.
- Topical antibiotics can be applied during the flap surgery.
- Barriers may be loaded with antiseptics (CHX) or antibiotics.

EMD-specific considerations.

- Several sites may be treated at the same appointment, and three to six sites can be treated with only one 0.7-mL syringe of Emdogain gel. Therefore, most treatments can be finished at a single appointment.
- Use of as small a mini-flap as possible is recommended to optimally enclose the gel in the defect and minimize the wound trauma.
- The effect of the gel is strongly correlated to the accessibility. Therefore, presurgical healing of the periodontal tissues and complete removal of the granulation tissue are very important to prevent bleeding and to allow chemical conditioning of the root surface (removal of debris).

Growth factors

Periodontal tissue engineering with growth factors applies advances in materials science and biology to regenerate alveolar bone, periodontal ligament, and cementum. The following growth factors may be of interest for periodontal regenerative therapy after meta-analyses of well-designed multicenter RCTs are conducted to ensure efficacy and safety:

- Transforming growth factor β (TGF-β) and particularly the bone morphogenetic proteins (BMPs), BMP-2 and BMP-7
- Fibroblast growth factors (FGFs)
- Platelet-derived growth factors (PDGFs)
- Insulin-like growth factors (IGFs)

Bone morphogenetic proteins

BMPs have shown potent effects in stimulating periodontal tissue repair in several experimental animal model systems (King et al, 1997; Kinoshita et al, 1997; Sigurdsson et al, 1995). In most of these studies of large, critical-sized alveolar bone defects, bone and cementum were predictably regenerated. Bowers et al (1991) demonstrated significant periodontal regeneration in humans after the use of DFDBA plus a partially purified extract of BMP (osteogenin, also called *BMP-3*). Pinpoint ankylosis was noted on submerged roots treated with DFDBA plus osteogenin.

Human trials using recombinant molecules have been completed to examine the efficacy of BMP-2 or BMP-7 for regeneration of chronic periodontitis lesions (from Genetics Institute and Stryker Biotech, respectively). To date, no local or systemic safety concerns have been noted in humans after local application of BMP-2 or BMP-7 in periodontal osseous defects.

Additional human clinical and histologic reports are needed to more fully elucidate the potential value and applicability of these agents in periodontal regeneration. The delivery system for growth factors may play a role in regenerative response. Of particular interest are surface area, surface properties for cell-surface interaction, inflammatory and immune reactions, and degradation kinetics. Reported delivery systems are collagen in sponge, membrane, gel, and gelatin forms. Bone and cementum formation occur in different time spans in animal models. This factor has to be considered during the drug delivery.

The degradation kinetics of bioresorbable carriers seems to influence the type of new tissue formation. A fast degradation and relapse of BMP-2–induced bone formation is significantly greater with slow-degrading and slow-releasing BMP gelatin carriers. Whether these findings apply to humans in an inflamed environment is unknown.

Fibroblast growth factors

FGFs are a family of structurally related polypeptides that are known to play a critical role in angiogenesis and mesenchymal cell mitogenesis. In normal adult tissues, the most abundant proteins are FGF-1 and FGF-2. FGF-2 is expressed by osteoblasts and is generally more potent than FGF-1.

The basic FGF (bFGF or FGF-2) is a member of a heparin-binding family that possesses potent angiogenic properties. FGF-2 is mitogenic and chemotactic for endothelial cells, fibroblasts, and periodontally derived cells. Among other origins, bFGFs are synthesized by inflammatory cells and are stored in the extracellular matrix by binding to heparin sulfate proteoglycans.

FGF-2 has been extensively studied for its role in dermal wound healing in both preclinical and human clinical trials. More recently, experimental animal periodontal models revealed a potential benefit of FGF-2 for closure of grade III furcations or for the regeneration of intrabony defects (Murakami et al, 1999; Rossa et al, 2000; Takayama et al, 2001). However, no human studies have been carried out so far.

Platelet-derived growth factors

PDGF is composed of two polypeptide chains and can exist in three different isoforms of two gene products (PDGF-AA, PDGF-BB, and PDGF-AB). There are two different PDGF receptors: PDGF-Rα (binds PDGF-AA, PDGF-BB, and PDGF-AB) and PDGF-Rβ (binds PDGF-BB and PDGF-AB). The capacity of certain cells to respond to these PDGFs depends on the presence of these specific α or β receptors on the cells.

PDGF has been isolated from a variety of cells and tissues, including monocytes, macrophages, fibroblasts, endothelial cells, and bone matrix. PDGF stimulates cells of mesenchymal origin, such as fibroblasts, glia, smooth muscle, and bone cells. PDGF has been identified as a competent growth factor and acts synergistically with progression growth factors, such as the IGFs. PDGF, however, also acts as a paracrine factor by stimulating certain cells to produce their own progression growth factors.

PDGF-BB is the most potent stimulator of mitogenesis, followed by PDGF-AA and PDGF-AB. PDGF-BB is twice as potent as PDGF-AA as a chemoattractant for connective tissue cells and promotes periodontal regeneration.

In animal experiments, GTR supplemented with PDGF has resulted in significantly greater regeneration of furcation defects than GTR alone (Cho et al, 1995; Park et al, 1995). Most interestingly, a large multicenter study involving 180 patients has been reported (Nevins et al, 2005). In that study, recombinant human PDGF-BB, with a β-tricalcium phosphate carrier, resulted in improved bone fill and enhanced rate of clinical attachment gain compared with carrier-only controls. This is probably the first large study in humans to assess the role of recombinant growth factor therapy, and these interesting results will need further evaluation over time (Reynolds and Aichelmann-Reidy, 2005).

Insulin-like growth factors

IGFs are a family of single-chain serum proteins that share 49% homology in sequence with proinsulin. IGF-1 and IGF-2 are two polypeptides from this group that have been well described. They are synthesized by multiple tissues, including liver, smooth muscle, and placenta, and are carried in plasma as a complex with specific binding proteins. These binding proteins may positively or negatively affect the biologic activities of IGF. IGFs and their receptors can also be locally produced by osteoblasts.

IGFs have a spectrum of activities similar to that of insulin. IGF-1 acts as progression factor.

IGFs have been shown to stimulate bone formation and to have a mitogenic effect on periodontal ligament cells. It is believed that PDGF and IGF-1 have a synergistic effect and that IGF-1 alone does not enhance bone repair.

The synergistic potential for periodontal regeneration by combination of PDGF and IGF has been shown in animal experiments and a few human studies. Lynch et al (1989, 1991) examined the effect of placing a combination of PDGFs and IGFs in naturally occurring periodontal defects in dogs. The control sites treated without growth factors healed with a long junctional epithelium and no new cementum or bone formation, while regeneration of a periodontal attachment apparatus occurred at the sites treated with growth factors. Similar results were reported by other investigators following application of a combination of PDGF and IGF in experimentally induced periodontal lesions in monkeys (Giannobile et al, 1996; Rutherford et al, 1993). One study examined the effect of PDGF and IGF in periodontal intrabony defects and grade II furcation involvements in humans (Howell et al, 1997). At reentry after 9 months, significantly increased bone fill was observed only at the furcation sites that had been treated with growth factors.

Outcomes

Because limited human clinical data are available, more studies will be needed to fully evaluate the potential of growth factors for enhancing periodontal regeneration (for review, see Giannobile and Somerman, 2003; Hughes et al, 2006).

Conclusions

The optimal goal after successful healing of infectious inflamed periodontal tissues is regeneration of all lost periodontal tissues (alveolar bone, periodontal ligament, and root cementum). At best, traditional periodontal treatment, whether nonsurgical or surgical, will result in *repair* of lost periodontal support: bone fill of periodontal osseous defects and formation of a long junctional epithelium attachment between the new alveolar bone and the root surface.

True regeneration, or formation of new acellular cementum and periodontal ligament with principal fibers that insert into the new root cementum as well as new alveolar bone, can only be confirmed by histologic analysis, which is impossible in clinical practice. On the other hand, animal studies and some human case reports have shown that true regeneration of lost periodontal tissues is possible by implementation of special regenerative methods and materials. During the last two decades, three different methods have been used alone or in combination for periodontal regeneration therapy: bone replacement grafts, barrier membranes for GTR, and EMD gels. Recently, some growth factors have been introduced for clinical use in humans after several animal experimental studies. All these materials are placed during open flap surgery and debridement.

Generally, all bone replacement grafts increase bone level and CAL better than OFD alone. However, this observation in reality means only bone fill and repair. Autografts and demineralized freeze-dried bone allografts may result in some regeneration, but the outcomes are not predictable (for review, see Reynolds et al, 2003; Trombelli et al, 2002).

Systematic reviews and meta-analyses of RCTs have shown that successful regenerative therapy can be achieved in two- and three-wall intrabony and mandibular grade II furcation defects. After removal of the barrier membrane and completion of healing, histologic evaluations in animals as well as humans have indicated that GTR procedures resulted in regeneration of new root cementum, periodontal ligament, and alveolar bone. Histologic analyses in animals as well as in humans have shown that regenerative therapy with EMD results in true periodontal regeneration. However, great variation has been observed in the clinical outcomes reported in different studies. To overcome this heterogeneity, all the steps—from patient selection and education in self-care to defect selection, presurgical professional treatment, regenerative surgical procedures, and postsurgical maintenance care—have to be of the highest quality because the outcome represents the sum of all these steps. The following are current recommendations for successful periodontal regenerative therapy:

- Patient selection: Well-motivated nonsmokers in good general health might represent the best prognosis.
- Defect selection: Narrow two- and three-wall intraosseous defects and mandibular grade II furcation defects are preferable.
- Professional presurgical treatment:
  - Needs-related oral hygiene habits based on self-diagnosis are established (for details, see Axelsson, 2004).
  - Comprehensive presurgical minimally invasive scaling, root planing, and debridement are supplemented with bactericidal irrigation with iodine solution.
  - PMTC is performed at needs-related intervals.
  - Subgingival microbiologic analysis and antibiotic sensitivity tests are performed for the sites scheduled for regenerative therapy.
  - Beginning 1 week presurgically, so-called complete-mouth disinfection is performed including PMTC, tongue scraping, subgingival debridement and irrigation, and twice-daily mouthrinsing with 0.2% CHX solution.
  - Antibiotics are administered systemically (amoxicillin, 375 mg, and metronidazole, 250 or 400 mg, three times daily for 10 days, starting 2 days presurgically) depending on the outcome of the microbiologic tests and the general health of the patient. An alternative could be topical use of a controlled slow-release antibiotic (doxycycline) 1 week presurgically.
- Regenerative surgical treatment:
  - Tailored mini-flap surgery is used.
  - All granulation tissues are eliminated.
  - Supplementary debridement is performed with minimally invasive and safe instrumentation to prevent iatrogenic removal of root cementum.
  - Debris is removed, and the root surface is conditioned with EDTA gel for 2 minutes.
  - Defect sites are irrigated with saline solution and dried.
  - In narrow two- and three-wall intraosseous defects, EMD gel is applied by itself.

- In wide intraosseous defects and furcation defects, Emdogain TS gel can be used alone or in combination with a trimmed bioresorbable barrier membrane.
  - The flaps are coronally repositioned and sutured for complete closure of the defect and stabilization of the wound and blood clot.
  - Supplementary EMD gel is applied in the sulcus and over the incision wounds.
- Professional postsurgical treatment:
  - Administration of four ibuprofen (analgesic and anti-inflammatory) tablets is recommended over the first 36 hours postsurgery.
  - The patient should rinse twice a day with 0.2% CHX solution for the first 6 weeks postsurgery.
  - The patient can begin cautious mechanical cleaning with an extrasoft toothbrush on the treated teeth 2 to 3 days postsurgery.
  - The clinician should perform cautious PMTC combined with application of iodine solution once a week for the first 4 weeks postsurgery. A schedule of regular PMTC once a month is recommended for the subsequent 5 to 6 months.
  - The sutures are removed 2 weeks postsurgery.
  - The first clinical and radiographic reexaminations are not recommended until 6 months postsurgery.
- The patient is maintained with needs-related intervals of supportive care and reexaminations (three to six times per year).

GTR and EMD seem to result in similar gain in CAL and reduction in probing depth in RCTs with 6 to 12 months' duration. So far, no long-term RCTs comparing GTR, EMD, and OFD have been carried out and thus no meta-analyses or systematic reviews are possible. Experimental histologic studies have shown that EMD may result in true regeneration of periodontal tissues with alveolar bone, acellular root cement, and principal fibers inserting into the root cementum as well as the alveolar bone, while GTR results in cellular root cementum. This observation may favor the long-term outcome of EMD over that of GTR.

In addition, EMD is a biomaterial with some specific characteristics that may enhance true periodontal regeneration:

- It increases migration of periodontal ligament cells, osteoblasts, gingival fibroblasts, and dermal fibroblasts.
- It increases cell proliferation.
- It suppresses the downgrowth of junctional epithelium onto root surfaces.
- It acts as a multipurpose growth factor stimulating the proliferation of mesenchymal cells while inhibiting cell division of epithelial cells.
- It contains TGF–β1.
- It expresses BMPs, which may enhance cementum as well as bone formation.
- It increases the attraction of periodontal ligament cells, cementoblasts, and fibroblasts to the root surface.
- It has antimicrobial effects on periopathogens.

In the near future, even grade III furcation defects, one-wall intraosseous defects, and suprabony defects with horizontal loss of periodontal tissues may be successfully regenerated by optimal combinations of:

- Root surface conditioning with EDTA followed by application of fibronectin, to enhance cellular attachment, and application of Emdogain gel.
- Three-dimensional scaffolds with appropriate cells or instruction messages (eg, growth factors and matrix-attachment factors). In particular, the combination of PDGFs and IGFs seems to have a synergistic enhancing effect on periodontal regeneration.
- Tailored barrier membranes loaded with antiseptics or antibiotics as space holders.

In addition, more advanced tissue engineering, including use of stem cells and nanotechniques, is waiting around the corner. For example, to regenerate both periodontal ligament and alveolar bone, the possibility exists of bilaterally seeding periodontal ligament cells on one side of a bioscaffold and osteoblasts on the opposite side. In a similar vein, a periodontal ligament–like matrix could be engineered from periodontal ligament fibroblasts; one side would then be seeded with cementoblasts and the opposite side seeded with osteoblasts. With such an approach, it might be possible to fully reconstitute various compartments of the periodontium in vitro and then implant such constructs into periodontal defects.

Advances in nanotechnology will also undoubtedly allow the synthesis of materials with desirable nanoscale structures. Nanotechnology is the science of engineering at the individual molecular level to produce materials with hitherto unthought-of properties. Already, self-assembly systems that simulate many features of the extracellular matrix have been described and fabricated (for reviews on periodontal regenerative therapy, see Al-Hamdan et al, 2003; Bartold et al, 2006; Cortellini and Tonetti, 2008; Giannobile and Somerman, 2003; Hughes et al, 2006; Hwang and Wang, 2006; Jepsen et al, 2002; Karring and Lindhe, 2008; Murphy and Gunsolley, 2003; Needleman et al, 2005; Polimeni et al, 2006; Reynolds et al, 2003; Sculean et al, 2008; Srisuwan et al, 2006; Trombelli, 2005; Trombelli et al, 2002; Wang et al, 2005; Zeichner-David, 2006).

CHAPTER 5

NEEDS-RELATED PERIODONTAL PREVENTIVE AND MAINTENANCE CARE

Prevention and control of periodontal diseases may be primary, secondary, or tertiary. The aim of primary prevention programs is to prevent the initiation and development of periodontal diseases. Primary prevention should be targeted toward populations with healthy periodontal tissues. Secondary prevention is aimed at preventing the recurrence of disease after successful treatment and is achieved through supportive (maintenance) care programs. Tertiary prevention is the elimination of disease through treatment, usually using nonsurgical or surgical periodontal treatment methods.

Worldwide, only a small percentage of young adults, adults, and particularly the elderly have had no experience of periodontal diseases. Thus, about 80% to 90% of the world's population will require secondary and/or tertiary preventive programs. However, the ratio between tertiary and secondary levels of prevention varies greatly among different countries, age groups, and individuals.

PRIMARY PREVENTION

If efficient primary prevention is established in young children, neither secondary nor tertiary prevention should be necessary during adulthood. This assertion is supported by the experience of my daughter, Eva, aged 47 years (Figs 243a and 243b), and my son, Torbjörn, aged 44 years (Figs 244a and 244b), who are caries and gingivitis free, despite the fact that both of their parents had caries lesions before adulthood.

Large-scale implementation of a needs-related preventive program for 1- to 19-year-old residents in the county of Värmland, Sweden, has resulted in a dramatic reduction of caries prevalence and excellent periodontal health. The goals for the subjects following the program from the age of 1 to 19 years were to:

- Have no approximal restorations
- Have no occlusal amalgam restorations
- Have no approximal loss of periodontal attachment
- Motivate and encourage individuals to assume responsibility for their own oral health

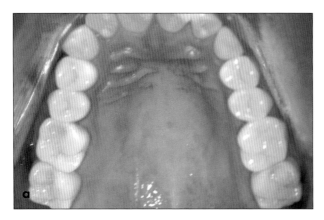
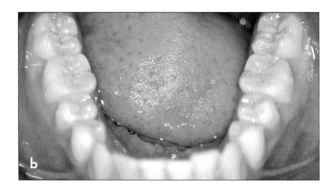

Figs 243a and 243b Dentition of a 47-year-old woman who is caries-free and exhibits excellent periodontal health.

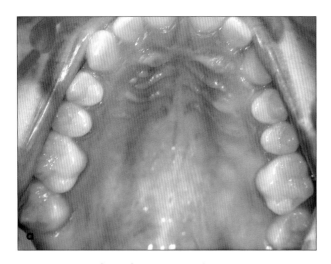
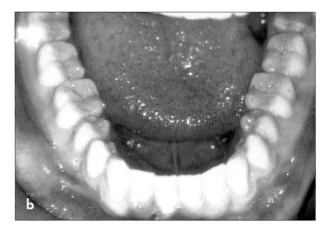

Figs 244a and 244b Dentition of a 44-year-old man who is caries-free with excellent periodontal health.

Most of the individualized preventive program was carried out by specially trained dental hygienists or dental assistants at clinics in the elementary schools. Since 1979, the effect of the program has been evaluated with a computer-aided epidemiologic program once every year for almost 100% of all 3- to 19-year-old participants.

Nearly 100% of the stated goals have been achieved, and results continue to improve. Caries prevalence in 19 year olds was reduced from more than 24 decayed or filled surfaces (DFSs) in 1979 to only 2 DFSs in 1999 (Axelsson, et al, 2004). On average, there was only 1 approximal DFS in 1999, and less than 1 was filled because the goal was for noncavitated dentin caries lesions diag-

nosed on bitewing radiographs to be arrested by "prevention instead of extension" or at least "prevention before extension."

Needs-related self-care habits based on self-diagnosis were established as early as possible. In addition, professional mechanical toothcleaning (PMTC) and chemical plaque control were provided for at-risk individuals at needs-related intervals. As a consequence, approximal loss of periodontal attachment was prevented. Thus, the goals set in 1979 were largely achieved by 1999 (Axelsson, 2004).

In addition, it seems realistic to anticipate that 20 year olds who have no lost teeth, only 2 DFSs, no loss of periodontal attachment, and well-established excellent self-care habits should maintain at least 25 healthy natural teeth for the rest of their life. This assumption has already been proven in a 30-year longitudinal study in adults; the 51- to 65- and 66- to 80-year-old participants in a needs-related preventive and supportive care program performed by dental hygienists lost, on average, only 0.4 and 0.7 teeth, respectively; experienced no periodontal attachment loss; and developed only 2 new decayed surfaces (DSs) per subject over 30 years (Axelsson et al, 2004).

Because of the implementation of continuous clinical research to improve and test new preventive materials and methods, the application of methods to predict risk for oral diseases, the adoption of new knowledge from other researchers, and the continued education of well-trained and highly motivated dental professionals, it seems reasonable to believe that the oral health of children and young adults in Sweden can be improved even further and at an even lower cost. However, the clinical evaluation of new methods, as well as the reevaluation of established methods, in the relevant population is essential before large-scale implementation, to avoid the hazards of direct implementation from animal and in vitro experiments. There are certain generally applicable methods, but preventive measures should be tailored to reflect trends in the pattern of dental disease in a specific population (for details on the aforementioned preventive programs for children and young adults, see chapter 7 in volume 4 of this series [Axelsson, 2004]).

SECONDARY AND TERTIARY PREVENTION

Goals

Secondary prevention is the method of choice in the adult population after initial cause-related treatment (tertiary prevention) because the majority of adults currently have or have experienced chronic periodontitis at some tooth sites. A minority (5% to 10%) of patients are estimated to be particularly susceptible to periodontal diseases and may exhibit aggressive periodontitis. Because adults represent more than two-thirds of the world's population, the importance of efficient secondary prevention of periodontal diseases cannot be overestimated.

The main objective of secondary prevention of periodontal diseases is to prevent recurrence of disease through a combination of self-care and professional preventive measures after initial cause-related therapy (tertiary prevention), including both nonsurgical and surgical treatment. The American Academy of Periodontology (Cohen, 2003) has recommended that periodontal secondary prevention, formerly referred to as *supportive periodontal therapy*, be termed *periodontal maintenance* (PM). PM should include an update of the patient's medical and dental histories, examination, radiographic review, evaluation of the patient's oral hygiene performance, periodontal evaluation, and risk assessment. In addition, supragingival and subgingival removal of bacterial plaque and calculus and re-treatment of disease must be performed when indicated. The therapeutic goals of PM are to:

- Prevent or minimize the recurrence and progression of periodontal disease in patients who have been previously treated for periodontitis, peri-implantitis, or some types of gingivitis (eg, drug-induced gingival diseases, gingivitis modified by systemic factors, hereditary gingival fibromatosis)
- Prevent or reduce the incidence of tooth or implant loss by monitoring the dentition and any prosthetic replacement of natural teeth
- Increase the probability that other conditions or diseases found within the oral cavity will be located and treated in a timely manner

Once initial cause-related therapy has been successfully completed, it is critical that the clinician consider risk factors for the recurrence of periodontitis and prescribe adequate treatments and intervals of treatment to fulfill the goals of PM.

The following case demonstrates the extreme need for secondary as well as tertiary prevention of periodontal disease. Figure 245a shows complete-mouth radiographs of a 50-year-old man in 1969.

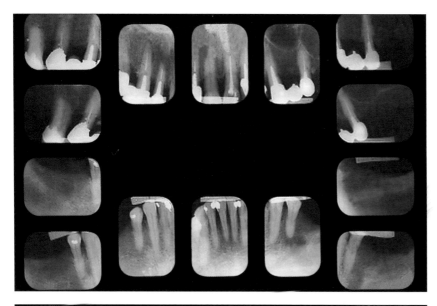

Fig 245a Complete-mouth radiographs of a 50-year-old man in 1969. The patient had undergone gingivectomy in all quadrants.

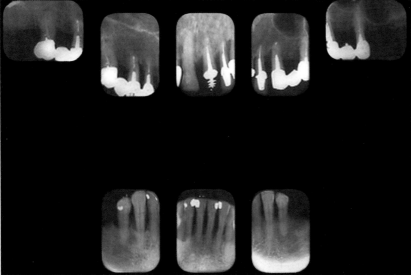

Fig 245b Same patient, exhibiting dramatic postoperative loss of alveolar bone, particularly at the maxillary left anterior teeth and the mandibular teeth, 3 years after surgery (1972). He had not been provided with any postoperative program to maintain plaque control.

While under the care of a general practitioner, the patient had undergone gingivectomy of all quadrants because of generalized pocketing of greater than 3 mm. He was enrolled in no postoperative maintenance program for gingival plaque control. In addition, the patient developed polyarthritis, for which anti-inflammatory drugs were prescribed.

Three years later (1972), complete-mouth radiographs showed dramatic postoperative loss of alveolar bone, particularly at the maxillary left anterior teeth and the mandibular teeth (Fig 245b). In the absence of preoperative and postoperative gingival plaque control programs, periodontal surgery will accelerate loss of periodontal support (Nyman et al, 1977).

In 1972, after detailed examination followed by education in comprehensive self-care and self-diagnosis, the patient received an initial, thorough nonsurgical scaling, root planing, debridement, and repeated PMTC. The effect of this initial treatment was evaluated after 1 month. A supplementary modified Widman flap surgery was then performed from the maxillary right central incisor to the left second premolar; this was combined with apicoectomy and retrograde root filling of the left canine, which had a periapical lesion and a mesiopalatal marginal-apical communication. At the same session, the maxillary right second premolar was extracted because of root fracture and marginal-apical communication.

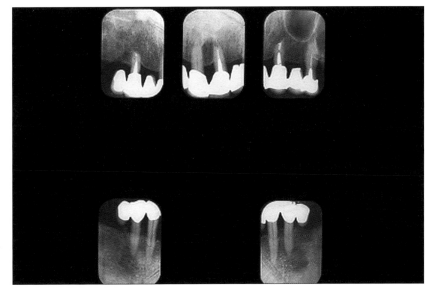

Fig 245c Same patient in 1985, 13 years after a second round of periodontal surgery and restoration of the dentition. This time, the patient was provided with a rigorous maintenance program to ensure excellent gingival plaque control.

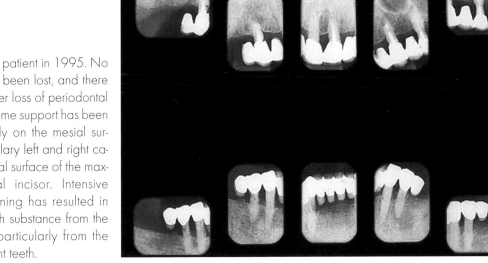

Fig 245d Same patient in 1995. No further teeth have been lost, and there has been no further loss of periodontal support. In fact, some support has been gained, especially on the mesial surfaces of the maxillary left and right canines and the distal surface of the maxillary left central incisor. Intensive mechanical cleaning has resulted in some loss of tooth substance from the exposed roots, particularly from the maxillary abutment teeth.

After a 2-month healing period, including excellent gingival plaque control by self-care (0.2% chlorhexidine [CHX] mouthrinse twice a day for 2 weeks and mechanical cleaning) and PMTC once every 2 weeks, the maxillary lateral incisors and the four mandibular incisors were extracted and provisional fixed partial dentures were made. Three months later, maxillary and mandibular fixed prostheses were made on the following abutments: the maxillary right central incisor and canine; the maxillary left central incisor, canine, and second premolar; the mandibular right canine and first premolar; and the mandibular left canine and first premolar.

Figures 245c and 245d show complete-mouth radiographs after 13 (1985) and 23 (1995) years, respectively. Excellent gingival plaque control was achieved by a maintenance program comprising self-care supplemented by PMTC and debridement at needs-related intervals. No further teeth were lost, nor was there any further loss of periodontal support. The radiographs show some gain of support, notably on the mesial surfaces of the maxillary left and right canines and the distal surface of the maxillary left central incisor. After 23 years of intensive mechanical cleaning by self-care, there had been some iatrogenic loss of tooth substance from the exposed roots, particularly from the maxillary abutment teeth.

Longitudinal studies of effectiveness

Longitudinal clinical studies have shown that gingival plaque control by self-care and supportive care based on frequent PMTC and needs-related subgingival debridement in patients with periodontal disease will result in reduction of probing depth; maintenance or gain of clinical attachment level; reduction of quantities of subgingival microflora; reduction of the range of subgingival periopathogenic microflora; improvement in the healing of periodontal soft tissues as well as intrabony pockets after periodontal surgery and regenerative therapy; and prevention of recurrent periodontal disease. Longitudinal clinical studies have also shown that supportive care performed by dental hygienists can prevent the recurrence of periodontitis as well as dental caries in adults because these strategies target the causes of the diseases. The range of effects reported in different clinical studies is strongly correlated to the materials and methods used, the sample size, and the incidence of the disease in the population. When needs-related plaque control habits for self-care are established and supplemented by needs-related intervals of PMTC, significant preventive effects are achieved, particularly in high-risk individuals, compared with a matched control group (for review, see Axelsson, 1994, 1998, 2004; Baehni and Tessier, 1994; Garmyn et al, 1998; Gaunt et al, 2008; Lang et al, 2008; Renvert and Persson, 2004).

The overall goals for maintenance programs in randomized samples of adults should be to prevent tooth loss and the recurrence of dental caries and periodontitis after initial active treatment of the diseases, ie, secondary prevention and control. However, for cost effectiveness, such programs must be based strictly on individual needs. For example, in a longitudinal study of 75 patients with extremely advanced periodontitis who had been successfully treated for the disease through initial cause-related therapy and modified Widman flap procedures (Lindhe and Nyman, 1984), recurrent infection occurred in only very few sites during a 14-year period of effective supportive periodontal treatment. Recurrent periodontitis was observed at completely unpredictable time intervals but was concentrated in about 25% of the patient population (15 of 61 patients). This suggests that, in a periodontitis-susceptible population, the majority of patients can be "cured" provided that optimally organized PM is performed, while a relatively small proportion of patients (20% to 25%) will suffer from occasional episodes of recurrent periodontal reinfection. It is obviously a challenge for the diagnostician to identify such patients with very high disease susceptibility and to monitor their dentitions for recurrent periodontitis on a long-term basis.

Microbiology has been used to determine the frequency of recalls. A longitudinal study examined treated periodontitis patients on two different maintenance program schedules. The control schedule was standard and consisted of recall every 3 months with professional prophylaxis. The experimental group followed the same program; however, the decision for active prophylaxis was determined by the outcome of subgingival plaque analysis. The results showed that in the experimental group, PM intervals could be increased from an average of 4.5 months after 1 year to 20.1 months after 4 years (Listgarten and Schifter, 1982; Listgarten et al, 1986). The researchers concluded that recalls every 3 months may not be adequate for all patients, and that some patients may still do well even with longer intervals.

The intervals of PM in test groups in most studies have been three to four times per year or even more frequent, irrespective of the individual patient's needs. Even for subjects with high susceptibility for periodontal disease, this frequent interval seems to be efficient. However, for subjects with low susceptibility and a high standard of gingival plaque control by self-care, three to four sessions of PM per year should be regarded as overtreatment. From a cost-effectiveness point of view, the materials, methods, and intervals for PM must be based on the individual's needs.

Few studies have compared the impact of different recall intervals. However, Rosén et al (1999) studied the effects of 3-, 6-, 12-, and 18-month intervals between supportive recall treatments. With the exception of a trend of some rebounding at sites that initially were 6.0 mm or greater and attachment loss at molar sites with furcation involvement in the 18-month recall group, no differences were found between the groups. The results suggest that recall intervals could be extended to at least 1 year in subjects with a history of limited susceptibility to periodontitis (for review on PM, see Cohen, 2003; Gaunt et al, 2008; Knowles et al, 1979, 1980; Lang et al, 2008; Mousquès et al, 1980; Ramfjord et al, 1968, 1975, 1982, 1987; Renvert and Persson, 2004; Westfelt et al, 1983a, 1983b).

There are very few longitudinal clinical studies in adults on the prevention of recurrence of both periodontal disease and dental caries. From 1971 to 1972, a clinical study was initiated in the city of Karlstad, in the county of Värmland, Sweden, to determine whether the development of caries and the progression of periodontitis could be prevented in adults and whether a high level of mechanical plaque control could be maintained by regularly repeated self-care education based on self-diagnosis, PMTC, and needs-related subgingival debridement. An attempt was also made to study the progression of dental disease in individuals who did not receive special self-care education but who regularly received conventional dental care.

Two groups of subjects from the same region were recruited for the study and assigned to test groups or control groups, stratified by age. During the first 6-year period, the control patients were examined regularly once a year with conventional dental care. After initial scaling and root planing (see chapter 1), the test group participants were recalled every second month during the first 2 years and once every third month during the following 4 years of the study for education in self-care, PMTC, and needs-related subgingival debridement by a dental hygienist.

The subjects were reexamined toward the end of the third and sixth years of the study. After 6 years, the number of new carious surfaces per subject was 14.0 in the control groups and only 0.2 in the test groups. On average, patients in the control groups lost 1.2 mm of periodontal attachment during the 6-year period, while those in the test groups had an average gain of 0.2 mm. It is important to note, however, that most of the subjects and sites in the control groups lost no or only very limited amounts of periodontal attachment, while some high-risk patients and sites lost considerably more periodontal attachment compared with the average.

After the 6-year reexamination, the control groups were disbanded: For ethical reasons, these subjects were also offered needs-related preventive programs, and most accepted. The few subjects in the test groups who developed new caries lesions and/or lost periodontal attachment during the 6-year period were classified as high-risk or at-risk individuals for caries and/or periodontitis.

During the following years, up to the 15- and 30-year reexaminations, all subjects in the test groups received a needs-related maintenance program from the same dental hygienist. To ensure maximum cost effectiveness, the recall intervals, as well as the preventive measures used, were based strictly on individual need. At the 15- and 30-year reexaminations, 317 and 257, respectively, of the original 375 test subjects from the baseline examination in 1972 were available for re-examination. Fewer than 10 subjects were unwilling to continue in the study, confirming high patient acceptance of the maintenance program. Only 0.2 teeth per individual were lost over 15 years (Axelsson et al, 1987a). During the same period, it was estimated that the randomized samples of the Swedish adult population lost, on average, 3.0 teeth per individual (Håkansson, 1991). From 1978 until 1987, the total cost per individual per year in the test groups was approximately 50% of the cost per Swedish adult recall patient.

At 30 years, except for a mean loss of 0.2 mm on the buccal surfaces in one age group as an iatrogenic effect of frequent mechanical cleaning, there was no marked change in probing attachment level on the buccal and lingual surfaces; on the approximal surfaces, in contrast, gains ranging from 0.3 to 0.4 mm were recorded in the study groups (Axelsson et al, 2004). Most likely, several approximal intrabony pockets at baseline had been "repaired" during the study. Although there was an overall gain of attachment in the sample, further attachment loss of 2.0 mm or more had occurred on a few of the sites (2% to 8%), mainly buccally, as an iatrogenic effect. For comparison, the annual mean loss of periodontal support was 0.1 mm in an 11-year (Håkansson, 1991) and two 20-year (Hugoson and Laurell, 2000; Jansson et al, 2002) longitudinal studies of Swedish adults—that is, an average 3.0-mm loss of periodontal support over 30 years.

The results of this study showed that a well-trained dental hygienist, supervised by a dentist and using established professional preventive

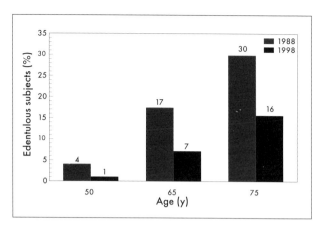

Fig 246a Percentage of edentulous 50-, 65-, and 75-year-old subjects in the county of Värmland, Sweden, in 1988 and 1998. (From Axelsson et al, 2000. Reprinted with permission.)

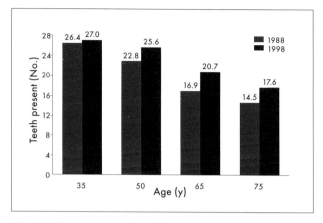

Fig 246b Mean number of teeth (excluding third molars) by age group in 1988 and 1998. (From Axelsson et al, 2000. Reprinted with permission.)

measures (eg, PMTC) to complement improved self-care, was able to prevent further loss of periodontal attachment and reduce the development of new caries lesions to fewer than 2 carious surfaces per subject over 30 years, irrespective of age. It was also shown that excellent self-care habits, including self-diagnosis, can be successfully established in adults; age does not matter. At the 30-year reexamination, 92% of the subjects brushed their teeth twice or more daily and 8% brushed either in the morning or before going to bed. In addition, 70% used toothpicks daily, 44% used dental tape daily, and 35% used interdental brushes daily. In addition, the percentage of smokers was reduced from 46% in 1972 to 10% in 2002.

Experience gained from this study is applied in the 2-year training program for dental hygienists at the University of Karlstad, Sweden, and in preventive programs for adults at the public dental health clinics and private dental practices in the county of Värmland, which has the highest ratio of dental hygienists per dentist (1:1) in Sweden. As a consequence, dental health status has improved considerably in the adult population, as shown in analytical epidemiologic studies in randomized samples of 35-, 50-, 65-, and 75-year-olds in 1988 and 1998 (Axelsson et al, 2000). The percentage of edentulous 50-, 65-, and 75-year-olds decreased from 4%, 17%, and 30%, respectively, in 1988 to 1%, 7%, and 16% in 1998 (Fig 246a). These data indicated that only about 2% of 65-year-olds and fewer than 10% of 75-year-olds would be eden-

tulous in 2008. The number of teeth (third molars excluded) increased from 26.4, 22.8, 16.9, and 14.5 to 27.0, 25.6, 20.7, and 17.6 in 35-, 50-, 65-, and 75-year-olds, respectively (Fig 246b). It was estimated that the mean number of teeth would increase to 26.0, 24.0, and 20.0 in 50-, 65-, and 75-year-olds, respectively, in 2008. Although the projected 2008 data have not been confirmed, they seem realistic because of the low numbers of teeth that have been lost per year.

The long-term effect of the 30-year comprehensive program of PM on tooth loss, caries prevalence, loss of periodontal support, gingival health status, and standard of oral hygiene may be illustrated by the following three cases.

Case 1

Figure 247a shows complete-mouth radiographs of a 50-year-old man at baseline in 1972. Figure 247b presents the radiographs taken at the 30-year reexamination in 2002. In 1972, the patient exhibited greater-than-average loss of periodontal attachment for his age, especially in the maxillary teeth. During the following 30 years, no teeth were lost, there was no further loss of attachment, and no new caries lesions developed. The margin of the alveolar crest was well mineralized, indicating periodontal health at the age of 80 years. The buccogingival status and standard of oral hygiene at the 30-year reexamination are shown in Figs 247c and 247d.

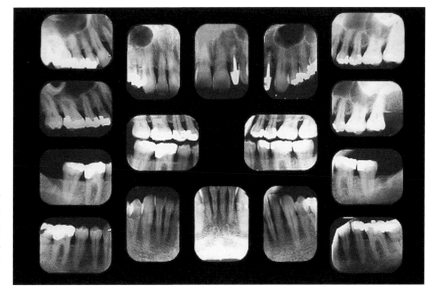

Fig 247a Complete-mouth radiographs of a 50-year-old man at the baseline examination (1972). He has greater-than-average periodontal attachment loss for his age, especially in the maxillary teeth.

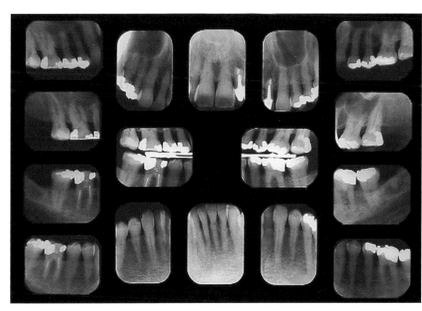

Fig 247b Complete-mouth radiographs of the same patient, aged 80 years, at the 30-year reexamination (2002). No teeth have been lost, there has been no further loss of probing attachment level, and no new caries lesions have developed. Note the well-mineralized margin of the alveolar bone, indicating an absence of active periodontitis.

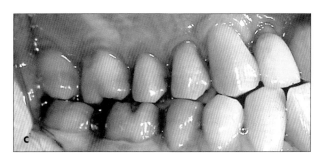
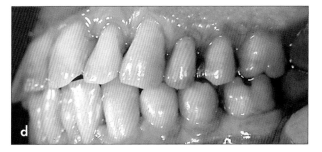

Figs 247c and 247d Buccogingival health and oral hygiene status of the same patient at the 30-year reexamination.

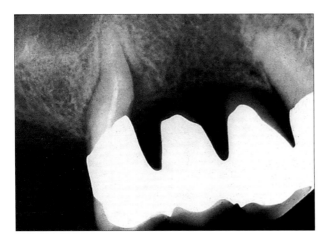

Fig 248a Radiograph of a maxillary right second premolar exhibiting advanced loss of alveolar bone in 1972.

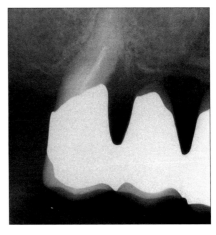

Fig 248b Radiograph of the same premolar 30 years later. Note the gain of alveolar bone mesially.

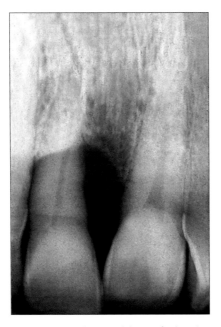

Fig 249a Advanced loss of alveolar bone mesial to the maxillary right central incisor in 1972.

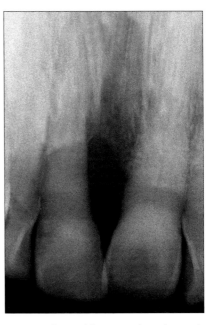

Fig 249b Stable periodontal attachment level 30 years later, with no further loss of alveolar bone.

Case 2

At the baseline in 1972, a 56-year-old woman exhibited far fewer remaining teeth (6 maxillary teeth and 10 mandibular teeth) and greater loss of periodontal support than the average for her age group. Figure 248a shows her maxillary second premolar, which exhibited advanced loss of alveolar bone in 1972. At the 30-year reexamination, some gain of alveolar bone had been achieved (Fig 248b), and no more teeth had been lost.

Case 3

A 59-year-old man exhibited advanced loss of alveolar bone in 1972, particularly mesial to the maxillary right central incisor (Fig 249a). In 2002, no more teeth or alveolar bone had been lost (Fig 249b).

GLOBAL ORAL HEALTH PERSONNEL RESOURCES AND TRENDS

The prevalence of moderate periodontal treatment needs (Community Periodontal Index of Treatment Needs [CPITN] score 1 to 3) is much higher in developing countries than in industrialized countries, despite a similar prevalence of advanced periodontal treatment needs (CPITN score 4). However, the dilemma is that the developing countries represent the majority of the world's population.

According to the World Health Organization (WHO) Data Bank, in 1994 Europe had more than 50% of the world's oral health personnel resources, although it had only 17.7% of the world's population (WHO, 1994). The extremes of the ratio of dentists to inhabitants are found in Scandinavia (1:1,000) and in China and India (1:120,000).

Increasing the availability of oral health personnel

Improving dental schools worldwide

Overcoming this imbalance in the ratio of oral health personnel, particularly of dentists, to the population in different countries is a major challenge. Many developing countries are experiencing either an actual increase in caries prevalence or an inability to reduce the existing level. Although the disease prevalence is, or threatens to be, only moderate, its impact is much more serious than would be the case in industrialized countries because of the almost total lack of effective care.

This predicament is not limited to developing countries. There is a wide divergence in dental school performance across the range of industrialized countries and within any country in which there are a number of dental schools. Even where schools may be judged to be similar in quality, strength and creativity may vary markedly from subject to subject. The profession is thus facing a challenge to minimize undesirable variation and

to provide up-to-date and high-quality education for all.

An answer lies in broad exploitation of new communication technology, which is versatile in keeping information at hand and in offering opportunities for interactive use by undergraduates and graduates as well as teaching staff. An obvious outcome will be the development of a new type of student as well as new types of teachers. Major elements of this new experience will be:

- Much greater ease in pooling intellectual resources
- Speedy exchange of information, especially in relation to effective new methodologies and materials
- Development of common assessment methods
- Access to a wide variety of databanks
- Greater opportunity to adapt careers over an extended period of time based on changes in society and the job market

Preparation of a broad set of modules, addressing oral health topics within a health sciences structure, will demonstrate what might be achieved and thus initiate a snowballing effect toward the ultimate objective of a complete computer-assisted curriculum. Already there are several centers of excellence around the globe that produce the type of interactive materials needed for computer-assisted training. The assortment of such programs is steadily increasing and available as CD-ROM and on the Internet. There is a need to direct that excellence toward the overall objective. This is what the WHO hopes to do, in collaboration with the International Federation of Dental Education Associations, which is enthusiastic about this approach (WHO, 1994).

Succinctly, empowerment of the learner is the principal aim of this concept, in both a variation on the theme of universities without walls and an attempt to make excellence available whatever the constraints of quantity and quality of the teaching staff. It will benefit dental schools where the resources needed to deliver an adequate and appropriate curriculum are very scarce. Every school will need a certain core of staff to administer, coordinate, guide, evaluate, and conduct practical exercises. The specific teaching and learning, however, would come largely from the students, the alumni, and the teachers interacting with the computer programs at their disposal.

The excellence of those programs would depend on having a "brain trust" group of the very best experts responsible for devising the programs. In this way, the best available courses would be offered to all students, everywhere, rather than the wide range of messages, often contradictory or outdated, that students currently receive. Whatever the definitive choice of approaches, an initiative of this type will streamline the training of health personnel, with sufficient flexibility to ensure that training of health personnel will keep pace with the leading edge of science more consistently than is the case today.

Expanding the role of dental hygienists

In addition to the overwhelming need for dental treatment by dentists, particularly in developing countries in Asia, Africa, and Latin America, which are home to the majority of the world's population, there is a clear indication for training of dental hygienists, who are committed exclusively to prevention and control of dental caries and periodontal diseases and nonsurgical periodontal treatment. In addition, their work is very cost effective, as discussed earlier (Axelsson, 1998; Axelsson et al, 1991, 2004).

The role and supply of dental hygienists are of increasing interest worldwide, mainly because of a growing acknowledgment of the importance of oral health as a part of general health, renewed emphasis on setting and attaining health policy goals, and recognition of dental hygienists as a major resource for attaining those goals. Dental hygienists today constitute one of the largest and fastest growing groups in oral health service. They practice, in collaboration with other health professionals, primarily as clinicians and health educators. Their work involves the use of preventive and therapeutic methods to promote good health and to prevent and control oral diseases.

According to Fédération Dentaire Internationale (FDI) surveys, dental hygienists are now trained in more than 25 countries (FDI, 1990). The pioneers were the United States (1906), followed by Norway (1924), Great Britain (1943), Canada (1947), Japan (1949), Nigeria (1958), Sweden (1968), and the Netherlands (1968). The United States has the highest ratio of dental hygienists per head of the population (1:2,500), followed by Japan, Sweden, and Canada (about 1:4,000). The United States also has the highest ratio of dental hygienists to dentists (0.75:1), followed by Japan (0.50:1), South Korea (0.50:1), Canada (0.50:1) and Sweden (0.30:1).

In most countries, the length of the dental hygienist training program is 2 years, but it may range from 1 to 4 years. The entrance requirement is qualification as a dental assistant or matriculation from high school. The occupation is held predominantly by women (more than 90%).

According to a survey in 13 countries (Australia, Canada, Denmark, Italy, Japan, Korea, the Netherlands, Nigeria, Norway, Sweden, Switzerland, Great Britain, and the United States), which comprise most of the world's dental hygienists, the legal scope of their clinical practice is remarkably similar (FDI, 1990). It is characterized by a common set of procedures and activities, including treatment planning for the dental hygiene stages of care; history taking on general health, socioeconomic, and oral health aspects; explanation of optimized self-care for individuals and groups; scaling, root planing, and debridement and PMTC; topical application of fluoride gels and varnishes; application of fissure sealants; finishing of restorations and removal of overhangs; dietary evaluations and counseling; and administration of salivary and oral microbiology tests. In some countries, including Sweden, the training program also emphasizes behavioral science. Dental hygienists are also trained in administration of local anesthesia (infiltration and regional block).

In Sweden, the training program for dental assistants also includes practical preventive dentistry. They are responsible for most of the preventive measures so successfully carried out in children and young adults, as discussed earlier in this chapter. Because the training program for these preventive dentistry assistants takes less than half the time required for the dental hygiene program, this personnel category could well be appropriate in other countries.

Future of oral health personnel

For too long, the oral cavity has been separated from the rest of the body and "donated" to dentists, a profession more or less independent from the general medical professions. At the beginning of this century, dentistry centered around extracting teeth and making complete and partial dentures with the assistance of technicians. Then came an era of "drilling, filling, and billing" in most industrialized countries and aggressive exploration of the tooth crown because of dental caries. In recent decades, in many industrialized countries, the roots of the teeth have also been exploited by subspecialists in periodontology and endodontics, and teeth have been moved around for functional and esthetic reasons by specialists in orthodontics.

Recently, successful reconstructions with implant technology have been achieved through the teamwork of oral surgeons, periodontists, prosthodontists, and dental technicians. Specialists in periodontology as well as general practitioners now offer regeneration of lost periodontal support (see chapter 4).

Integrated education

Modern knowledge and experience obliges dental professionals to focus on prevention and control of dental caries, periodontal diseases, and other oral diseases concurrently with elimination of existing treatment needs.

Increasing numbers of individuals worldwide will have intact tooth crowns and no loss of periodontal support. Therefore, the tooth crowns and the roots have to be reunited in the oral cavity, and the oral cavity must be returned to its rightful place in the body. This requires a more holistic approach, centered on the owner of the oral cavity. Preventive dentistry and oral health promotion have to be integrated with general health promotion in collaboration with general health personnel. Dental education has to be comprehensively reoriented to serve the changing needs of oral health and be linked more closely to the requirements of the whole health sector.

As an alternative to existing schools, which are specific to medicine, dentistry, nursing, and pharmacy, the aim should be to create an integrated system for educating all health personnel within a health sciences school structure. Elimination of separate training of auxiliary and professional personnel categories is also desirable. A "ladder" system of education is envisaged, in which, for the oral health team, the oral physician, instead of today's dentist, is seen as the highest category, at parity with other medical specialties. Other oral health personnel categories, such as dental assistants, preventive dentistry assistants, and dental hygienists would leave this ladder at various levels, corresponding to defined lists of duties, as would be the case for personnel focusing on any other health area. A number of dental schools, predominantly but not exclusively in Europe, have already begun to move toward this type of structure.

Integrated health teams

At the community and city levels, integrated local health teams should be established to improve oral health as well as general health among the population. Such a team should consist of well-trained professionals highly experienced in prevention and health promotion rather than treatment:

- *General physician:* Leader of the team; the most highly qualified and experienced in leadership and communication, general medicine, general health promotion, and epidemiology
- *Psychologist:* Highly qualified and experienced in behavioral science, with special reference to establishing good, healthy lifestyle habits and eliminating bad habits, such as smoking
- *Nutritionist:* Highly qualified and experienced in the concept of "input and output" related to eating at the cellular level as well as the individual level; emphasis should be placed on the consequences of healthy versus unhealthy dietary habits
- *Sociologist:* Well educated and experienced in the influence of socioeconomic conditions on health status
- *Physiotherapist:* Well educated and experienced in how to prevent the development (primary prevention) and the recurrence (secondary pre-

Box 5 WHO's international oral health goals for
the year 2000

- The WHO databases for oral health will be further developed. Coordinated national database systems will be established. A WHO personal computer card for oral health recordings will be defined and produced.
- 50% of 5- to 6-year-old children will be caries free.
- Children will have no more than three decayed, missing, or filled teeth at 12 years.
- 85% of the population will have all their teeth left at 18 years.
- The levels of edentulousness at ages 35 to 44 years will be 50% less than the levels reported in 1969.
- The levels of edentulousness at ages 65 years and older will be 25% less than the levels reported in 1969.

vention) of musculoskeletal orthopedic problems (such as back pain), as well as diagnosis and early rehabilitation of such problems

- *Physical education teacher:* Well educated and experienced in the consequences of physical training and activity versus physical inactivity for general health and how to activate all members of the population
- *Engineer:* Well educated and experienced in the effects of the external and internal environment on health and how to diagnose and eliminate unhealthy environments
- *Oral physician:* Leader of the oral health personnel team and highly qualified and experienced in preventive dentistry and oral health promotion as an integrated part of general health promotion
- *General health nurse:* Responsible for education of the population in self-diagnosis and self-care, with special reference to prevention and control of diseases
- *Dental hygienist:* Well educated and experienced in optimizing oral self-diagnosis and self-care for prevention and control of dental caries, periodontal diseases, and other oral diseases, supplemented by needs-related professional preventive measures

The local health team should be supported, at the county level by a central resource team with a great variety of specialists and subspecialists. Most should have a scientific background at the doctoral level:

- Physicians, all specialties
- Psychologists
- Sociologists
- Nutritionists
- Oral physicians
- Epidemiologists
- Statisticians
- Economists

The remainder should have extensive research experience:

- Physiotherapists
- Sports professionals
- Engineers
- General nurses
- Dental hygienists
- Public relations officers (art directors and copywriters)

The effects of such teams on the health status of the population and the costs should be repeatedly evaluated in terms of the following:

- Absence from work because of disease
- Internationally (WHO) accepted, disease-specific variables
- Cost effectiveness and cost-to-benefit ratio

GLOBAL GOALS FOR ORAL HEALTH

Governments and communities should recognize the need to develop and maintain preventive programs for oral diseases. Communities will be responsible for these activities. All communities should be able to afford and manage basic, health-promoting oral care so that adult teeth will be retained throughout life.

Box 6 International oral health goals for the years 2010 and 2025

Goals for the year 2010	Goals for the year 2025
• A complete electronic global, nation-based WHO database for oral health and a coordinated general health database will be established.	• A global electronic database for automatic oral and general health evaluation, including possibilities for health economy analysis, will be established.
• 90% of 5-year-old children will be caries free.	• 90% of 5-year-old children will be caries free.
• Children will have no more than two decayed, missing, or filled teeth at 12 years of age.	• Children will have no more than one decayed, missing, or filled tooth at 12 years of age.
• 75% of 20-year-old adults will be caries inactive.	• 90% of 20-year-old adults will be caries inactive.
• 75% of 20-year-old adults will not develop destructive periodontal diseases.	• 90% of the whole population will not develop destructive periodontal diseases.
• More than 75% of all children and young adults will have sufficient knowledge of the etiology and prevention of oral diseases to motivate self-diagnosis and self-care.	• More than 75% of the total population will have sufficient knowledge of the etiology and prevention of oral diseases to motivate self-diagnosis and self-care.

Realistic goals for the effects of all preventive dental care programs should be set up at global as well as national, county, district, and clinic levels. Such goals should also be updated in accordance with improved oral health status at certain intervals. As discussed earlier in this chapter, the goals set in the county of Värmland, Sweden, in 1979, were almost 100% achieved by 1999 for those individuals who had followed the needs-related program from the age of 1 to 19 years.

Oral health for life should be approaching reality for all. To promote improved oral health worldwide, the WHO's Oral Health Unit drew up international oral health goals for severity of oral disease involvement at various key ages—12, 35 to 44, and 65 years and older—by the year 2000 (Box 5). However, in 2000 there was still significant heterogeneity amongst countries. For example, the

oral health status was far ahead of these goals in the Scandinavian countries (Sweden, Denmark, Norway, and Finland), while the eastern European countries and most Latin American countries were far from the WHO goals.

In 1988, the first International Conference on Preventive Dentistry and Epidemiology was held in Karlstad, Sweden, in collaboration with the WHO, the FDI, and the Swedish Board of Health and Welfare. Among other topics discussed at the workshops were goals that could be realistically achieved by the years 2010 and 2025 (Box 6), to follow the WHO's goals for the year 2000; what was known about already existing preventive measures; and the future potential of large-scale implementation of recent clinical research (Axelsson et al, 1988). The proposed goals involve:

- Creation of gradually better-developed computerized analytical epidemiologic systems for quality control of oral and general health programs and cost effectiveness
- Focusing on education of all the population in self-diagnosis and self-care, which are the most cost-effective forms of oral health care
- Prevention and control of the development and progression of caries and periodontitis in the vast majority of the adult population (secondary prevention), in parallel with efficient primary prevention in children, so that about 90% of young children will be caries free

More detailed and rigorous goals can be established at national, county, city, and clinic levels, depending on the actual oral health status of the population and the availability of dental care resources.

ESTABLISHMENT OF NEEDS-RELATED PREVENTIVE AND SUPPORTIVE CARE PROGRAMS BASED ON RISK PREDICTION AND RISK PROFILES

In countries with high prevalence and incidence of dental caries and/or periodontal diseases and limited resources of dentists, a so-called whole-population strategy for preventive programs, performed by other oral health personnel such as dental hygienists and preventive dentistry assistants, should still be cost effective.

In populations with poor oral hygiene standards and limited oral health care resources, most children have gingivitis, and most adults have gingivitis and untreated chronic periodontitis. Under these conditions, until the existing treatment needs are met, a whole-population strategy for general oral health promotion should be applied. School-based education in self-diagnosis and daily oral hygiene should be very cost effective because periodontitis always is preceded by gingivitis. In addition, such a program is very rational because "clean teeth never decay."

There are several similarities between periodontal diseases and dental caries. Both are multifactorial infectious diseases. Besides etiologic, preventive, and control factors, many other factors may modify the prevalence, onset, and progression of both diseases. These modifiers may be divided into external (environmental) and internal (endogenous) factors.

Probabilities statements

For cost effectiveness, the methods used to select and predict groups and individuals at "true" risk for disease development should be as sensitive as possible. The optimal *sensitivity* for a diagnostic risk test is 100%; that is, of 100 individuals selected as "at-risk individuals," all are true at-risk individuals. Similarly, for methods used to select true "nonrisk individuals," specificity should be as high as possible; that is, of selected nonrisk individuals, 100% are truly nonrisk.

Usually, the higher the sensitivity, the lower the specificity. Thus, the clinician is usually forced to choose a test based on the consequences of making an error. A test method with high sensitivity and low specificity is likely to err in the direction of false positives. For a disease such as periodontitis, the implications are not usually serious when people are incorrectly identified as having active disease: They do not suffer extreme anxiety or undergo radical treatment. They may undergo intensified preventive treatment and incur increased treatment costs.

The consequence of a false-negative result, when a person with disease is incorrectly identified as healthy, is that the disease may progress further before it is diagnosed at a subsequent examination. This may be serious in the case of aggressive disease and of major consequence when there are prolonged intervals between examinations. For periodontal disease, as well as dental caries, the consequences of a false-positive diagnosis are less serious than those of a false-negative diagnosis. Alternatively, multiple tests, one highly sensitive and one highly specific, may be combined.

The probability of development of dental caries or periodontitis, given the result of a test method, is known as the *predictive value*. The positive predictive value is the probability that a patient with a positive test result actually has active caries or periodontitis. Similarly, the negative predictive value is the probability that a patient with a negative test result actually has inactive dental caries or periodontal disease.

Likelihood ratios can be used to evaluate the performance of a diagnostic test that is dichotomous or has interval properties. In addition, likelihood ratios can be used to calculate the probability of disease after a positive or negative test result.

Sensitivity, specificity, and predictive values are probability statements representing the proportion of people with disease who have a positive test. Likelihood ratios are based on odds, which is the ratio of two probability values that contain the same information but express it differently. The relationship between the two is expressed in the following formulas:

$$Odds = \frac{Probability\ of\ event}{1 - Probability\ of\ event}$$

$$Probability = \frac{Odds}{1 + Odds}$$

The likelihood ratio for any value of a diagnostic test method is the probability of getting that test result when disease is present, divided by the probability of the result when disease is absent. Thus, likelihood ratios express how many times more or less likely a test result is to be found in diseased test subjects than it is in nondiseased test subjects.

This type of calculation can be done with different values of an interval scale diagnostic test. The resulting distribution of likelihood ratios can then provide the clinician with information on the likelihood of disease for a range of values.

Risk categories

For the clinician, accurate prediction of patients or sites at high risk of developing caries or periodontitis is of fundamental importance. Because of the particular nature of dental caries as well as periodontal diseases, prediction of disease progression is important. Diagnostic tests differentiate whether or not a person has a specific disease at the time. *Risk indicators* (RIs) are factors that

have proved to be significantly associated with the occurrence of a specific disease but only in cross-sectional studies.

Risk factors (RFs), on the other hand, are those that significantly increase the likelihood that people without disease, if exposed to these factors, will succumb to the disease within a specified time interval. Although diagnostic tests and RIs can be evaluated by cross-sectional research design, longitudinal studies are necessary to confirm RFs.

The term *risk factor* is rather loosely used and can refer to an attribute or exposure associated with increased probability of disease (not necessarily causal); any type of determinant (cause); or a determinant that can be modified. This loose terminology may cause confusion when multivariate aspects of diseases are considered. Use of the term should be restricted as follows: Risk factors are characteristics of the person or environment that, when present, directly result in an increased likelihood that a person will get a disease and, when absent, directly result in a decreased likelihood.

Exposure to a risk factor means that a person has been exposed to or manifested the factor prior to the onset of the disease. There may be continuous exposure, an isolated episode, or multiple exposures over a period of time. Clinicians must recognize that risk factors, like etiologic factors (the periopathogens and the cariogenic microflora), are based on the current state of knowledge about a direct relationship: In light of further knowledge, a current risk factor for a specific disease may in the future be excluded. Because periodontal diseases are the result of multiple etiologic factors (different species of periopathogens) and modifying factors, removal of a risk factor, such as the cessation of smoking in a patient with periodontal disease, does not necessarily cure the disease. It should reduce the likelihood of disease development, but once a person has the disease, removal of the risk factor may or may not result in cure.

Prognostic risk factors (PRFs) are factors that increase the risk that an already existing disease will progress. For example, in patients with existing periodontal disease, smoking will increase the risk for progression of the disease. Thus in adults, it is more practical to assess PRFs instead of RFs.

Risk markers and *risk predictors* (eg, advanced attachment loss and deep diseased pockets in periodontal disease) are usually biologic markers that indicate either disease or disease progression but currently are thought not to be causal or that represent historical evidence of the disease, such as past evidence of periodontal disease. If a risk predictor is more strongly associated with the disease than a risk factor, and the risk predictor and risk factor are also associated with each other, then the risk predictor will appear in the multivariate model instead of the risk factor.

For example, baseline periodontal status is usually strongly associated with the occurrence of new disease because it is a measure of past disease and thus is a risk predictor. Microorganisms are the etiologic risk factors and are also associated with new disease. Microorganisms are also associated with baseline periodontal status because they are partially responsible for this status. Thus, baseline periodontal status may replace microorganisms in the multivariate model. Having a risk predictor in the model results in a prediction model rather than a risk model.

Periodontal diseases have multiple levels of measurement: person, tooth, and site. A person can have disease, although many teeth and even more tooth sites may be disease free. Thus, the same person can have sites with onset of disease as well as sites with established disease exhibiting progression. If the risk factor for disease onset is different from the prognostic factors for disease outcome, established sites should be evaluated under prognosis and not under risk prediction. Currently, however, both types of sites tend to be considered together when risk factors are delineated. In the future, it may be useful to consider the two as separate entities.

In addition to etiologic and preventive factors, many other factors may modify the prevalence, onset, and progression (incidence) of periodontal diseases. Such factors are divided into external (environmental) and internal (endogenous) factors.

External modifiers

Examples of external modifying RIs, RFs, and PRFs for periodontal diseases are smoking, use of smokeless tobacco, irregular dental care, low socioeconomic (particularly low educational) level, infectious and other acquired diseases, side ef-fects of medication, and poor dietary habits. The most important are smoking, poor oral hygiene, and irregular attendance habits.

Internal modifiers

Internal RIs, RFs, and PRFs related to periodontal disease include genetic factors, impaired host factors, chronic diseases, and reduced salivary flow and quality. Most studies of genetic factors in periodontal disease have concerned the aggressive forms of disease. Family studies suggest that susceptibility to the aggressive forms of disease, particularly in prepubertal and adolescent children, is at least in part influenced by host genotype. Inherited phagocytic cell deficiencies appear to confer risk for aggressive periodontitis in prepubertal children. The prevalence and distribution of aggressive periodontitis in affected families are most consistent with an autosomal-recessive mode of inheritance. Comparisons between adult monozygous twins reared together and twins reared apart indicate that early family environment has no appreciable influence on probing depth and attachment loss in adults (Michalowicz et al, 1991).

A number of apparently genetically determined syndromes or diseases appear to carry an associated increased risk for periodontal destruction. Defects of phagocytic cell function, especially polymorphonuclear leukocytes (PMNLs), but also mononuclear phagocytes, is common in patients with aggressive periodontitis.

Genetic polymorphism of proinflammatory cytokines, particularly interleukin 1 (IL-1), has been shown to be an RF and a PRF for periodontal diseases (Kornman et al, 1997). It has also been shown that the combination of genetic polymorphism of IL-1 and a smoking habit has a synergistic negative effect (Axelsson et al, 2001; McGuire and Nunn, 1999). It is estimated that about 80% of the most severe forms of periodontal diseases could be explained by these two joint factors.

Of the chronic diseases, poorly controlled diabetes (type 1 as well as type 2) is the most important RF and PRF for periodontal disease (for review, see Salvi et al, 2008; for more details on etiologic factors and external and internal RIs, RFs, and PRFs related to periodontal diseases, see volume 3 of this series [Axelsson, 2002]).

Individual periodontitis risk assessment

The relative risk for developing periodontal disease can be evaluated by combining clinical examination; preventive factors; etiologic factors; the absence or presence of environmental (external) and host-related (internal) RIs, RFs, and PRFs; risk markers; and risk predictors. Periodontal risk increases in accordance with the severity and number of these factors to which the individual is exposed. Criteria for grading individual risk into one of four classes, from no risk to high risk (P0 to P3), have been proposed for children, young adults, adults, and the elderly (Table 6). The colors, from green to red, symbolize escalated risk. The criteria are based on history taking, established clinical diagnostic criteria, and supplementary bacterial sampling and laboratory tests, where indicated.

During the last 10 years, nearly 100% of the adult patients at the Public Dental Health Clinics, representing about 50% of the adult population in the county of Värmland, Sweden, and the majority of the adult patients in private clinics have been assigned to one of four classes of general risk, periodontal risk, caries risk, and iatrogenic risk: 0 = no risk; 1 = low risk; 2 = risk; 3 = high risk. This assessment was developed to improve the needs-related preventive program for adults, which was initiated in 1985.

General risk includes general health problems, physiologic compliance problems, physical disabilities, and so on. Iatrogenic risk includes the risk for cuspal fractures because of complicated restorative dentistry and root fractures because of the presence of posts and complicated fixed prostheses. The fee per year for needs-related maintenance or so-called supportive care is based on the sum of the individual patient's general, periodontal, caries, and iatrogenic risk classes.

Risk profiles

Risk profiles for tooth loss, dental caries, and periodontal diseases can be presented graphically by combining symptoms (risk markers) of disease (eg, prevalence, incidence, treatment needs); etiologic factors; external modifying risk indicators, risk factors, and prognostic risk factors; internal modifying risk indicators, risk factors, and prognostic risk factors; and preventive factors. This can be done manually or by computer. Degrees of risk, 0, 1, 2, or 3, are displayed in green, blue, yellow, or red, respectively. The graphs are very useful tools for communication with the patient during discussions about oral health status, etiology, modifying factors, prevention, possibilities, responsibilities, and reevaluations.

Risk profiles for tooth loss

A profile of risk for future tooth loss can be compiled by combining several RIs, RFs, and PRFs (Fig 250). Among these are age, estimated risk for periodontal diseases (P0 to P3) and dental caries (C0 to C3), poor socioeconomic conditions, chronic diseases, iatrogenic root fractures, trauma, genetics and impaired host response, medication, and irregular dental care habits.

In many industrialized countries, elderly people have heavily restored dentitions because of high caries incidence 30 to 50 years previously, when dental treatment was invasive. In such populations, the most frequent reason for tooth loss would be iatrogenic root fractures caused by posts in endodontically treated teeth. On the other hand, in developing countries with very limited oral health care resources, the main reasons for tooth loss would be untreated periodontal diseases and dental caries among elderly people and untreated dental caries and trauma among young people.

Detailed risk profiles for periodontal diseases

An example of a detailed risk profile for a patient at high risk, predominantly for periodontal diseases, is shown in Fig 251. The abbreviations in Fig 251 are explained in Box 7. The risk profile illustrates graphically how high periodontal risk (P3) has been reduced to low risk (P1) by improved needs-related plaque control measures via self-care and supplementary professional treatment. The greater the difference between the solid line (baseline) and the dotted line (maintenance phase), the greater the improvement. The absence of any change suggests that this par-

Table 6 Criteria for evaluating individual periodontal risk in children, young adults, adults, and the elderly

No periodontal risk (P0; green)

I	Children
I:1	Healthy gingivae
I:2	Excellent oral hygiene habits
I:3	No approximal probing loss of attachment
I:4	No internal or external risk indicators or risk factors

No periodontal risk (P0; green)

II	Young adults
II:1	Healthy gingivae
II:2	Excellent oral hygiene habits
II:3	No approximal probing loss of attachment
II:4	No internal or external risk indicators or risk factors

No periodontal risk (P0; green)

III	Adults
III:1	No diseased periodontal pockets
III:2	Excellent oral hygiene habits
III:3	No approximal probing loss of attachment
III:4	No internal or external risk indicators or risk factors

No periodontal risk (P0; green)

IV	Elderly
IV:1	No diseased periodontal pockets
IV:2	Excellent or good oral hygiene habits
IV:3	Mean approximal probing loss of attachment < 1 mm
IV:4	No internal or external risk indicators or risk factors

Low periodontal risk (P1; blue)

I	Children
I:1	Gingival bleeding index < 10% (CPITN 1)
I:2	Good oral hygiene habits
I:3	No approximal probing loss of attachment
I:4	No internal or external risk indicators or risk factors

Low periodontal risk (P1; blue)

II	Young adults
II:1	Gingival bleeding index < 10% (CPITN 1)
II:2	Good oral hygiene habits
II:3	No approximal probing loss of attachment
II:4	No internal or external risk indicators or risk factors

Low periodontal risk (P1; blue)

III	Adults
III:1	Fewer than five diseased approximal pockets > 3 mm (CPITN 3–4)
III:2	Good oral hygiene habits
III:3	Mean approximal probing loss of attachment < 1 mm
III:4	No internal or external risk indicators or risk factors

Low periodontal risk (P1; blue)

IV	Elderly
IV:1	Chronic periodontitis: fewer than five diseased approximal pockets > 5 mm (CPITN 4)
IV:2	Good oral hygiene habits
IV:3	Mean approximal probing loss of attachment < 2 mm
IV:4	No tooth loss caused by periodontal disease
IV:5	No internal or external risk indicators or prognostic risk factors

Periodontal risk (P2; yellow)

I	Children
I:1	Gingival bleeding index < 20% (CPITN 1)
I:2	Poor oral hygiene habits
I:3	Internal risk indicators, risk factors, and prognostic risk factors
I:4	External risk indicators, risk factors, and prognostic risk factors (eg, low educational level of parents)

Periodontal risk (P2; yellow)

II	Young adults
II:1	One to five diseased approximal pockets > 3 mm (CPITN 3–4)
II:2	Poor oral hygiene habits
II:3	Mean approximal probing loss of attachment < 1 mm
II:4	Internal risk indicators, risk factors, and prognostic risk factors
II:5	External risk indicators, risk factors, and prognostic risk factors (eg, low socioeconomic level, smoking)

Periodontal risk (P2; yellow)

III	Adults
III:1	Chronic periodontitis: more than five diseased approximal pockets > 5 mm (CPITN 4)
III:2	Poor oral hygiene habits
III:3	Mean approximal probing loss of attachment > 2 mm
III:4	Internal risk indicators, risk factors, and prognostic risk factors (eg, type 1 or 2 diabetes)
III:5	External risk indicators, risk factors, and prognostic risk factors (eg, smoking, low educational level, irregular dental care)

Table 6 *(cont)* Criteria for evaluating individual periodontal risk in children, young adults, adults, and the elderly

Periodontal risk (P2; yellow)

IV Elderly

IV:1 More than 15 approximal sites with chronic periodontitis (CPITN 4)

IV:2 Poor oral hygiene habits

IV:3 Mean approximal probing attachment loss > 4 mm

IV:4 More than four teeth lost because of periodontal disease

IV:5 Internal risk indicators, risk factors, and prognostic risk factors (eg, type 1 or 2 diabetes)

IV:6 External risk indicators, risk factors, and prognostic risk factors (eg, smoking, low educational level, irregular dental care)

High periodontal risk (P3; red)

I Children

I:1 Localized or generalized aggressive periodontal diseases (0.1% to 0.3% of the Scandinavian population)

I:2 Very poor oral hygiene

I:3 Most diseased sites infected with bacteria associated with aggressive periodontitis (eg, *Aggregatibacter actinomycetemcomitans*)

I:4 Internal risk indicators, risk factors, and prognostic risk factors, such as genetic interleukin 1 polymorphism, dysfunction of the polymorphonuclear leukocytes, reduced immunoglobulin G2 response, type 1 diabetes, Down syndrome, and leukemia

I:5 External risk indicators, risk factors, and prognostic risk factors (eg, low educational level of parents, AIDS, irregular dental care)

High periodontal risk (P3; red)

II Young adults

II:1 Localized or generalized aggressive periodontal diseases

II:2 High periodontal incidence (annual probing loss of attachment) and several sites related to aggressive periodontitis

II:3 Very poor oral hygiene

II:4 Most diseased sites infected with bacteria associated with aggressive periodontitis (eg, *Aggregatibacter actinomycetemcomitans*, *Porphyromonas gingivalis*)

II:5 Internal risk indicators, risk factors, and prognostic risk factors, such as genetic interleukin 1 polymorphism, dysfunction of the polymorphonuclear leukocytes, reduced immunoglobulin G2 response, type 1 diabetes, and leukemia

II:6 External risk indicators, risk factors, and prognostic risk factors (eg, smoking, low educational level, AIDS, irregular dental care)

High periodontal risk (P3; red)

III Adults

III:1 Aggressive periodontitis: high periodontal incidence (annual probing loss of attachment) and several sites with aggressive periodontitis

III:2 More than four teeth lost because of periodontal disease

III:3 Very poor oral hygiene; most diseased sites infected by *Porphyromonas gingivalis*, *Tannerella forsythia*, and other periopathogens

III:4 Internal risk indicators, risk factors, and prognostic risk factors (eg, type 1 or 2 diabetes, genetic interleukin 1 polymorphism)

III:5 External risk indicators, risk factors, and prognostic risk factors (eg, smoking, low educational level, AIDS, irregular dental care)

High periodontal risk (P3; red)

IV Elderly

IV:1 Aggressive periodontitis (periodontitis gravis and complications involving most teeth)

IV:2 More than 10 teeth lost because of periodontal disease

IV:3 Very poor oral hygiene; most diseased sites infected by *Porphyromonas gingivalis*, *Tannerella forsythia*, and other periopathogens

IV:4 Internal risk indicators, risk factors, and prognostic risk factors (eg, type 1 or 2 diabetes, genetic interleukin 1 polymorphism)

IV:5 External risk indicators, risk factors, and prognostic risk factors (eg, smoking, low educational level, irregular dental care)

CPITN = Community Periodontal Index of Treatment Needs.

257

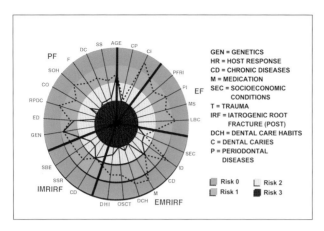

Fig 250 Risk profile for tooth loss.

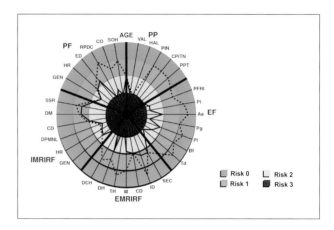

Fig 251 Risk profile for periodontal diseases: *(solid line)* baseline, P3; *(dotted line)* 2 years later, P1. (For explanation of abbreviations, see Box 7.)

ticular factor cannot be influenced (for example, genetic factors, host response, and some chronic diseases).

The patient in question was a 50-year-old man with the following clinical diagnosis and anamnestic data at his initial assessment.

Clinical variables related to periodontal disease.

- Eight teeth had been lost because of periodontal disease (four maxillary molars, two maxillary premolars, and two mandibular molars).
- The mean decrease in vertical attachment level on the approximal surfaces was 4 mm more than the average for his age group. In addition, several posterior teeth had two- and three-wall intrabony pockets. All of the remaining molars had grade I to II furcation involvement (loss of horizontal attachment level).
- Retrospective radiographs and diagnoses of vertical attachment loss from the referring dentist showed irregular but advanced loss of periodontal support during the last few years (periodontal incidence).
- More than 60% of the approximal sites were diseased, with greater than 5-mm probing depths (CPITN score 4). Purulent exudate was frequent. Analysis of the gingival crevicular fluid showed high levels of prostaglandin E_2, IL-1β, aspartate aminotransferase, and other endogenous metalloproteinases, particularly from PMNLs,

which together indicated active lesions with advanced breakdown of periodontal tissues.
- The periodontal pocket temperature was elevated in all pockets deeper than 3 mm, which also indicated active lesions.

Etiologic factors.

- He was a very fast plaque former (Plaque Formation Rate Index [PFRI] = 5).
- The standard of oral hygiene was very poor (Plaque Index = 76%).
- DNA probe analyses from the deepest pockets showed the following values, on a scale of 0 to 5: *Aggregatibacter actinomycetemcomitans* = score 3 (> 10^5); *Porphyromonas gingivalis* = score 5 (> 10^6); *Prevotella intermedia* = score 3 (> 10^5); *Tannerella forsythia* = score 4 (10^6); and *Treponema denticola* = score 5 (> 10^6).

External modifiers.

- His socioeconomic condition, including education, was about average.
- He had a history of urinary infection (infectious diseases).
- He had diagnosed hypertension and had experienced some minor heart infarcts (chronic inflammatory diseases).
- He was taking medication for his cardiovascular disease.

Box 7 Abbreviations related to periodontal risk used in Fig 251

- **Periodontal risk**
  - PO = No periodontal risk
  - P1 = Low periodontal risk
  - P2 = Periodontal risk
  - P3 = High periodontal risk
- **Clinical periodontal diagnosis**
  - PP = Periodontitis prevalence (experience)
  - VAL = Vertical attachment level
  - HAL = Horizontal attachment level (furcation involvement)
  - PIN = Periodontitis incidence (activity)
  - CPITN = Community Periodontal Index of Treatment Needs
  - PPT = Periodontal pocket temperature
- **Etiologic factors (EF)**
  - PFRI = Plaque Formation Rate Index
  - PI = Plaque Index (scores and pattern)
  - Aa = Aggregatibacter actinomycetemcomitans
  - Pg = Porphyromonas gingivalis
  - Pi = Prevotella intermedia
  - Tf = Tannerella forsythia
  - Td = Treponema denticola

- **External modifying risk indicators, risk factors, and prognostic risk factors (EMRIRF)**
  - SEC = Socioeconomic conditions
  - D = Infectious diseases
  - CD = Chronic diseases
  - M = Medication
  - TH = Tobacco habits
  - DH = Dietary habits
  - DCH = Dental care habits
- **Internal modifying risk indicators, risk factors, and prognostic risk factors (IMRIRF)**
  - GEN = Genetic factors
  - HR = Host response
  - DPMNL = Defective PMNL function
  - CD = Chronic diseases
  - DM = Diabetes mellitus
  - SSSR = Stimulated salivary secretion rate
- **Preventive factors (PF)**
  - GEN = Genetic factors
  - HR = Host response
  - ED = Educational level
  - RPDC = Regular preventive dental care habits
  - CO = Compliance
  - SOH = Standard of oral hygiene

- He had smoked more than 20 cigarettes a day since the age of 15 years (more than 35 pack years).
- His dietary habits (DH) were poor, including frequent snacks between meals, sweets, and sweet drinks. His body mass index was high (> 30).
- His dental care habits were very irregular.

Internal modifiers.

- Use of the Periodontal Susceptibility Test revealed that he was positive for the polymorphic IL-1 gene cluster; ie, he was genetically predisposed. It has been shown that this genetic defect is strongly correlated to increased susceptibility to periodontal diseases (Kornman et al, 1997), particularly in combination with smoking (Axelsson et al, 2001; Axelsson, 2002, 2004; McGuire and Nunn, 1999).

- His host response was also reduced because of defective PMNL function, an effect of regular smoking. The importance of aggressive, phagocytosing PMNLs as the first line of nonspecific defense in periodontal pockets should not be underestimated.
- As stated previously, he had a diagnosis of cardiovascular disease, which could be attributable to the presence of several diseased pockets, from which gram-negative microorganisms and their lipopolysaccharides continuously entered the connective tissue and the vascular system. Other contributing factors could be 35 years of smoking, poor dietary habits, hereditary factors, and physical inactivity.
- He occasionally experienced symptoms of type 2 diabetes.
- Because of regular medication with saliva-depressive effects, his stimulated salivary secretion rate was low (< 0.7 mL/min).

Preventive factors.

- He was genetically predisposed to periodontal disease.
- Instead of having an effective host response, his first line of defense was impaired because of smoking.
- His educational level was slightly above average.
- He sought preventive dental care only irregularly.
- His compliance on oral hygiene, smoking, and dietary habits was very poor, resulting in a very low standard of oral hygiene. He used a toothbrush and toothpaste only irregularly.

During the case presentation, a graphic illustration (see Fig 251) was used as a tool for communication with the patient. Concurrently, the patient was educated in self-diagnosis to confirm the diagnosis of his own oral health status and treatment needs. Thereafter, an agreement was reached by the patient and the oral health personnel with respect to a treatment strategy in which responsibility for the patient's oral health was shared between the patient and the oral health personnel (dentist and dental hygienist) at the clinic. This was followed by an initial intensive preventive period, including education in needs-related plaque control measures based on self-diagnosis.

The dentist and dental hygienist, working in cooperation, eliminated all supragingival and subgingival plaque-retentive factors. Conservative, minimally invasive methods were used for scaling and root planing to achieve smooth root cementum without exposing dentinal tubules, which would have led to bacterial invasion. The subgingival biofilm and nonattaching microflora were comprehensively removed by minimally invasive debridement and powered irrigation with bactericidal chemical plaque control agents (iodine solution). During this initial intensive period, the entire oral cavity was treated according to the so-called complete-mouth disinfection strategy: Three times in 1 week, the dental hygienist cleaned the tongue and all tooth surfaces (supragingival as well as subgingival) both mechanically (PMTC) and chemically with chemical plaque control agents (CHX and iodine).

Thereafter, the patient practiced needs-related plaque control measures twice a day, based on self-diagnosis and self-evaluation. Plaque disclosure before and after cleaning was performed every day during the first week and weekly thereafter. Needs-related plaque control measures included use of selected mechanical toothcleaning aids and a tongue scraper, as well as a toothpaste that contained fluoride and triclosan. For the first 4 weeks, the patient also used a CHX mouthrinse twice a day. Because CHX is cationic, the patient was instructed not to use toothpastes containing anions (eg, sodium lauryl sulfate and monofluorophosphate) within an hour before or after rinsing with CHX.

The first reevaluation was carried out after 3 months. Thereafter, the patient began a maintenance program tailored to his individual requirements. Maintenance included needs-related intervals of clinical evaluation, PMTC, minimally invasive debridement of diseased pockets, and control of the oral hygiene standard.

The 1-year recall assessment involved comprehensive clinical examination, digitized computer-aided radiographs, DNA probe analyses, pocket temperature measurement, and gingival crevicular fluid analysis. Only three remaining deep pockets (deeper than 5 mm) exhibited signs of activity: Prostaglandin E_2, IL-1, and aspartate aminotransferase levels in gingival crevicular fluid were still high, and the pocket temperature was elevated. The levels of *A actinomycetemcomitans*, *P gingivalis*, and *T forsythia* remained high. Use of millimeter-graded probes in combination with the digitized radiographs disclosed the presence of two-wall intrabony pockets at all three active sites.

At this stage, the patient was highly motivated, and his standard of oral hygiene was excellent. After a "case presentation," including reevaluation of the risk profile, the patient decided to stop smoking if the remaining three active lesions could be healed and arrested by regenerative therapy.

One week before regenerative therapy, any remaining subgingival biofilms were mechanically removed by minimally invasive debridement, followed by comprehensive powered irrigation with iodine solution. Because the sites contained high levels not only of the anaerobes *P gingivalis* and *T forsythia* but also the exogenous pathogen *A actinomycetemcomitans*, a fiber that delivered controlled, slow release of tetracycline was placed in the pockets for 1 week. In addition to the needs-related mechanical plaque control measures and the use of fluoride toothpaste that contained triclosan, the patient began a CHX rinsing program 1 week before surgery.

Tailor-made mini-flap surgery was used both to gain accessibility to the three different periodontal lesions and to execute regenerative therapy in one surgical session. After minimally invasive mechanical cleaning of the root surfaces with curettes (used with a negative angle) and PER-IO-TOR reciprocating instruments (Dentatus), followed by chemical cleaning and surface conditioning with ethylenediaminetetraacetic acid gel (PrepGel, Straumann), a matrix-guided regenerative material (Emdogain gel, Straumann) was placed on the root surfaces. The mini-flaps were resutured (see chapter 4).

For the first postoperative month, only chemical plaque control by rinsing twice a day with CHX solution and the use of an extrasoft toothbrush was allowed around the treated sites to prevent disruption of healing by mechanical trauma, particularly from interdental cleaning aids. After 4 weeks, the patient resumed needs-related mechanical plaque control measures and the needs-related maintenance program, based on evaluations, PMTC, and minimally invasive debridement at sites where subgingival biofilms had re-formed, despite the concerted efforts at gingival plaque control by both patient and hygienist.

The second detailed reexamination was carried out after 2 years. At these reexaminations it is most important that the patient participate in self-evaluation. Digitized radiographs, an intraoral camera, and a lighted mouth mirror are very useful tools for this purpose. The risk profile (see Fig 251) was again used as a tool for communication with the patient and to supplement self-evaluation in the mouth and on radiographs. The changes in the risk profile show how successfully the patient and the dental personnel fulfilled their responsibilities:

- Etiologic factors were dramatically reduced by improved mechanical plaque control and intermittent use of CHX by self-care, supplemented at needs-related intervals by PMTC and debridement.

- The PFRI was reduced from 5 to 2 (indicating that the gingivae had healed following the establishment of meticulous gingival plaque control).
- The Plaque Index was reduced from 76% to 8%.
- The exogenous periopathogens *A actinomycetemcomitans* and *P gingivalis*, as well as the opportunistic periopathogens *T forsythia*, *P intermedia*, and *T denticola*, were almost totally eliminated.
- The urinary infection and the periodontal pockets healed. The patient stopped smoking and improved his dietary habits. The need for medication for infection as well as for cardiovascular disease was reduced.
- For 2 years, the patient had participated in a needs-related maintenance program, which included regular dental care habits and regular professional preventive care.
- The reduced need for medication for cardiovascular disease eased the saliva-depressive effects of the drugs. Together with changes in dietary habits (such as increased intake of fiber-rich vegetables), this led to improved salivary function: The stimulated salivary secretion rate increased from < 0.7 to 1.2 mL/min.
- Because the patient stopped smoking, the PMNL function and thereby the host response seemed to improve.
- The patient's educational level, that is, knowledge of dental diseases, self-diagnosis, and self-care, increased considerably over 2 years.
- High motivation, based on self-diagnosis, knowledge, and training, resulted in establishment of excellent needs-related plaque control habits and compliance.

The outcome of these efforts and improvement by self-care and needs-related professional preventive treatment was that there was no further loss of periodontal support during the 2-year period. Instead, a mean 6-mm gain of vertical attachment was achieved at three sites, as a result of successful regenerative therapy. All periodontal sites were healthy (CPITN = 0), and no increase in periodontal pocket temperature was observed. The patient's periodontal risk was therefore reassessed: Although the risk lessened, the patient tested positive (Periodontal Susceptibility Test)

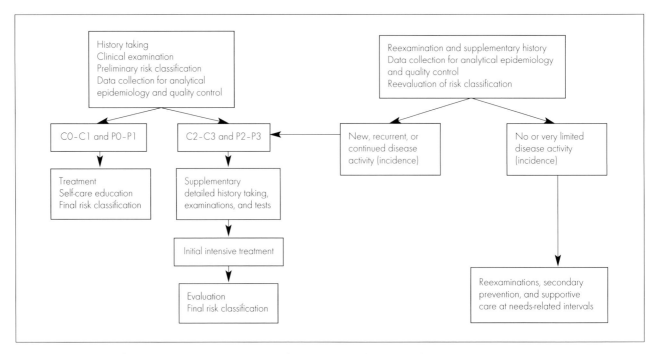

Fig 252 Schedule for needs-related preventive and maintenance (supportive) care.

for the polymorphic IL-1 gene cluster; therefore, he will continue in a maintenance program with recall at needs-related intervals. The aim will be to gradually prolong the intervals between recalls.

This example illustrates the usefulness of the risk profile as a tool for:

• Case presentation and communication with the patient
• Establishment of needs-related self-care habits
• Detailed evaluation of self-care and professional preventive treatment, even in individuals assessed as high risk according to current knowledge

In the United States, a computer-aided risk calculator (PreViser) has been frequently used for prediction of periodontal diseases (Page et al, 2003). Lang and Tonetti (2003) have also presented a graphic model for risk prediction of periodontal diseases (for details on risk prediction of periodontal disease, see Axelsson, 2002).

Schedules for needs-related preventive programs based on risk prediction

In countries with ample oral health personnel, oral health resources, and relatively high standards of living and oral health, by far the most cost-effective strategy for improvement of oral health status is needs-related self-care based on self-diagnosis supplemented with PMTC and topical application of fluoride agents at needs-related intervals. Figure 252 illustrates a schedule for needs-related preventive and maintenance care for new and maintenance patients. All new patients should be introduced to a needs-related preventive program in the following order.

Screening and history taking

At the very first appointment, these are the goals:

• To obtain a brief overview of oral health status by screening diagnosis, supplemented with necessary radiographic examinations
• To gain an impression of the owner of the oral cavity by taking an oral and a general history

For the oral history, an evaluation of the patient's dental care, oral hygiene, fluoride, dietary and smoking habits, and attitudes to oral health are of great importance. The most important variables for general history evaluations are level of education, occupation, lifestyle, systemic diseases, use of medicines, attitudes to general health, and body mass index.

It is important to remember that the diagnosis reveals only the present oral status, but the history discloses the reasons for that status. On the basis of the results of screening and history taking, appropriate detailed supplementary examinations and tests are selected.

Examinations and tests

Supplementary examinations and tests are carried out with the following goals:

- To obtain detailed information on oral health status
- To obtain detailed information on etiologic and modifying factors related to the patient's oral health status

The most important clinical variables related to periodontal diseases are vertical probing attachment loss (millimeters); horizontal attachment loss (furcation involvement, grades 0 to III); Gingival Index, probing depth, alveolar bone level, shape, and structure, based on complete-mouth radiographs, conventional or computer digitized; bleeding on probing; purulent exudate; periodontal pocket temperature; amount and content of gingival crevicular fluid; and subgingival plaque-retentive factors (eg, calculus, rough root surfaces, restoration overhangs). If retrospective data are available, the incidence of periodontal attachment loss is estimated.

From an etiologic point of view, the PFRI, the Plaque Index, and the occurrence of subgingival plaque biofilms and specific periopathogens such as *A actinomycetemcomitans, P gingivalis,* T *forsythia, T denticola,* and *P intermedia* (diagnosed via checkerboard DNA-DNA hybridization technique) are of great importance. The most important external and internal modifying factors for periodontal diseases are oral and dental care habits, smoking habits, ed-

ucational level, systemic diseases (particularly type 1 and type 2 diabetes), and genetic susceptibility.

Risk classification

Based on all data from the diagnosis and history taking, the patient is classified according to risk for periodontal diseases: no risk (P0), low risk (P1), risk (P2), or high risk (P3). The individual risk profile is established as a tool for case presentation and communication with the patient, as discussed earlier in this chapter.

Initial intensive treatment

The number of visits and the materials and methods used are strictly related to patient's classification and predicted risk. The initial intensive treatment has the following main goals:

- To establish needs-related self-care habits based on self-diagnosis and education
- To heal diseased periodontal tissues as soon as possible, resulting in a reduction in probing depths, Gingival Index, and PFRI
- To eliminate plaque-retentive factors such as restoration overhangs, unpolished restorations, calculus, rough root surfaces, and cavitated caries lesions

For nonrisk (P0) and low-risk (P1) patients without any treatment need, the initial preventive treatment may be limited to one or two visits. For risk (P2 and P3) patients, the initial intensive treatment may range from three to six visits. These visits will be concentrated in as short a period as possible (7 to 10 days) at about 2-day intervals. However, the first two should take place at exactly a 24-hour interval for evaluation of PFRI and establishment of needs-related oral hygiene habits based on PFRI and education in self-diagnosis (see chapter 2).

To facilitate mechanical plaque control by self-care as well as PMTC, plaque-retentive factors will be eliminated as early as possible. The most severe plaque-retentive factors are remaining roots that are untreatable because of caries and teeth that are untreatable because of advanced periodontal disease. Such teeth should be extracted as soon as possible. Overhangs and undercuts of restorations and crowns must be eliminated. Rough surfaces of restorations are finished and polished. Cavitated caries lesions are excavated and restored at least semipermanently with glass-ionomer cement or resin-modified glass-ionomer cement. This should be extra beneficial in caries-risk patients because glass-ionomer cement may act as a slow-release fluoride agent, which can be recharged by daily use of fluoride toothpaste and professional use of fluoride varnish and gels.

Subgingival and supragingival calculus are eliminated, and rough root surfaces are planed with a minimally invasive technique that will not result in exposure of the dentinal tubules. With these procedures, subgingival biofilms should be removed as well. Recontouring can reduce the plaque retention in root grooves and furcation-involved teeth (see chapters 1 and 3.)

The so-called complete-mouth disinfection method (see chapter 2 and Axelsson, 2004) should be implemented in risk patients during this initial intensive treatment period. This means mechanical cleaning of *all* tooth surfaces by PMTC, scraping of the dorsum of the tongue, and interproximal placement of CHX gel or the use of CHX varnish on the key-risk tooth surfaces at every office visit, and subsequent rinsing by the patient with 0.1% or 0.2% CHX solution twice a day. In these patients, complete-mouth disinfection also includes subgingival mechanical removal of the biofilm in combination with irrigation with iodine solution (bactericidal). Depending on the outcome of the analyses of the subgingival microflora, topical use of doxycycline gels or systemic use of antibiotics (amoxicillin and/or metronidazole) may be indicated in especially susceptible patients with impaired general health, such as those with severe cardiovascular problems or poorly controlled diabetes (see chapter 3).

As an effect of this intensive combination of mechanical and chemical plaque control, the periodontal tissues—particularly the free gingivae—will heal. In addition, the PFRI will be dramatically reduced and thus facilitate daily oral hygiene procedures.

Reevaluation

Reevaluation has the following goals:

- To evaluate the results of the initial intensive treatment
- To assess patient compliance
- To evaluate supplementary need for regenerative therapy because of lost periodontal support and restorative treatment
- To determine the materials and methods needed for the maintenance period and the optimal recall intervals

Patients assessed as P2 or P3 should be recalled within 3 to 6 months after the initial intensive treatment for evaluation of the effect on the symptoms of gingivitis and periodontitis. Inflamed gingival sites should be healed and probing depths significantly reduced in P2 and P3 patients. Repeated oral microbiology tests may be indicated in P2 and P3 patients who had high levels of periopathogens in deep diseased pockets at baseline.

At this reevaluation, the dentist decides whether supplementary restorative dentistry or regenerative periodontal therapy is indicated. Through interviews and questionnaires, the patient's knowledge, attitude, and compliance are evaluated. The quality of the patient's self-performed oral hygiene is evaluated by plaque disclosure. It is of great importance to motivate the patient to participate in the evaluation by self-diagnosis at every visit. Based on the outcome of the initial intensive treatment and risk classification, the materials and methods needed for the maintenance period and the optimal recall intervals are determined.

Maintenance program

Intervals, materials, and methods of the maintenance (supportive care) program are strictly related to the patient's classification and predicted risk. The maintenance program has these optimal goals:

- To ensure that healthy individuals with no experience of oral diseases remain healthy (primary prevention)
- To prevent recurrence of oral disease (secondary prevention) after initial successful symptomatic treatment (tertiary prevention); that is, to prevent new infectious inflamed periodontal tissues and further loss of periodontal attachment
- To encourage continuous improvement in self-care habits to prolong the intervals and reduce the need for professional preventive measures

All these goals have been proven to be successfully achieved by a dental hygienist in adults for 30 years, as discussed earlier in this chapter (Axelsson et al, 2004). However, if the maintenance care is failing and the patient exhibits new or further loss of periodontal attachment, he or she will undergo a new sequence of detailed history taking, clinical diagnosis, and testing to evaluate the reasons for new continued disease activity. Based on the outcome of these detailed analyses, another phase of needs-related intensive treatment will be carried out according to the flowchart in Fig 252.

Recall examination

Recall intervals, diagnosis, and supplementary history taking are strictly related to the patient's classification and predicted risk. The reexamination has several goals:

- To evaluate the effect of the PM program
- To prolong the intervals of the PM program and the recall examinations, provided that the patient's self-care has improved and there is no oral disease activity
- To evaluate whether there are new treatment needs
- To repeat an intensive treatment period and introduce a more comprehensive PM program if the previous program has proved unsuccessful

The recall examination should always be carried out by a dentist, at least in P2 and P3 patients. An alternative standard might be evaluation by a dentist specializing in periodontal diseases in at least P3 patients.

Implementation

These principles for needs-related preventive and maintenance programs are based on an ideal ratio of dental professionals, well-developed oral health care systems, high economic and educational standards among the population, and recent knowledge about diagnosis and preventive materials and methods. Local conditions may limit full implementation of this state-of-the-art program.

For example, in Sweden, almost all children and young adults and 80% to 90% of adults are so-called recall patients; they receive some kind of regular maintenance care, but only a minority receive a strictly needs-related preventive program. In many other countries, however, PM programs are still nonexistent, at least for adults.

Table 7 shows in detail a recommended schedule for needs-related preventive and maintenance programs for different age groups based strictly on risk classification, an ideal ratio of dental professionals, and well-developed oral health care systems in a well-educated population with high economic standing. Box 8 provides definitions of the abbreviations used in Table 7.

ANALYTICAL COMPUTERIZED ORAL EPIDEMIOLOGY FOR QUALITY CONTROL

A great deal of time, effort, and money are spent on oral health care each year, so it is reasonable that the government agency responsible for health care have an audit system that regularly evaluates the total effect of the national oral care and dental insurance systems on the oral health status and treatment needs of the population. At the same time, this review encourages and motivates dentists to continuously evaluate the efficiency of their own preventive program at surface, tooth, and individual levels, as well as for their total patient population. Furthermore, a

Table 7 Schedules for needs-related preventive programs (see Box 8 for explanation of abbreviations)

Screening		History taking		Examination/test		Patient category	Initial intensive treatment			Reevaluation		Maintenance period				Reexamination		
EX	DP	HT	DP	EX	DP	PR	PMM	DP	Intervals	EX	DP	EX	PMM	DP	Intervals	EX	DP	Intervals
Children (CH)																		
EX	D	GHT OHT	D	SDE, DEX, PLI, PFRI, OMT, PP, PI, CPITN, CPR, CCITN, PST	D	CH 12–13Y: P2, P3	SCE, OHMT, OHMD, SFD, OHC, OHME, DEB, PMTC	DH, D	2×D, 1×2D	SDE, DEX, 3M	D	SDE, DEX	SCE, OHC, PMTC, DEB, PLI, TAB, SAB	DH	3M	SDE, DEX, CI, PLI, CCITN, PI, CPITN, OMT	D	1Y
EX		GHT OHT	D	SDE, DEX, PLI, PFRI, OMT, PP, PI, CPITN	D	CH 14–19Y: P2, P3	SCE, OHMT, OHMD, SFD, OHC, SC, RP, PCI, PMTC	DH, D	2×D, 1×2D	SDE, DEX, 3M	D, DH	SDE, DEX	SCE, DEB, PCI, PMTC, PFV	DH	3M	SDE, DEX, CI, PLI, PI, CPITN, OMT, PPT	DSP	1Y
Adults (AD)																		
EX	D	GHT OHT	D	SDE, EX, CPR, CCITN, CPITN	D	AD: P0	SCE, OHMT, OHMD, SFD, DEB, PMTC	DH	1×D			SDE, EX	SCE, DEB, PMTC	PDA, DH	1Y	SDE, EX, CCITN	D, DH	2–3Y
EX	D	GHT OHT	D	SDE, EX, PLI, PFRI, CPR, PP, CPITN, CCITN	D	AD: P1	SCE, OHMT, OHMP, SFD, SC, DEB, PMTC	DH	2×D	SDE, EX, 6M	DH	SDE, EX	SCE, DEB, PMTC	DH	6M	SDE, EX, PI, PLI, CPITN, CCITN	D, DH	2Y

EX						AD												
EX	D	GHT OHT	D	SDE, DEX, PP, PI, CPITN, PLI, PFRI, OMT, CPR, CCITN, PPT	D	AD: P2	SCE, OHMT, OHMP, SFD, SC, RP, PCI, PMTC, PFV, OHC	DH	2×D + 2×2D	SDE, DEX, 3M	D / DH	SDE, EX	SCE, OHC, PCI, DEB, PMTC	DH	4–6M	SDE, DEX, PI, PLI, CPITN, CCITN	D	1Y
EX	GHT OHT, DSP		D, DSP	SDE, DEX, PP, PI, CPITN, PLI, PFRI, OMT, CPR, CCITN, PPT, PST	D, DSP	AD: P3	SCE, OHMT, OHMP, OHMI, OHME, SFD, SC, RP, PCI, PMTC, PFV, OHC, TAB, SAB	DH, DSP	2×D + 2–3×2D	SDE, DEX, 3M	D	SDE, DEX	SCE, OHC, DEB, CI, PMTC, TAB, SAB	DH, DSP	3–4M	SDE, DEX, PI, CPITN, CCITN, OMT, PPT	DSP	1Y
EX	D	GHT OHT	D	SDE, DEX, PP, CPR, PI, CI, CPITN, PFRI, PLI, CCITN, OMT, DHE, SSR, PPT	D	AD: C2 P2	SCE, OHMT, OHMP, OHMI, OHME, SFD, SC, RP, PCI, PMTC, PCV, PFV, SFCM, FCG, DHR, SS	D	2×D + 2×2D	SDE, DEX, 3M	DSP, D, DH	SDE, DEX	SCE, FCG, SFCM, DEB, PCI, PMTC, PCV, PFV, SS, DHR	DH, D	4M	SDE, DEX, PI, CI, PLI, PFRI, CPITN, CCITN, DHE, SS, SBC, PPT, OMT	D	1Y
EX	DSC DSP	GHT OHT	DSC DSP	SDE, DEX, PP, CPR, CI, PI, CPITN, PFRI, PLI, CCITN, OMT, DHE, SSR, SBC, PPT, PST	D, DSP, DSC	AD: C3 P3	SCE, OHMT, OHMP, OHMI, OHME, SFD, SC, RP, PCI, PMTC, PCV, PFV, SFCM, FCG, SS, DHR, TAB, SAB	DSC DSP	2×D + 3×2D	SDE, DEX, 2–3M	DSC, DSP, D, DH	SDE, DEX	SCE, FCG, SFCM, DEB, PCI, PMTC, PCV, PFV, SS, DHR, SAB, TAB	DH, D, DSC, DSP	2–3M	SDE, DEX, PI, CI, PLI, PFRI, CPITN, CCITN, DHE, SS, SBC, PPT, OMT	DSC, DSP	6M–1Y

Box 8 Abbreviations used in Table 7

Dental professionals (DP)
D = Dentist
DH = Dental hygienist
DSP = Dentist specialized in periodontology
DSC = Dentist specialized in cariology
PDA = Preventive dentistry assistant

Patient category
AD = Adults
CH = Children

Predicted risk (PR)
C2 = Caries risk
C3 = High caries risk
P0 = No periodontal risk
P1 = Low periodontal risk
P2 = Periodontal risk
P3 = High periodontal risk

History taking (HT)
GHT = General history taking
OHT = Oral history taking

Examinations and tests (EX)
CCITN = Community Caries Index of Treatment Needs
CI = Caries incidence (decayed surfaces/year)
CPITN = Community Periodontal Index of Treatment Needs
CPR = Caries prevalence (decayed, missing, or filled surfaces)
DEX = Detailed examination
DHE = Dietary habits evaluation
EX = Examination
OMT = Oral microflora test
PFRI = Plaque Formation Rate Index
PI = Periodontitis incidence (attachment loss/year)
PLI = Plaque Index
PP = Periodontitis prevalence (attachment loss)
PPT = Periodontal pocket temperature
PST = Genetic periodontal susceptibility test
SBC = Salivary buffer capacity test
SDE = Self-diagnosis education
SSR = Salivary secretion rate

Intervals
$1 \times D$ = One single visit
$2 \times D$ = One visit per day on 2 consecutive days
$2-3 \times 2D$ = Two to three visits at 2-day intervals
$1 \times 2D$ = One visit 2 days after the first two visits
$2 \times 2D$ = Two visits at 2-day intervals after the first two visits
$3 \times 2D$ = Three visits at 2-day intervals after the first two visits
2M = Every 2 months
3M = Every 3 months
4M = Every 4 months
6M = Every 6 months
1Y = Every year
2Y = Every 2 years
3Y = Every 3 years

Preventive materials and methods (PMM)
DEB = Debridement
DHR = Dietary habit recommendation
FCG = Fluoride chewing gum
OHC = Oral hygiene by chemical plaque control
OHMD = Oral hygiene by mechanical plaque control with fluoridated dental tape
OHME = Oral hygiene by mechanical plaque control with electric toothbrush
OHMI = Oral hygiene by mechanical plaque control with interdental brush
OHMP = Oral hygiene by mechanical plaque control with fluoridated wooden toothpick
OHMT = Oral hygiene by mechanical plaque control with toothbrush
PCI = Antimicrobial irrigation of diseased pockets
PCV = Chlorhexidine varnish
PFV = Fluoride varnish
PMTC = Professional mechanical toothcleaning
RP = Root planing
SAB = Systemic use of antibiotics
SC = Scaling
SCE = Self-care education
SFCM = Fluoride antimicrobial mouthwash
SFD = Fluoride dentifrice
SS = Salivary stimulation
TAB = Topical use of antibiotics

national dental insurance scheme should promote preventive dentistry and analytical epidemiology for quality control.

According to Lindskog and Zetterberg (1975), the definition of *epidemiology* is "the medical science of the spread, etiology, and prevention of the epidemic (infectious) diseases." Because certain types of transmissible microorganisms that colonize the tooth surfaces are implicated in the etiology of both caries and periodontal diseases, these diseases are regarded as epidemic diseases.

As discussed earlier, the WHO, in collaboration with the FDI, international dental associations, and ministries of health, established goals for the level of oral health to be attained by the year 2000 for selected indicator age groups in children and adults (see Box 5). One goal recommends that computer-based epidemiologic systems be established to monitor whether these goals are being attained. Epidemiologic surveys in randomized samples of the population are recommended; these should be repeated at 5-year intervals.

Oral health variables

Very powerful personal computers are now available, and portable computers are suitable for field surveys. Today, large volumes of epidemiologic data may be collected, and direct statistical evaluation and graphic presentation of the results are readily accomplished with computer processing. In contrast to other medical disciplines, dentistry has well-established and measurable variables for evaluation of oral health. These variables should be stratified according to their importance. The main reasons for loss of teeth are dental caries and periodontal diseases. Variables associated with these conditions should be given priority in oral health epidemiology. The masticatory efficiency of the dentition and the condition of the oral mucosa should also be included in these surveys.

Tooth loss

The final outcome of untreated caries and periodontal disease is total edentulousness. According to the WHO's goals, edentulousness in 35- to 44- and 65-year-olds should have been reduced from 1969 levels by 50% and 25%, respectively, by the year 2000, and this goal was achieved in most industrialized countries.

In field surveys, retrospective determination of the reasons that teeth are missing is frequently difficult and uncertain. Information with respect to which teeth are most frequently missing and the reason for extraction is important for planning appropriate preventive measures. Important questions that arise are:

- Why are the maxillary molars the most frequently missing teeth?
- Why are maxillary premolars missing more frequently than mandibular premolars?
- Why are the mandibular canines the most resistant of all the teeth?

Loss of occlusal contacts

Mastication is the primary function of the teeth. Masticatory efficiency, that is, chewing capacity, may be expressed in terms of the Eichner index, which is based on the number of occlusal contacts in the molars and premolar areas (Eichner, 1955; Österberg and Landt, 1976).

Dental caries and periodontal diseases

There is a strong correlation between oral health status and the occurrence of dental caries and periodontal diseases. The prevalence of these diseases is therefore the most important dental health variable. Many parallels may be drawn between these two diseases: The etiologies are known in both diseases; pathogenic microorganisms that colonize the tooth surfaces are implicated; and both diseases are site related, that is, not evenly distributed among the teeth and tooth surfaces. For example, the difference in prevalence of both caries and marginal periodontitis at the distal surface of the maxillary first molars and the distal surface of the mandibular canines is usually more significant than the difference in total prevalence between individuals: There are specific, highly susceptible, key-risk teeth and surfaces. If the standard of oral health is to be improved by preventive measures, such facts must be acknowledged and the mechanisms explained.

The prevalence of both caries and periodontal disease should be presented at the individual level as well as at tooth-surface levels. The prevalence of both diseases represents the end result of all incidences and does not progress linearly. In other words, prevalence represents the results of unpredictable site-specific exacerbations and periods of disease quiescence.

Apical periodontitis

In most countries, the prevalence of apical periodontitis has not been determined because complete-mouth intraoral radiographs or panoramic radiographs are required for diagnosis.

Endodontic treatment

Data on the prevalence of endodontic treatment should also be collected. In an adult population, the number of root fractures is strongly correlated with the number of endodontically treated teeth with posts. Most coronal fractures also occur in endodontically treated teeth.

Mucosal diseases

From the oral health aspect, diagnosis and collection of data on diseases of the oral mucosa are very important. In many countries, the prevalence of serious diseases, such as precancerous and cancerous lesions and human immunodeficiency virus–associated lesions, is increasing.

Treatment needs

To allow planning and organization of the resources necessary to meet the need for oral treatment, an estimate must be made of treatment needs, not only for marginal periodontal diseases but also for caries, apical periodontitis, malocclusion, oral mucosal diseases, and bone diseases. Some new indices for treatment needs have therefore been designed: the Community Caries Index of Treatment Needs (CCITN) and the Apical Periodontitis Index of Treatment Needs (APITN; Axelsson, 1988a, 1988b). These indices are analogous to the well-established CPITN (Ainamo et al,

1982; see chapter 9 in volume 4 of this series [Axelsson, 2004]).

Etiologic and modifying factors

In addition to epidemiologic data on prevalence and treatment needs, epidemiologic studies should also include causal and modifying factors (such as systemic diseases and smoking), in terms of the previously mentioned definition of epidemiology.

Computerized epidemiologic survey

Objectives

Based on the experiences of a longitudinal preventive clinical study in adults in Karlstad, county of Värmland, Sweden (Axelsson and Lindhe, 1978, 1981a; Axelsson et al, 1991, 2004), discussed earlier in this chapter, a needs-related preventive program for the adult population of county of Värmland was designed in 1985. This program is continuously updated in accordance with the principles already discussed.

In 1988 a new computer-aided analytic epidemiologic system was designed to evaluate the effects of this preventive program at population, individual, tooth, and surface levels as well as the role of etiologic and modifying factors (Axelsson et al, 1988, 1990, 2000). In 1988 the baseline examination was carried out in randomized samples of 35-, 50-, 65-, and 75-year-olds (N = 1,086) in the county of Värmland, Sweden. They were stratified into living areas (50% rural area and 50% urban area), gender, and dental care system (public dental health care, private practice, and nonpatients). The largest proportion of the study group was 50-year-old subjects (more than 400), the mean age of the adult population; these individuals were followed longitudinally for 10 years to the age of 60 years. New cross-sectional studies were scheduled every 5 years.

A specially designed computer program was used to collect the data. Table 8 shows, in ranking order, the variables included in the new analytical oral epidemiologic system.

Table 8   Variables included in the analytical computer-based oral epidemiologic system

Code	Variable
1	**Oral epidemiology**
1:1	Percent edentulous
1:2	Number of teeth
1:3	Function of teeth: Modified Eichner index
2	**Prevalence**
2:1	Dental caries; decayed, missing, and filled teeth (DMFT); decayed and filled teeth (DFT); decayed, missing, and filled surfaces (DMFSs); decayed and filled surfaces (DFSs)
2:2	Marginal periodontitis
2:2:1	Vertical loss of attachment (mm)
2:2:2	Horizontal loss of attachment (furcation involvement grade 0, I, II, III)
2:3	Apical periodontitis index (Axelsson, 1988b)
2:4	Oral mucosal lesions and bone diseases
2:5	Malocclusion
3	**Treatment needs**
3:1	Dental caries: CCITN (Axelsson, 1988a)
3:2	Marginal periodontitis: CPITN
3:3	Apical periodontitis: APITN (Axelsson, 1988b)
3:4	Oral mucosal lesions and bone diseases
3:5	Malocclusion
4	**Etiologic factors**
4:1	Nonspecific oral microflora: PLI and PFRI (Axelsson, 1987, 1991)
4:2	Specific microflora
5	**Modifying factors**
5:1	External modifying risk indicators, risk factors, and prognostic risk factors: eg, poor oral hygiene and dietary habits, smoking and snuffing habits (other unhealthy lifestyle habits), socioeconomic background (particularly low educational level), use of medicines, infectious and other acquired diseases
5:2	Internal modifying risk indicators, risk factors, and prognostic risk factors: eg, chronic diseases (eg, diabetes mellitus, cardiovascular diseases, Sjögren syndrome), impaired host response (particularly reduced PMNL function), genetic susceptibility to periodontal diseases, reduced salivary secretion rate

Questionnaire

Prior to the clinical examination, the participants answered a questionnaire about their dental care habits, oral hygiene habits, dietary and smoking habits, systemic diseases and use of medicines, socioeconomic background, lifestyle, knowledge of causes and prevention of oral diseases, and other factors. In addition, complete-mouth radiographs were taken.

Some results of the preventive programs for adults were presented earlier in this chapter (see Figs 246a and 246b; for detailed results, see chapter 9 in volume 4 of this series [Axelsson, 2004]).

IMPORTANCE OF CHANGING ATTITUDES TOWARD ORAL HEALTH

If the goal of oral health care is to maintain a natural dentition throughout life, the loss of all teeth is the ultimate failure, closely followed by the high percentage of people with only 20 or fewer remaining teeth. The relevant question is why such a high failure rate has been accepted by the public and the dental profession. Intact teeth and healthy gingiva are simply beautiful, attractive, functional parts of the body and should be much more highly regarded by the population. On the other hand, carious teeth, swollen, red, bleeding gingiva, and foul-smelling breath are most unattractive.

Under similar conditions, patients would never accept destruction of other parts of the body: An ugly false nose or other part of the body normally covered by clothes would never be accepted. Why should anyone accept false teeth? Patients would not accept having even 1% of the nose replaced by amalgam or gold. Imagine having to amputate a finger once every 5 years and replace it with a gold finger, in spite of regular checkups once or twice a year, because of an infectious disease—in an age when this disease, with a well-known etiology, could be successfully prevented.

It is the duty of dental professionals to educate and motivate the public, health personnel, and politicians to regard intact teeth and healthy gingiva as highly as, for example, a healthy nose, eyes, or ears and a justifiable external mode of dress. It is all a matter of changing attitudes and priorities. Famous clothing designers change fashion annually, and people accept the extra costs without hesitation.

A healthy and well-cared-for mouth facilitates communication and human relationships. In addition, the boost in health, well-being, and self-confidence not only is very important for quality of life but also contributes at a very basic biologic level to protection from systemic infection and other general health problems. For example, analytical studies have disclosed a clear relationship between periodontal diseases and cardiovascular diseases (Beck et al, 1996; Kolltveit and Eriksen, 2001; Persson and Persson, 2008), as well as preterm low–birth weight deliveries (Offenbacher et al, 1996, 1998, 1999; Wimmer and Pihlstrom, 2008), diabetes mellitus (Grossi and Genco, 1998; Salvi et al, 2008), and other general health problems. Therefore, when oral health is compromised, the overall health and quality of life are also compromised.

Patient responsibility

Motivation is defined as readiness to act or the driving force behind a person's actions (see chapter 2). Greater responsibility has been described as the motivating factor of longest duration. Optimized responsibility may sometimes result in lifelong motivation, in contrast to the limited durations of encouragement provided by, for example, commendation or a salary increase.

Adults should believe, "No dentist or dental hygienist should accept more responsibility for my oral status than I do myself, because it is my mouth." However, in many industrialized countries with well-organized social health and welfare systems, the population is more or less passive; patients regard the dentist and dental hygienist as responsible for their oral health, the physician as responsible for their general health, and the politicians as responsible for their social welfare.

With the current level of knowledge about the etiology, prevention, and control of dental caries and periodontal diseases, patients who are well motivated and well educated in self-diagnosis and self-care can prevent and control these diseases by themselves. Much more important to general health, quality of life, and costs for health and welfare are the following examples: It is estimated that, among external (environmental) carcinogenic factors, an unhealthy diet accounts for about 30% of cancers, smoking for about 20%, and viruses for about 10%. The simple message on diet is reduction of animal fat and increased intake of fiber-rich vegetables and fruits, which are the cheapest and most accessible food products in tropical and subtropical climates, where most of the world's population lives. For cardiovascular diseases, unhealthy diet and smoking, along with physical inactivity and chronic infectious diseases such as periodontal diseases, are also highly ranked as external (environmental) risk factors.

Physical inactivity may also result in skeletal disorders, particularly back pain.

The important question is: "Who is responsible for what you eat or whether you smoke, exercise, and clean your teeth?" Health maintained and controlled by self-diagnosis and self-care is not only cost effective but also an important factor in quality of life to maintain independence and health.

Practitioner responsibility

The principles of *lege artis* require clinicians to practice dentistry according to modern science and established, well-tried methods, ie, the state of the art. From experimental and well-controlled longitudinal clinical studies in humans, the following conclusions may be drawn:

- Dental caries and periodontal diseases can successfully be prevented and controlled by self-care supplemented by needs-related professional preventive measures.
- Noncavitated caries lesions affecting enamel, root, and even dentin can be arrested successfully (for details see volume 4 of this series [Axelsson, 2004]).
- Regeneration of periodontal attachment is a reality.

Members of the profession are obliged to be continuously updated and to implement state-of-the-art practices (the most recent level of science and evidence-based methods). Therefore, the profession must concentrate on prevention, control, and arrest of dental caries and periodontal diseases. For dental caries, "prevention instead of extension," or at least "prevention before extension," should be given priority. By the same token, aggressive treatment of periodontal diseases with aggressive scaling, extensive flap surgery, extractions, and replacement of teeth with very expensive implant therapy must be regarded as outdated and more or less unjustified.

Oral health and general health are strongly correlated with the level of education. All over the world, the level of education is improving. Eventually, increasingly well-educated patients will learn the implications of high-quality dentistry and will request more preventive dentistry. Dentists who are not wiling to comply with their patients' requests will find that their practices decline.

Improving access to oral care

In all countries, economic restraints, changes in demand for oral health care, political pressures to extend services to underprivileged groups, and concerns about quality, costs, and effectiveness of care demand that alternative ways of organizing oral health care be examined and implemented. Cost and lack of access for underprivileged and low-income groups constrain all oral health care systems. What actions can be taken to combat this neglect, break down the barriers of costs, and improve access to oral health care? Alternative oral care systems must be developed so that a maximum number of people can have access to and can afford oral health care.

Several recent advances give great scope for the transformation of the delivery and quality of oral care:

- New educational technologies via interactive training (eg, the Internet) that make learning both knowledge and skills simpler and faster for all types of personnel
- Simplified and logical design of oral clinics that improve the workplace and substantially reduce the capital cost of equipment and the need for maintenance
- Better materials that are easier and simpler to use

Based on these technological advances, three types of care can be defined: *(1)* simple low-technology care, which is very cost effective; *(2)* moderate-technology care, which is rather expensive; and *(3)* high-technology care, which is often extremely expensive. The first level of oral care includes education of the population in self-diagnosis and self-care on an individual and a group basis, PMTC; use of fluoride varnish and fissure sealants, scaling, root planing, and debridement; and low-technology treatment of single-surface cavitated caries lesions with the so-called atraumatic restorative technique, which has the potential to revolutionize the type of care that can be given in developing countries with a low ratio of dentists. The aim of the first level of oral care is to prevent the need for more traditional and costly invasive oral care; thus PM care should be regarded as level 1.

The second level includes multiple-surface restorations, extractions, simple periodontal surgery, and removable prostheses; that is, traditional invasive oral care practiced by most dentists worldwide. The third and most complex, high-technology level of oral care includes precision prosthetics; implants; laminates and ceramic inlays and onlays; orthodontics; regenerative periodontal treatment; and complex oral surgery and medicine; in other words, costly and complex procedures that require highly qualified specialists. Therefore, in any society, the availability of high-technology oral care will be limited.

A rational, health-promoting, affordable mix of oral care should be planned and implemented in all countries. Emphasis on prevention and control of oral diseases will minimize the need for intervention at the moderate- and high-technology levels. As a consequence of improving oral health in most industrialized countries, the need for moderately complex care is decreasing. With further emphasis on prevention, the need and demand for first-level interventions will increase slightly, while the need for high-technology care will probably increase for several decades because of the desire to preserve natural teeth and the increasing numbers of elderly people who have some natural teeth and edentulous people who want implant treatment.

In developing countries, the low-technology, noninvasive level of oral care will continue to be the major need. In those developing countries where the prevalence of caries is increasing, a rising demand for moderate-technology care will continue over the next few decades. High-technology oral care must, on the other hand, still be limited. In most countries, total coverage is an unrealistic goal, but steps should be taken to ensure that oral care is available to all those who need it.

INFLUENCE OF DENTAL INSURANCE SYSTEMS ON ORAL HEALTH

There is no doubt that different financing and insurance systems will significantly influence oral health status. Some of the different approaches to financing oral care are quality control guidelines, fixed fee agreements, capitation schemes, health maintenance organizations, rewards for increased preventive care, and public health funding.

Quality control guidelines

Information about the duration of treatment methods and acceptable care products is being used to prepare quality control guidelines, indicating the average number of years each type of care should last. If care procedures do not last the specified time, the clinician is then obliged to provide re-treatment free of charge. Such guidelines are intended to reduce unnecessary treatment that results in progressive destruction of tooth substance and periodontal support and higher costs for oral care. Such a system should promote periodontal maintenance care.

Fixed fees

In some countries, for most procedures, dentists may charge only fixed fees agreed on by the health authorities and the professionals. These fees may be exceeded only for special treatment and after a review of the diagnosis and proposed procedure. In countries using this system, the costs of oral care are not rising, and costs are even decreasing in some countries.

Capitation schemes

Capitation schemes pay the dentist a fixed sum for each person enrolled as a patient in the practice. For this fixed annual fee, a dentist contracts to maintain the oral health of all the enrolled patients. However, patients must undertake to attend checkups on a regular basis, or they lose their rights and have to pay for treatment needed to restore their oral health. It seems likely that costs will be reduced and the oral health status improved by this type of program, and this system promotes PM care.

Health maintenance organizations

Health maintenance organizations contract with a group of oral care professionals to provide care to a group of communities or individuals at agreed fees. Health maintenance organizations are usually organized and managed by companies that are specialized in health insurance. This has proved an effective way to limit the costs of providing comprehensive oral care and to promote PM care.

Rewards for increased preventive care

In some countries, projects to encourage preventive care give dental care managers a financial reward if disease levels are reduced in the patients in their geographic area. Such a system will also promote PM care.

Public health funding

During the last decades, in most Scandinavian countries, oral health care programs for children and young adults, including school-based preventive programs, have been organized free of charge by the department of health. For example in Sweden, the Public Dental Health Service has been granted a fixed annual allowance by the Department of Health to carry out needs-related dental care for all individuals up to 20 years of age. This has encouraged and motivated the Public Dental Health Service to focus on preventive dentistry and to delegate preventive treatment to dental hygienists and preventive dentistry assistants, to minimize costly restorative dentistry by dentists; as a result, the oral health status among children and young adults has been dramatically improved.

Proposed oral health insurance system

In 1973, a national dental insurance was introduced for all adults in Sweden, irrespective of whether they chose the public Dental Health Service (40%) or private practice (60%). About 80% to 90% of the Swedish adult population visits dental clinics reg-

ularly for maintenance programs. Until 1999, restorative dentistry, including crown and prostheses, had been based on an itemized fee schedule, but preventive dentistry and periodontal treatment were based on an hourly fee, with different rates for specialized periodontists, general dental practitioners, dental hygienists, and preventive dental assistants. In 1999 the insurance system was reviewed. A capitation system based on the individual's predicted risk combined with analytical epidemiology for quality control was introduced parallel to a modified version of the earlier system.

As discussed earlier in this chapter, oral health professionals must practice according to modern scientific principles and well-established methods. The causes of both dental caries and periodontal diseases are known, as are efficient preventive measures (Axelsson et al, 2004). Therefore, high-quality oral health care must focus on prevention and control of dental caries, periodontal diseases, and other oral diseases, ie, primary and secondary prevention. Existing treatment needs (tertiary prevention) must also be addressed.

In this context, it seems that all national dental health insurance schemes and finance systems should promote prevention and control of oral diseases and include provisions for analytical epidemiology for quality control and analyses of cost effectiveness by the ministry of health, in accordance with national and global oral health goals. In other words, dental professionals should expect to be well paid for successful prevention and control of oral diseases. Ancient Chinese doctors were said to be very well paid as long as they were able to keep their patients healthy. If they failed, they received no reimbursement at all.

The following proposal for an oral health insurance system is based on the state of the art.

The insurance would involve a capitation system based on the predicted risk, including needs-related primary, secondary, and tertiary prevention. The individual annual fee would be combined with a punitive fee based on the effect of the needs-related maintenance program on disease progression. For example, if the patient developed a new caries lesion, the patient's annual fee would be increased by $60 and the dentist's reimbursement would be reduced by $60. Likewise, the annual fee would be increased by a certain amount for the patient and reduced by the same amount for the dentist if the patient exhibited further loss of periodontal support in spite of regular PM care.

For quality control of such an oral health insurance system, a computer-aided analytical oral epidemiologic system should be introduced (as earlier shown in this chapter). The dentist could present beautiful graphs in the waiting room to show the success of the practice in improving the oral health status and eliminating treatment need among the patients. It would significantly increase the dentist's reputation and good will. The patients would feel privileged to belong to the practice and pleased with the effects of their own efforts in self-care; they would be willing to pay a reasonable fee for the high quality of oral health care they were being offered. Old-fashioned colleagues focused on drilling, filling, and billing fear that they are cutting the branch they are sitting on and will lose patients if they practice preventive dentistry. On the contrary, such dentists will lose patients as the public becomes better educated about the benefits of prevention.

Undoubtedly, no single preventive measure or combination of preventive measures would have such a significant impact on the improvement of oral health status as the aforementioned proposal:

- Patients will be motivated to learn and enhance self-diagnosis and self-care to improve their oral health status and prevent increased annual fees for oral health care.
- Dentists will have a reasonable opportunity to practice state-of-the-art dentistry, and as a consequence, their annual reimbursement will not be reduced.

CONCLUSIONS

Primary prevention is mainly performed in children and young adults, who still have no experience of periodontal disease and dental caries or only a few carious tooth surfaces. Large-scale studies have shown that needs-related preventive programs in children and young adults performed by

dental hygienists and specially trained dental assistants are very cost effective. In adults, secondary prevention or so-called maintenance (supportive) care dominates. However, particularly among the elderly, much tertiary prevention is also necessary.

A 30-year longitudinal study revealed that a needs-related PM program carried out by a dental hygienist almost completely prevented tooth loss, loss of periodontal support, and caries development, irrespective of the patient's age. Based on the experiences from this study, a needs-related secondary preventive program for the entire adult population in the county of Värmland, Sweden, was introduced. These large-scale needs-related preventive and supportive care programs for children and adults have shown that periodontal diseases and dental caries can be prevented and controlled successfully with well-known materials and methods. Therefore, it is the duty of dental professionals to implement such programs as much as possible in light of local personnel and economic resources as well as the oral health status and socioeconomic conditions of the population.

It seems improbable that the world will achieve a needs-related distribution of dentists because the resources of teachers and dental schools are very limited in most developing countries. New technology and global interactive training programs may help to overcome this problem. However, training programs for dental hygienists and preventive dentistry assistants are much shorter and less expensive than training programs for dentists. In addition, dental hygienists and preventive dentistry assistants are 100% focused on preventive dentistry, including education of the population in self-care as well as low-cost, low-technology professional preventive treatment and nonsurgical periodontal treatment. Therefore, training programs for these two categories of oral health personnel should be prioritized not only in developing countries but also in most industrialized countries to improve the oral health status of the world population as soon as possible.

In countries with a high prevalence and incidence of dental caries and/or periodontal diseases and limited resources of dentists, a so-called whole-population strategy for preventive programs, performed by other oral health personnel such as dental hygienists and preventive dentistry assistants, should still be cost effective.

On the other hand, in countries with a relatively good oral health status, well-organized dental care systems, and abundant resources, needs-related preventive programs based on predicted risk have to be implemented to improve cost effectiveness. Criteria for classification of caries and periodontitis risk in different age groups should be established in relation to the oral health status and dental care resources. Such criteria should be reevaluated at certain intervals.

Evaluation of the individual patient's risk profile is of great importance. The risk profile is a very useful tool for case presentation and communication with the patient, establishment of needs-related self-care habits, and detailed evaluation of self-care and professional preventive treatment. All new patients should be introduced to a needs-related preventive program in the following order:

- Screening, history taking, and preliminary risk classification
- Supplementary examinations, history taking, and tests in selected risk and high-risk individuals
- Final risk classification
- Initial intensive treatment, in which the number of visits, materials, and methods are related to the individual risk classification
- Reevaluation

In risk and high-risk patients, the effect of the initial intensive treatment should be evaluated after 3 to 6 months. At this evaluation, the materials and methods of the maintenance program and the intervals of reexaminations are determined (see Fig 252 and Table 7).

According to the WHO's goals for the year of 2000, the ministries of health worldwide should support computer-aided oral epidemiology programs to collect data on the oral health status of the population at the national level. Surveys at, for example, 5-year intervals are recommended in randomized samples of specific age groups to evaluate the effect of national oral health programs and to facilitate international comparison. In every county or district, similar surveys should be carried out for comparison at the national level. For ex-

ample, a detailed analytic epidemiologic computer program has been designed to evaluate the effect of a needs-related preventive program for adults, which was introduced in the county of Värmland, Sweden, in 1985. These data allow analysis of outcomes and methods so that oral health care resources can be distributed optimally.

However, all dentists should also be eager to monitor the oral health status of their own patients at group, individual, tooth, and surface level for quality control. Otherwise, clinicians who are optimistic remember only the successful cases, and those who are pessimistic remember only the failures. Furthermore, practitioners who introduce a needs-related preventive program in accordance with the main principles described in this chapter can present yearly, simplified graphs in the waiting room to give patients feedback and to prove how successfully the patients' oral health status is improving. These patients will, in turn, tell their relatives and friends about the successful outcome of the practice.

For successful oral health promotion and improvement of oral health levels, it is necessary to change attitudes toward oral health among patients, oral health personnel, and politicians. Intact, well-functioning teeth and healthy gingiva should be appreciated as much as other healthy and intact parts of the body. Patients must be well educated in self-diagnosis and self-care so that they have the ability to be responsible for their own oral health. Oral health personnel are obliged to be continuously updated about the most recent science and evidence-based new materials and methods, not only to treat but more importantly to prevent and control oral diseases. Likewise, the government and politicians should give priority to prevention of oral diseases.

A rational, health-promoting, affordable mix of oral care should be planned and implemented in all countries. Emphasis on prevention and control of oral diseases will minimize the need for intervention at the moderate- and high-technology levels. As a consequence of improving oral health in most industrialized countries, the need for moderately complex care is decreasing.

In developing countries, the low-technology, noninvasive level of oral care will continue to be the major need. In those developing countries where the prevalence of caries is increasing, a rising demand for moderate-technology care will continue over the next few decades. High-technology oral care must, on the other hand, still be limited.

Because dental insurance and fee systems have a great impact on the content of dental care, they should be specially designed to focus on preventive dentistry. Therefore, a yearly fee based on individual risk prediction has been proposed, combined with increased fees if the outcome of the individualized preventive program is failing (ie, if the patient still develops caries or periodontitis).

REFERENCES

Adriaens PA, Loesche WJ, de Boever JA (1986). Bacteriological study of the microbial flora invading the radicular dentin of periodontally diseased caries-free human teeth. In: Lehner T, Cimasoni G (eds). Borderland Between Caries and Periodontal Disease, vol 3. Geneva: Editions Médecine et hygiène: 383.

Adriaens PA, De Boever JA, Loesche WJ (1988a). Bacterial invasion in root cementum and radicular dentin of periodontally diseased teeth in humans. A reservoir of periodontopathic bacteria. J Periodontol 59:222–229.

Adriaens PA, Edwards CA, De Boever JA, Loesche WJ (1988b). Ultrastructural observations on bacterial invasion in cementum and radicular dentin of periodontally diseased human teeth. J Periodontol 59:493–503.

Adriaens PA, Adriaens LM (2004). Effects of nonsurgical periodontal therapy on hard and soft tissues. Periodontol 2000 36:121–145.

Aimetti M, Romano F, Torta I, Cirillo D, Caposio P, Romagnoli R (2004). Debridement and local application of tetracycline-loaded fibres in the management of persistent periodontitis: Results after 12 months. J Clin Periodontol 31:166–172.

Ainamo J, Barmes D, Beagrie G, Cutress T, Martin J, Sardo-Infirri J (1982). Development of the WHO community periodontal index of treatment needs (CPITN). Int Dent J 32:281–291.

Albandar JM, Rise J, Abbas D (1987). Radiographic quantification of alveolar bone level changes. Predictors of longitudinal bone loss. Acta Odontol Scand 45:55–59.

Albandar JM (1990). A 6-year study on the pattern of periodontal disease progression. J Clin Periodontol 17:467–471.

Al-Hamdan K, Eber R, Sarment D, Kowalski C, Wang H-L (2003). Guided tissue regeneration-based root coverage: Meta-analysis. J Periodontol 74:1520-1533.

American Academy of Periodontology (1996). Proceedings of the 1996 World Workshop in Periodontics. Ann Periodontol 1996;1:1–947.

American Academy of Periodontology (2001). Glossary of Periodontal Terms. Chicago: American Academy of Periodontology.

Aoki A, Sasaki KM, Watanabe H, Ishikawa I (2004). Lasers in nonsurgical periodontal therapy. Periodontol 2000 36:59–97.

Araújo MG, Berglundh T, Lindhe J (1997). On the dynamics of periodontal tissue formation in degree III furcation defects. An experimental study in dogs. J Clin Periodontol 24:738–746.

Araújo MG, Berglundh T, Lindhe J (1998). GTR treatment of degree III furcation defects with 2 different resorbable barriers. An experimental study in dogs. J Clin Periodontol 25:253–259.

Araújo MG, Lindhe J (1998). GTR treatment of degree III furcation defects following application of enamel matrix proteins. An experimental study in dogs. J Clin Periodontol 25:524–530.

Araújo M, Hayacibara R, Sonohara M, Cardaropoli G, Lindhe J (2003). Effect of enamel matrix proteins (Emdogain) on healing after re-implantation of "periodontally compromised" roots. An experimental study in the dog. J Clin Periodontol 30:855–861.

Asikainen S, Dahlén G, Klinge B, Westergaard J (2002). Antibiotika vid paradontala behandlingar [Antibiotic periodontal therapy]. Tandläkartidningen 94:26–33.

Atkinson DR, Cobb CM, Killoy WJ (1984). The effect of an air powered abrasive on in vitro root surfaces. J Periodontol 55:13–18.

Axelsson P, Lindhe J (1974). The effect of a preventive program on dental plaque, gingivitis and caries in schoolchildren. Results after 1- and 2 years. J Clin Periodontol 1:126–138.

Axelsson P, Lindhe J (1977). The effect of a plaque control programme on gingivitis and dental caries in schoolchildren. J Dent Res 56 (special issue):C142–C148.

Axelsson P (1978). The Effect of Plaque Control Procedures on Gingivitis, Periodontitis and Dental Caries [thesis]. Gothenburg: Univ of Gothenburg.

Axelsson P, Lindhe J (1978). Effect of controlled oral hygiene procedures on caries and periodontal disease in adults. J Clin Periodontol 5:133–151.

Axelsson P, Lindhe J (1981a). Effect of controlled oral hygiene procedures on caries and periodontal disease in adults. Results after six years. J Clin Periodontol 8:239–248.

Axelsson P, Lindhe J (1981b). The significance of maintenance care in the treatment of periodontal disease. J Clin Periodontol 8:281–294.

Axelsson P (1987). Placknybildningsindex PFRI—Indikator för karies- och parodontitprevention, munhygien-frekvens och ytrelaterad munhygien. Tandlakartidningen 79:387–391.

Axelsson P, Lindhe J (1987). Efficacy of mouthrinses in inhibiting dental plaque and gingivitis in man. J Clin Periodontol 14:205–212.

Axelsson P, Paulander J, Nordqvist K, Karlsson R (1987a). The effect of fluoride containing dentifrice, rinsing and varnish on interproximal dental caries. A 3-year clinical trial. Community Dent Oral Epidemiol 15:177–180.

Axelsson P, Kristoffersson K, Karlsson R, Bratthall D (1987b). A 30-month longitudinal study of the effects of some oral hygiene measures on Streptococcus mutans and approximal dental caries. J Dent Res 66:761–765.

Axelsson P (1988a). The Community Caries Index of Treatment Needs (CCITN). Presented at the 1st International Conference on Preventive Dentistry and Epidemiology, Karlstad, Sweden, 8–10 Aug 1988.

References

Axelsson P (1988b). The Apical Periodontal Index of Treatment Needs (APITN). Presented at the 1st International Conference on Preventive Dentistry and Epidemiology, Karlstad, Sweden, 8–10 Aug 1988.

Axelsson P, Paulander J, Tollskog G (1988). A new computer-based oral epidemiology system. Presented at the 1st International Conference on Preventive Dentistry and Epidemiology, Karlstad, Sweden, 8–10 Aug 1988.

Axelsson P, Paulander J, Tollskog G (1990). A new computer-based oral epidemiology system. Presented at the 2nd International Conference on Preventive Dentistry and Epidemiology, Karlstad, Sweden, 8–10 Aug 1988.

Axelsson P (1991). A four-point scale for selection of caries risk patients, based on salivary *S. mutans* levels and plaque formation rate index. In: Johnson NW (ed). Risk Markers for Oral Diseases, vol 1. Dental Caries. Cambridge, NY: Cambridge University Press: 158–170.

Axelsson P, Lindhe J, Nyström B (1991). On the prevention of caries and periodontal disease. Results of a 15-year-longitudinal study in adults. J Clin Periodontol 13:182–189.

Axelsson P (1993). New ideas and advancing technology in prevention and nonsurgical treatment of periodontal disease. Int Dent J 43:223–238.

Axelsson P (1994). Mechanical plaque control. In: Lang N, Karring T (eds). Proceedings of the 1st European Workshop on Periodontology, 1993. London: Quintessence: 219–243.

Axelsson P (1998). Needs-related plaque control measures based on risk prediction. In: Lang NP, Attström R, Löe H (eds). Proceedings of the European Workshop on Mechanical Plaque Control. Berlin: Quintessence: 190–247.

Axelsson P, Paulander J, Svärdström G, Kaijser H (2000). Effects of population based preventive programs on oral health conditions. J Parodontol Implantol Orale 19:255–269.

Axelsson P, Paulander J, Nordström L, Jonsson AS, Appel B (2001). The Role of Genetic Interleukin-1 Polymorphism on Tooth Loss and Periodontal Support Loss in 50- to 60-year-old Smokers and Non-smokers [abstract]. Gothenburg, Sweden: Scientific Congress, Dept of Periodontology, Univ of Gothenburg.

Axelsson P (2002). Axelsson Series on Preventive Dentistry, vol 3. Diagnosis and Risk Prediction of Periodontal Diseases. Chicago: Quintessence.

Axelsson P (2004). Axelsson Series on Preventive Dentistry, vol 4. Preventive Materials, Methods, and Programs. Chicago: Quintessence.

Axelsson P, Nyström B, Lindhe J (2004). The long-term effect of a plaque control program on tooth mortality, caries and periodontal disease in adults. Results after 30 years of maintenance. J Clin Periodontol 31:749–757.

Badersten A, Nilvéus R, Egelberg J (1981). Effect of nonsurgical periodontal therapy. 1. Moderately advanced periodontitis. J Clin Periodontol 8:57–72.

Badersten A, Nilvéus R, Egelberg J (1984a). Effect of nonsurgical periodontal therapy. 2. Severely advanced periodontitis. J Clin Periodontol 11:63–76.

Badersten A, Nilvéus R, Egelberg J (1984b). Effect of nonsurgical periodontal therapy. 3. Single versus repeated instrumentation. J Clin Periodontol 11:114–124.

Badersten A, Nilvéus R, Egelberg J (1985a). Effect of nonsurgical periodontal therapy. 4. Operator variability. J Clin Periodontol 12:190–200.

Badersten A, Nilvéus R, Egelberg J (1985b). Effect of nonsurgical periodontal therapy. 5. Patterns of probing attachment loss in non-responding sites. J Clin Periodontol 12:270–282.

Badersten A, Nilvéus R, Egelberg J (1985c). Effect of nonsurgical periodontal therapy. 6. Localization of sites with probing attachment loss. J Clin Periodontol 12:351–359.

Badersten A, Nilvéus R, Egelberg J (1985d). Effect of nonsurgical periodontal therapy. 7. Bleeding, suppuration and probing depth in sites with probing attachment loss. J Clin Periodontol 12:432–440.

Badersten A, Nilvéus R, Egelberg J (1987a). Effect of nonsurgical periodontal therapy. 8. Probing attachment changes related to clinical characteristics. J Clin Periodontol 14:425–432.

Badersten A, Nilvéus R, Egelberg J (1987b). 4-year observations of basic periodontal therapy. J Clin Periodontol 14:438–444.

Baehni P, Thilo B, Chapuis B, Pernet D (1992). Effects of ultrasonic and sonic scalers on dental plaque microflora in vitro and in vivo. J Clin Periodontol 19:455–459.

Baehni PC, Tessier JF (1994). Supportive periodontal care. In: Lang NP, Karring T (eds). Proceedings of the 1st European Workshop on Periodontology, 1993. London: Quintessence: 274–288.

Bardet P, Suvan J, Lang N (1999). Clinical effects of root instrumentation using conventional steel or non-tooth substance removing plastic curettes during supportive periodontal therapy (SPT). J Clin Periodontol 26:742–747.

Bartold PM, Xiao Y, Lyngstaadas SP, Paine ML, Snead ML (2006). Principles and applications of cell delivery systems for periodontal regeneration. Periodontol 2000 41:123–135.

Bass CC (1954). An effective method of personal oral hygiene. J La State Med Soc 106:100–112.

Beck J, Garcia R, Heiss G, et al (1996). Periodontal disease and cardiovascular disease. J Periodontol 67(suppl):1123–1137.

Becker W, Becker BE, Prichard JF, Caffesse R, Rosenberg E, Gian-Grasso J (1987). Root isolation of new attachment procedures. A surgical and suturing method. Three case reports. J Periodontol 58:819–826.

Becker W, Becker B, Ochsenbein C, et al (1988). A longitudinal study comparing scaling, osseous surgery and modified Widman procedures. Results after one year. J Periodontol 59:351–365.

Becker W, Becker BE, Caffesse R, et al (2001). A longitudinal study comparing scaling, osseous surgery and modified Widman procedures: Results after 5 years. J Periodontol 72:1675–1684.

Björn AL, Björn H, Grkovic B (1969). Marginal fit of restorations and its relation to periodontal bone level. 1. Metal fillings. Odontol Rev 20:311–321.

Björn AL, Björn H, Grkovic B (1970). Marginal fit of restorations and its relation to periodontal bone level. 2. Crowns. Odontol Rev 21:337–346.

Blomlöf L, Lindskog S, Appelgren R, Jonsson B, Weintraub A, Hammarström L (1987). New attachment in monkeys with experimental periodontitis with and without removal of the cementum. J Clin Periodontol 14:136–143.

Blomlöf L, Friskopp J, Appelgren R, Lindskog S, Hammarström L (1989). Influence of granulation tissue, dental calculus and contaminated root cementum on periodontal wound healing. An experimental study in monkeys. J Clin Periodontol 16:27–32.

Blomlöf J, Lindskog S (1995). Root surface texture and early cell and tissue colonization after different etching modalities. Eur J Oral Sci 103:17–24.

Blomlöf J, Blomlöf L, Lindskog S (1996). Smear removal and collagen exposure after nonsurgical root planing followed by etching with an EDTA gel preparation. J Periodontol 67:841–845.

Bogren A, Teles RP, Torresyap G, Haffajee AD, Socransky SS, Wennström JL (2008). Locally delivered doxycycline during supportive periodontal therapy: A 3-year study. J Periodontol 79:827–835.

Bollen CML, Mongardini, C, Papaioannou W, Van Steenberghe D, Quirynen M (1998). The effect of a one-stage full-mouth disinfection on different intra-oral niches. Clinical and microbiological observations. J Clin Periodontol 25:56–66.

Bonito AJ, Lux L, Luhr KN (2005). Impact of local adjuncts to scaling and root planing in periodontal disease therapy: A systematic review. J Periodontol 76:1227–1236 [erratum 2006;77:326].

Bosman CW, Powell RN (1977). The reversal of localized experimental gingivitis. A comparison between mechanical toothbrushing procedures and a 0.2% chlorhexidine mouth rinse. J Clin Periodontol 4:161–172.

Bosshardt DD (2008). Biological mediators and periodontal regeneration: A review of enamel matrix proteins at the cellular and molecular levels. J Clin Periodontol 35(8 suppl):87–105.

Bouwsma O, Yost K, Baron H (1992). Comparison of a chlorhexidine rinse and a wooden interdental cleaner in reducing interdental gingivitis. Am J Dent 5:143–146.

Bowers G, Felton F, Middleton C, et al (1991). Histologic comparison of regeneration in human intrabony defects when osteogenin is combined with demineralized freeze-dried bone allograft and with purified bovine collagen. J Periodontol 62:690–702.

Braun A, Krause F, Nolden R, Frentzen M (2003). Subjective intensity of pain during the treatment of periodontal lesions with the Vector-system. J Periodontal Res 38:135–140.

Braun A, Krause F, Frentzen M, Jepsen S (2005). Removal of root substance with the Vector-system compared with conventional debridement in vitro. J Clin Periodontol 32:152–157.

Brunsvold MA, Lane JJ (1990). The prevalence of overhanging dental restorations and their relationship to periodontal disease. J Clin Periodontol 17:67–72.

Brunsvold MA, Mellonig JT (1993). Bone grafts and periodontal regeneration. Periodontol 2000 1:80–91.

Buchanan SA, Robertson PB (1987). Calculus removal by scaling and root planing with and without surgical access. J Periodontol 58:159–163.

Caffesse RG, Sweeney PL, Smith BA (1986). Scaling and root planing with and without periodontal flap surgery. J Clin Periodontol 13:205–210.

Cairo F, Pagliaro U, Nieri M (2008). Treatment of gingival recession with coronally advanced flap procedures: A systematic review. J Clin Periodontol 35(8 suppl):136–162.

Cardaropoli G, Araújo M, Hayacibara R, Sukekava F, Lindhe J (2005). Healing of extraction sockets and surgically produced–augmented and non-augmented–defects in the alveolar ridge. An experimental study in the dog. J Clin Periodontol 32:435–440.

Carey HM, Daly CG (2001). Subgingival debridement of root surfaces with a micro-brush: Macroscopic and ultrastructural assessment. J Clin Periodontol 28:820–827.

Castellanos A, de la Rosa MR, de la Garza M, Caffesse RG (2006). Enamel matrix derivative and coronal flaps to cover marginal tissue recessions. J Periodontol 77:7–14.

Caton J, Nyman S (1980). Histometric evaluation of periodontal surgery. 1. The modified Widman flap procedure. J Clin Periodontol 7:212–223.

Caton J, Nyman S, Zander H (1980). Histometric evaluation of periodontal surgery. 2. Connective tissue attachment levels after four regenerative procedures. J Clin Periodontol 7:224–231.

Cattabriga M, Pedrazzoli V, Wilson G Jr (2000). The conservative approach in the treatment of furcation lesions. Periodontol 2000 22:133–153.

Chen J, Burch J, Beck F, Horton J (1987). Periodontal attachment loss associated with proximal tooth restorations. J Prosthet Dent 57:416–420.

Cho MI, Lin W-L, Genco RJ (1995). Platelet-derived growth factor–modulated guided tissue regenerative therapy. J Periodontol 66:522–530.

Christersson LA, Albini B, Zambon J, Wikesjö U, Genco R (1987). Tissue localization of *Actinobacillus actinomycetemcomitans* in human periodontitis. 1. Light immunofluorescence and electron microscopic studies. J Periodontol 58:529–539.

Claffey N, Polyzois I, Ziaka P (2004). An overview of non-surgical and surgical therapy. Periodontol 2000 36:35–44.

Cohen RE, Research, Science and Therapy Committee, American Academy of Periodontology (2003). Position paper: Periodontal maintenance. J Periodontol 74:1395–1401.

Coldiron NB, Yukna RA, Weir J, Caudill RF (1990). A quantitative study of cementum removal with hand curettes. J Periodontol 61:293–299.

Contreras A, Slots J (2000). Herpesviruses in human periodontal disease. J Periodontal Res 35:3–16.

Cortellini P, Prato GP, Baldi C, Clauser C (1990). Guided tissue regeneration with different materials. Int J Periodontics Restorative Dent 10(2):137–151.

Cortellini P, Prato GP, Tonetti MS (1993). Periodontal regeneration of human infrabony defects. 1. Clinical measures. J Periodontol 64:254–260.

Cortellini P, Prato GP, Tonetti M (1994). Periodontal regeneration of human infrabony defects. 5. Effects of oral hygiene on long-term stability. J Clin Periodontol 21:606–610.

Cortellini P, Bowers GM (1995). Periodontal regeneration at intrabony defects: An evidence-based treatment approach. Int J Periodontics Restorative Dent 15:128–145.

Cortellini P, Prato GP, Tonetti MS (1995). The modified papilla preservation technique. A new surgical approach for interproximal regenerative procedures. J Periodontol 66:261–266.

Cortellini P, Prato GP, Tonetti MS (1999). The simplified papilla preservation flap. A novel surgical approach for the management of soft tissues in regenerative procedures. Int J Peridontics Restorative Dent 19:589–599.

Cortellini P, Tonetti MS (2000). Focus on intrabony defects: Guided tissue regeneration (GTR). Periodontol 2000 22:104–132.

Cortellini P, Tonetti MS (2004). Long-term tooth survival following regenerative treatment of intrabony defects. J Periodontol 75:672–678.

Cortellini P, Tonetti MS (2008). Regenerative therapy. In: Lindhe J and Lang NP (eds). Clinical Periodontology and Implant Dentistry, ed 5, vol 2. Oxford: Blackwell Munksgaard: 901–954.

Costerton JW, Lewandowski Z, Caldwell D, Korber D, Lappin-Scott H (1995). Microbial biofilms. Ann Rev Microbiol 49:711–745.

Cury PR, Sallum E, Nociti FH, Sallum AW, Jeffcoat MK (2003). Long-term results of guided tissue regeneration therapy in the treatment of class II furcation defects: A randomized clinical trial. J Periodontol 74:3–9.

Dahlén G, Lindhe J, Sato K, Hanamura H, Okamoto H (1992). The effect of supragingival plaque control on the subgingival microbiota in subjects with periodontal disease. J Clin Periodontol 19:802–809.

References

Demolon IA, Persson GR, Moncla BJ, Johnson RH, Ammons WF (1993). Clinical and bacterial investigation of the guided tissue regeneration procedure. J Periodontol 64:609–616.

Demolon IA, Persson R, Ammons WA, Johnson RH (1994). Effect of antibiotic treatment on clinical conditions with guided tissue regeneration: One-year results. J Periodontol 65:713–717.

DeSanctis M, Murphy C (2000). The role of resective periodontitis surgery in the treatment of furcation defects. Periodontol 2000 22:154–168.

De Soete M, Mongardini C, Peuwels M, et al (2001). One-stage full-mouth disinfection. Long-term microbiological results analyzed by checkerboard DNA-DNA hybridization. J Periodontol 72:374–382.

Dragoo MR, Kaldahl WB (1983). Clinical and histological evaluation of alloplasts and allografts in regenerative periodontal surgery in humans. Int J Periodontics Restorative Dent 3(2):8–29.

Drisko CH, Lewis LH (1996). Ultrasonic instruments and antimicrobial agents in supportive periodontal treatment and retreatment of recurrent or refractory periodontitis. Periodontol 2000 12:90–115.

Dzink J, Gibbons R, Childs W, Socransky S (1989). The predominant cultivable microbiota of crevicular epithelial cells. Oral Microbiol Immunol 4:1–5.

Ehnevid H, Jansson L, Lindskog S, Weintraub A, Blomlöf L (1995). Endodontic pathogens: Propagation of infection through patent dentinal tubules in traumatized monkey teeth. Endod Dent Traumatol 11:229–234.

Eichner K (1955). Über eine Gruppeneinteilung des Lückengebisses für die Prothetik. Dtsch Zahnärztl Z 10:1831–1834.

Eickholz P, Kim TS, Bürklin T, et al (2002). Non-surgical periodontal therapy with adjunct topical doxycycline: A double blind randomized controlled multicenter study. 1. Study design and clinical results. J Clin Periodontol 29:108–111.

Eickholz P, Krigar DM, Prezl B, Steinbrenner H, Dörfer C, Kim TS (2004). Guided tissue regeneration with bioabsorbable barriers. 2. Long-term results in infrabony defects. J Periodontol 75:957–965.

Eickholz P, Pretzl B, Holle R, Kim TS (2006). Long-term results of guided tissue regeneration therapy with nonresorbable and bioabsorbable barriers. 3. Class II furcations after 10 years. J Periodontol 77;88–94.

Eickholz P, Krigar DM, Reitmeir P, Rawlinson A (2007). Stability of clinical and radiographic results after guided tissue regeneration in infrabony defects. J Periodontol 78:37–46.

Eid M (1986). Relationship between overhanging amalgam restorations and periodontal disease. Odontostomatol Trop 9:220–226.

Eide B, Lie T, Selvig KA (1983). Surface coatings on dental cementum incident to periodontal disease. 1. A scanning electron microscopic study. J Clin Periodontol 10:157–171.

Eide B, Lie T, Selvig KA (1984). Surface coatings on dental cementum incident to periodontal disease. 2. Scanning electron microscopic confirmation of a mineralized cuticle. J Clin Periodontol 11:565–575.

Ellegaard B, Karring T, Listgarten M, Löe H (1973). New attachment after treatment of interradicular lesions. J Periodontol 44:209–217.

Ellegaard B, Karring T, Davies R, Löe H (1974). New attachment after treatment of intrabony defects in monkeys. J Periodontol 45:368–377.

Esposito M, Coulthard P, Worthington HV (2003). Enamel matrix derivative (Emdogain) for periodontal tissue regeneration in intrabony defects. Cochrane Database Syst Rev 2:CD003875 [update: Esposito M, Grusovin MG, Coulthard P, Worthington HV (2005). 4:CD003875].

Fédération Dentaire International (1990). Basic Facts 1990: Dentistry around the world. Ferney-Voltaire, France: FDI.

Fine DH, Hammond BF, Loesche WJ (1998). Clinical use of antibiotics in clinical practice. Int J Antimicrob Agents 9:235–238.

Fives-Taylor PM, Meyer DH, Mintz KP, Brissette C (1999). Virulence factors of Actinobacillus actinomycetemcomitans. Periodontol 2000 20:136–167.

Fleischer HC, Mellonig JT, Brayer WK, Gray JL, Barnett JD (1989). Scaling and root planing in multirooted teeth. J Periodontol 60:402–409.

Flemmig TF, Petersilka GJ, Mehl A, Hickel R, Klaiber B (1998a). The effect of working parameters on root substance removal using a piezoelectric ultrasonic scaler in vitro. J Clin Periodontol 25:158–163.

Flemmig TF, Petersilka GJ, Mehl A, Hickel R, Klaiber B (1998b). Working parameters of a magnetostrictive ultrasonic scaler influencing root substance removal in vitro. J Periodontol 69:547–553.

Frank RM, Voegel J (1978). Bacterial bone resorption in advanced cases of human periodontitis. J Periodontal Res 13:251–261.

Frentzen M, Braun A, Aniol D (2002). Er:YAG laser scaling of diseased root surfaces. J Periodontol 73:524–530.

Froum SJ, Kushner L, Scopp IW, Stahl SS (1982). Human clinical and histologic responses to Durapatite implants in intraosseous lesions. Case reports. J Periodontol 53:719–725.

Froum S, Stahl SS (1987). Human intraosseous healing responses to the placement of tricalcium phosphate ceramic implants. 2. 13 to 18 months. J Periodontol 58:103–109.

Galloway SE, Pashley DH (1987). Rate of removal of root structure by the use of the Prophy-Jet device. J Periodontol 58:464–469.

Ganeles J, Listgarten MA, Evian CI (1986). Ultrastructure of Durapatite-periodontal tissue interface in human intrabony defects. J Periodontol 57:133–140.

Garmyn P, van Steenberghe D, Quirynen M (1998). Efficacy of plaque control in the maintenance of gingival health: Plaque control in primary and secondary prevention. In: Lang NP, Attström R, Löe H (eds). Proceedings of the European Workshop on Mechanical Plaque Control. Chicago: Quintessence: 107–120.

Garrett S, Johnson L, Drisko CH, et al (1999). Two multi-center studies evaluating locally delivered doxycycline hyclate, placebo control, oral hygiene, and scaling and root planing in the treatment of periodontitis. J Periodontol 70:490–503.

Gaunt F, Devine M, Pennington M, et al (2008). The cost-effectiveness of supportive periodontal care for patients with chronic periodontitis. J Clin Periodontol 35(8 suppl):67–82.

Gestrelius S, Andersson C, Johansson AC, et al (1997a). Formulation of enamel matrix derivative for surface coating. Kinetics and cell colonization. J Clin Periodontol 24:678–684.

Gestrelius S, Andersson C, Lidström D, Hammarström L, Somerman M (1997b). In vitro studies on periodontal ligament cells and enamel matrix derivative. J Clin Periodontol 24:685–692.

Gestrelius S, Lyngstadaas SP, Hammarström L (2000). Emdogain—Periodontal regeneration based on biomimicry. Clin Oral Investig 4:120–125.

Giannobile WV, Hernandez RA, Finkelman RD, et al (1996). Comparative effects of platelet-derived growth factor-BB and insulin-like growth factor-I, individually and in combination, on periodontal regeneration in *Macaca fascicularis*. J Periodontal Res 31:301–312.

Giannobile WV, Somerman MJ (2003). Growth and amelogenin-like factors in periodontal wound healing. A systematic review. Ann Periodontol 8:193–204.

Gilmore N, Sheiham A (1971). Overhanging dental restorations and periodontal disease. J Periodontol 42:8-12.

Giuliana G, Ammatuna P, Pizzo G, Capone F, D´Angelo M (1997). Occurrence of invading bacteria in radicular dentin of periodontally diseased teeth: Microbiological findings. J Clin Periodontol 24:478-485.

Gjermo P, Flötra L (1970). The effect of different methods of interdental cleaning. J Periodontal Res 5:230-236.

Glavind L (1977). Effect of monthly professional mechanical tooth cleaning on periodontal health in adults. J Clin Periodontol 4: 100-106.

Goodson J, Holborow D, Dunn R, Hogan P, Dunham S (1983). Monolithic tetracycline containing fibers for controlled delivery to periodontal pockets. J Periodontol 54:575-579.

Goodson JM, Haffajee AD, Socransky SS (1984). The relationship between attachment level loss and alveolar bone loss. J Clin Periodontol 11:348-359.

Goodson JM, Cugini MA, Kent RL, et al (1991a). Multi-center evaluation of tetracycline fiber therapy. 2. Clinical response. J Periodontal Res 26:371-379.

Goodson JM, Tanner A, McArdle S, Dix K, Watnabe SM (1991b). Multicenter evaluation of tetracycline fiber therapy. 3. Microbiological response. J Periodontal Res 26:440-451.

Gordon J, Walker C, Lamster I, et al (1985). Efficacy of clindamycin hydrochloride in refractory periodontitis: 12-month results. J Periodontol 56 (suppl):75-80.

Gordon J, Walker C, Hovliaras C, Socransky S (1990). Efficacy of clindamycin hydrochloride in refractory periodontitis: 24-month results. J Periodontol 61:686-691.

Gorzo I, Newman HN, Strahan JD (1979). Amalgam restorations, plaque removal and periodontal health. J Clin Periodontol 6: 98-105.

Gottlow J, Nyman S, Karring T, Lindhe J (1984). New attachment formation as the result of controlled tissue regeneration. J Clin Periodontol 11:494-503.

Gottlow J, Nyman S, Lindhe J, Karring T, Wennström J (1986). New attachment formation in the human periodontium by guided tissue regeneration. Case reports. J Clin Periodontol 13:604-616.

Gottlow J, Nyman S, Karring T (1992). Maintenance of new attachment gained thorough guided tissue regeneration. J Clin Periodontol 19:315-317.

Gottlow J (1994). Periodontal regeneration. In: Lang N, Karring T (eds). Proceedings of the 1st European Workshop on Periodontology, 1993. London: Quintessence: 172-192.

Gottlow J, Laurell L, Teiwik A, Genon P (1994). Guided tissue regeneration using a bioresorbable matrix barrier. Pract Periodontics Aesthet Dent 6(2):71-78.

Graziani F, Laurell L, Tonetti M, Gottlow J, Berglundh T (2005). Periodontal wound healing following GTR therapy of dehiscence-type defects in the monkey: Short-, medium- and long-term healing. J Clin Periodontol 32:905-914.

Greenstein G, Rethman M (1996). The role of tetracycline impregnated fibers in retreatment. Periodontol 2000 12:130-140.

Greenstein G, Polson A (1998). The role of local drug delivery in the management of periodontal diseases: A comprehensive review. J Periodontol 69:507-520.

Greenstein G, Tonetti M (2000). The role of controlled drug delivery for periodontitis. The Research, Science and Therapy Committee of the American Academy of Periodontology. J Periodontol 71:125-140.

Greenstein G (2006). Local drug delivery in the treatment of periodontal diseases: Assessing the clinical significance of the results. J Periodontol 77:565-578.

Gröndahl HG, Gröndahl K (1983). Subtraction radiography for the diagnosis of periodontal bone lesions. Oral Surg Oral Med Oral Pathol 55:208-213.

Gröndahl K, Gröndahl HG, Wennström J, Heijl L (1987). Examiner agreement in estimating changes in periodontal bone from conventional and subtraction radiographs. J Clin Periodontol 14:74-79.

Gröndahl HG (1997). Radiographic examination. In: Lindhe J, Karring T, Lang N (eds). Clinical Periodontology and Implant Dentistry. Copenhagen: Munksgaard: 873-889.

Grossi S, Genco R (1998). Periodontal disease and diabetes mellitus: A two-way relationship. Ann Periodontol 3:51-61.

Guerrero A, Griffiths GS, Nibali L, et al (2005). Adjunctive benefits of systemic amoxicillin and metronidazole in non-surgical treatment of generalized aggressive periodontitis: A randomized placebo controlled clinical trial. J Clin Periodontol 32:1096-1107.

Gutknecht N, Zimmerman R, Lampert F (2001). Lasers in periodontology: State of the art. J Oral Laser Appl 1:169-179.

Gutmann JL (1978). Prevalence, location and patency of accessory canals in the furcation region of permanent molars. J Periodontol 49:21-26.

Gwinnett AJ, Golub LM, Kleinberg I (1975). Effect of a repeated prophylaxis on plaque accumulation and gingival crevicular fluid flow [abstract 605]. J Dent Res 54(special issue A).

Haffajee AD, Cugini MA, Dibart S, Smith C, Kent RL Jr, Socransky SS (1997). The effect of SRP on the clinical and microbiological parameters of periodontal diseases. J Clin Periodontol 24: 324-334.

Haffajee AD, Bogren A, Hasturk H, Feres M, Lopez N, Socransky SS (2004). Subgingival microbiota of chronic periodontitis subjects from different geographic locations. J Clin Periodontol 31: 996-1002.

Haffajee AD, Teles RP, Socransky SS (2006). The effect of periodontal therapy on the composition of the subgingival microbiota. Periodontol 2000 42:219-258.

Håkansson R (1991). Dental Care Habits and Dental Status in 1974-1985 Among Adults in Sweden. Comparative Cross-Sectional and Longitudinal Investigations [thesis]. Lund, Sweden: Lund Univ.

Hakkarainen K, Ainamo J (1980). Influence of overhanging posterior tooth restorations on alveolar bone height in adults. J Clin Periodontol 7:114-120.

Hammarström L (1997). Enamel matrix, cementum development and regeneration. J Clin Periodontol 24:658-668.

Hanes PJ, Purvis JP (2003). Local anti-infective therapy: Pharmacological agents. A systematic review. Ann Periodontol 8:79-98.

Hänggi D, Ritz L, Rateitschak KH (1991). The Perioplaner/Periopolisher. The loss of substance on the root surface and the initial clinical experiences [in German]. Schweiz Monatsschr Zahnmed 101: 1535-1541.

Harper DS, Robinson PJ (1987). Correlation of histometric, microbial, and clinical indicators of periodontal disease status before and after root planing. J Clin Periodontol 14:190-196.

Heden G, Wennström JL (2006). 5-year follow-up of regenerative periodontal therapy with enamel matrix derivative at sites with angular bone defects. J Periodontol 77:295-301.

References

Heijl L, Heden G, Svardstrom G, Ostgren A (1997). Enamel matrix derivative (Emdogain) in the treatment of intrabony periodontal defects. J Clin Periodontol 24:705–714.

Heijl L, Gestrelius S (2001). Treatment of intrabony defects with periodontal surgery and adjunctive Emdogain. A review and meta-analysis involving all studies with at least 10 patients published between 1998 and January 2001 [unpublished report submitted to the US Food and Drug Administration].

Heitz-Mayfield L, Trombelli L, Heiltz F, Needleman I, Moles D (2002). A systematic review of the effect of surgical debridement vs non-surgical debridement for the treatment of chronic periodontitis. J Clin Periodontol 29(suppl 3):92–102.

Heitz-Mayfield L, Tonetti MS, Cortellini P, Lang NP (2006). On behalf of European Research Group on Periodontology (ERGOPERIO). Microbial colonization patterns predict the outcomes of surgical treatment of intrabony defects. J Clin Periodontol 33:62–68.

Hellström M, Ramberg P, Krok L, Lindhe J (1996). The effect of supragingival plaque control on the subgingival microflora in human periodontitis. J Clin Periodontol 23:934–940.

Hellwig E, Attin T (1994). Fluoride retention in dentin after topical application of fluoride varnishes [abstract 67]. Caries Res 28:199.

Herrera D, Sanz M, Jepsen S, Needleman I, Roldan S (2002). A systematic review on the effect of systemic antimicrobials as an adjunct to scaling and root planing in periodontitis patients. J Clin Periodontol 29(suppl 3):136–159.

Herrera D, Alonso B, León R, Roldán S, Sanz M (2008). Antimicrobial therapy in periodontitis: The use of systemic antimicrobials against the subgingival biofilm. J Clin Periodontol 35(8 suppl):45–66.

Hirsch RS, Clarke NG, Shrikandi W (1989). Pulpal pathosis and severe alveolar lesions: A clinical study. Endod Dent Traumatol 5:48–54.

Hoffmann T, Richter S, Meyle J, et al (2006). A randomized clinical multicenter trial comparing enamel matrix derivate and membrane treatment of buccal class II furcation involvement in mandibular molars. 3. Patient factors and treatment outcome. J Clin Periodontol 33:575–583.

Horning GM, Cobb CM, Killoy WJ (1987). Effect of an air-powder abrasive system on root surfaces in periodontal surgery. J Clin Periodontol 14:213–220.

Howell TH, Fiorellini JP, Paquette DW, Offenbacher S, Giannobile WV, Lynch SE (1997). A phase I/II clinical trial to evaluate a combination of recombinant human platelet-derived growth factor-BB and recombinant human insulin-like growth factor–I in patients with periodontal disease. J Periodontol 68:1186–1193.

Hughes FJ, Smales FC (1986). Immunohistochemical investigation of the presence and distribution of cementum-associated lipopolysaccharides in periodontal disease. J Periodontal Res 21:660–667.

Hughes FJ, Turner W, Belibasakis G, Martuscelli G (2006). Effects of growth factors and cytokines on osteoblast differentiation. Periodontol 2000 41:48–72.

Hugoson A, Laurell L (2000). A prospective longitudinal study on periodontal bone height changes in a Swedish population. J Clin Periodontol 27:665–674.

Hung H-C, Douglass CW (2002). Meta-analysis of the effect of scaling and root planing, surgical treatment and antibiotic therapies on periodontal probing depth and attachment loss. J Clin Periodontol 29:975–986.

Hwang D, Wang H-L (2006). Flap thickness as a predictor of root coverage: A systematic review. J Periodontol 77:1625–1634.

Isidor F, Karring T (1986). Long-term effect of surgical and non-surgical periodontal treatment. A 5-year clinical study. J Periodontal Res 21:462–472.

Jacobson L, Blomlöf J, Lindskog S (1994). Root surface texture after different scaling modalities. Scand J Dent Res 102:156–160.

Jansson L, Lavstedt S, Zimmerman M (2002). Marginal bone loss and tooth loss in a sample from the County of Stockholm—A longitudinal study over 20 years. Swed Dent J 26:21–29.

Jansson H, Bratthall G, Söderholm G (2003). Clinical outcome observed in subjects with recurrent periodontal disease following local treatment with 25% metronidazole gel. J Periodontol 74:372–377.

Jeffcoat MK, Howell TH (1980). Alveolar bone destruction due to overhanging amalgam in periodontal disease. J Periodontol 51:599–602.

Jeffcoat M (1992). Radiographic methods for the detection of progressive alveolar bone loss. J Periodontol 63:367–372.

Jeffcoat M, Reddy M (1993). Digital subtraction radiography for longitudinal assessment of peri-implant bone change; method and validation. Adv Dent Res 7:196–201.

Jeffcoat MK, Chung Wang I, Reddy M (1995). Radiographic diagnosis in periodontics. Periodontol 2000 7:54–68.

Jeffcoat MK, Bray KS, Ciancio SG, et al (1998). Adjunctive use of a subgingival controlled-release chlorhexidine chip reduces probing depth and improves attachment level compared with scaling and root planing alone. J Periodontol 69:989–997.

Jepsen S, Eberhard J, Herrera D, Needleman I (2002). A systematic review of guided tissue regeneration for periodontal furcation defects. What is the effect of guided tissue regeneration compared with surgical debridement in the treatment of furcation defects? J Clin Periodontol 29:103–116.

Jepsen S, Heinz B, Jepsen K, et al (2004). A randomized clinical trial comparing enamel matrix derivative and membrane treatment of buccal class II furcation involvement in mandibular molars. 1. Study design and results for primary outcomes. J Periodontol 75:1150–1160.

Jotikasthira NE, Lie T, Leknes KN (1992). Comparative in vitro studies of sonic, ultrasonic and reciprocating scaling instruments. J Clin Periodontol 19:560–569.

Kaldahl WB, Kalkwarf KL, Patil K, Dyer J, Bates RE Jr (1988). Evaluation of four modalities of periodontal therapy. Mean probing depth, probing attachment level and recession changes. J Periodontol 59:783–793.

Kaldahl WB, Kalkwarf KL, Patil KD, Molvar M, Dyer J (1996). Long-term evaluation of periodontal therapy. 1. Response to four therapeutic modalities. J Periodontol 67:93–102.

Kalpidis CD, Ruben MI (2002). Treatment of intrabony periodontal defects with enamel matrix derivative: A literature review. J Periodontol 73:1360–1376.

Kaner DK, Christian C, Dietrich T, Bernimoulin JP, Kleber BH, Friedmann A (2007). Timing affects the clinical outcome of adjunctive systemic therapy for generalized aggressive periodontitis. J Periodontol 78:1201–1208.

Karring T, Nyman S, Lindhe J (1980). Healing following implantation of periodontitis affected roots into bone tissue. J Clin Periodontol 7:96–105.

Karring T, Nyman S, Gottlow J, Laurell L (1993). Development of the biological concept of guided tissue regeneration—Animal and human studies. Periodontol 2000 1:26–35.

Karring T (2000). Regenerative periodontal therapy. J Int Acad Periodontol 2:101–109.

Karring T, Lindhe J (2008). Concepts in periodontal tissue regeneration. In: Lindhe J, Lang NP, Karring T (eds). Clinical Periodontology and Implant Dentistry, ed 5, vol 1. Oxford: Blackwell Munksgaard: 541–569.

Katsanoulas T, Renée I, Attström R (1992). The effect of supragingival plaque control on the composition of the subgingival flora in periodontal pockets. J Clin Periodontol 19:760–765.

Kepic TJ, O'Leary TJ, Kafrawy AH (1990). Total calculus removal: An attainable objective? J Periodontol 61:16–20.

Keszthelyi G, Szabo I (1984). Influence of Class II amalgam fillings on attachment loss. J Clin Periodontol 11:81–86.

Kinane DF, Radvar M (1999). A six-month comparison of three periodontal local antimicrobial therapies in persistent periodontal pockets. J Periodontol 70:1–7.

King GN, King N, Cruchley AT, Wozney JM, Hughes FJ (1997). Recombinant human bone morphogenetic protein-2 promotes wound healing in rat periodontal fenestration defects. J Dent Res 76:1460–1470.

Kinoshita A, Oda S, Takahashi K, Yokota S, Ishikawa I (1997). Periodontal regeneration by application of recombinant human bone morphogenetic protein-2 to horizontal circumferential defects created by experimental periodontitis in beagle dogs. J Periodontol 68:103–109.

Knowles JW, Burgett FG, Nissle R, Schick R, Morrison E, Ramfjord S (1979). Results of periodontal treatment related to pocket depth and attachment level, 8 years. J Periodontol 50:225–233.

Knowles JW, Burgett FG, Morrison EC, Nissle RR, Ramfjord SP (1980). Comparison of results of following three modalities of periodontal therapy related tooth type and initial pocket depth. J Clin Periodontol 6:32–47.

Kocher T, Plagmann HC (1997). The diamond-coated sonic scaler tip. 2. Loss of substance and alteration of root surface texture after different scaling modalities. Int J Periodontics Restorative Dent 17:484–493.

Kocher T, Langenbeck M, Rühling A, Plagmann HC (2000). Vigorous versus gentle subgingival debridement as assessed on extracted teeth 1. Residual deposits. J Clin Periodontol 27:243–249.

Kocher T, Fanghanel J, Sawaf H, Litz R (2001a). Substance loss caused by scaling with different sonic scaler inserts—An in vitro study. J Clin Periodontol 28:9–15.

Kocher T, Rosin M, Langenbeck N, Bernhardt O (2001b). Subgingival polishing with a Teflon-coated sonic scaler insert in comparison to conventional instruments as assessed on extracted teeth 2. Subgingival roughness. J Clin Periodontol 28:723–729.

Kocher T, Fanghanel J, Schwahn C, Rühling A (2005). A new ultrasonic device in maintenance therapy: Perception of pain and clinical efficacy. J Clin Periodontol 32:425–429.

Kolltveit KM, Eriksen HM (2001). Is the observed association between periodontitis and atherosclerosis causal? Eur J Oral Sci 109:2–7.

Kornman KS, Crane A, Wang H-Y, et al (1997). The interleukin-1 genotype as a severity factor in adult periodontal disease. J Clin Periodontol 24:72–77.

Ladner J, Lin P, Beck F, Mitchell J, Horton J (1992). An SEM study of root surfaces following planing by hand and two distinct types of ultrasonic instruments [abstract 947]. J Dent Res 71(special issue):224.

Lamont RJ, Jenkinson HF (2000). Subgingival colonization by Porphyromonas gingivalis. Oral Microbiol Immunol 15:341–349.

Lang NP, Cumming BR, Löe H (1973). Toothbrushing frequency as it relates to plaque development and gingival health. J Periodontol 7:396–405.

Lang NP, Karring T (eds) (1994). Proceedings of the 1st European Workshop on Periodontology, 1993. London: Quintessence.

Lang NP, Karring T, Lindhe J (eds) (1996). Proceedings of the 2nd European Workshop on Periodontology–Chemicals in Periodontics. Berlin: Quintessence.

Lang NP, Tonetti MS (2003). Periodontal risk assessment (PRA) for patients in supportive periodontal therapy (SPT). Oral Health Prev Dent 1:7–16.

Lang NP, Tan WC, Krahenmann MA, Zwahlen M (2008). A systematic review of the effects of full-mouth debridement with and without antiseptics in patients with chronic periodontitis. J Clin Periodontol 35(8 suppl):8–21.

Laurell L, Gottlow J, Zybutz M, Persson R (1998). Treatment of intrabony defects by different surgical procedures. A literature review. J Periodontol 69:303–313.

Lavespere JE, Yukna RA, Rice DA, LeBlanc D (1996). Root surface removal with diamond-coated ultrasonic instruments: An in vitro and SEM study. J Periodontol 67:1281–1287.

Leiknes T, Leknes KN, Böe OE, Skavland RJ, Lie T (2007). Topical use of a metronidazole gel in the treatment of sites with symptoms of recurring chronic inflammation. J Periodontol 78:1538–1544.

Leknes KN, Lie T, Wikesjö UME, Bogle GC, Selvig KA (1994). Influence of tooth instrumentation roughness on subgingival microbial colonization. J Periodontol 65:303–308.

Leknes KN (1997). The influence of anatomic and iatrogenic root surface characteristics on bacterial colonization and periodontal destruction: A review. J Periodontol 68:507–515.

Lie T, Meyer K (1977). Calculus removal and loss of tooth substance in response to different periodontal instruments. A scanning electron microscope study. J Clin Periodontol 4:250–262.

Lie T, Leknes KN (1985). Evaluation of the effect on root surfaces of air turbine scalers and ultrasonic instrumentation. J Periodontol 56:522–531.

Lindhe J, Hamp SE, Löe H (1975). Plaque-induced periodontal disease in beagle dogs. J Periodontal Res 10:243–255.

Lindhe J, Westfelt E, Nyman S, Socransky SS, Heijl L, Bratthall G (1982). Healing following surgical/non-surgical treatment of periodontal disease. A clinical study. J Clin Periodontol 9:115–128.

Lindhe J, Nyman S (1984). Long-term maintenance of patients treated for advanced periodontal disease. J Clin Periodontol 11:504–514.

Lindhe J, Westfelt E, Nyman S, Socransky SS, Haffajee AD (1984). Long-term effect of surgical/non-surgical treatment of periodontal disease. J Clin Periodontol 11:448–458.

Lindhe J, Nyman S (1985). Scaling and granulation tissue removal in periodontal therapy. J Clin Periodontol 12:374–388.

Lindskog BI, Zetterberg BL (1975). Medicinsk Terminologi. Stockholm, Sweden: Nordiska Bokhandeln.

Listgarten MA, Mayo H, Tremblay R (1975). Development of dental plaque on epoxy resin crowns in man. A light and electron microscopic study. J Periodontol 46:10–26.

Listgarten MA (1976). Structure of the microbial flora associated with periodontal health and disease in man. A light and electron microscopic study. J Periodontol 47:1–18.

Listgarten MA, Schifter C (1982). Differential dark field microscopy of subgingival bacteria as an aid in selecting recall intervals; results after 18 months. J Clin Periodontol 9:305–316.

Listgarten MA, Levin S, Schifter CC, Sullivan P, Evian CI, Rosenberg ES, Laster L (1986). Comparative longitudinal study of 2 methods of scheduling maintenance visits; 2-year data. J Clin Periodontol 13:692–700.

Löe H, Theilade E, Jensen SB (1965). Experimental gingivitis in man. J Periodontol 36:177–187.

References

Löe H, Anerud A, Boysen H, Smith M (1978). The natural history of periodontal disease in man. The rate of periodontal destruction before 40 years of age. J Periodontol 4:240–249.

Lövdal A, Arno A, Schei O, Waerhaug J (1961). Combined effect of subgingival scaling and controlled oral hygiene on the incidence of gingivitis. Acta Odontol Scand 19:537–555.

Lowman JV, Burke RS, Pelleu GB (1973). Patent accessory canals: Incidence in molar furcation region. Oral Surg Oral Med Oral Pathol 36:580–584.

Lynch SE, Williams RC, Polson AM, et al (1989). A combination of platelet-derived and insulin-like growth factors enhances periodontal regeneration. J Clin Periodontol 16:545–548.

Lynch M, Jandinski J, Fenesey K, Murray P (1991). Crevicular fluid interleukin-1 levels in HIV-associated periodontal disease [abstract]. J Dent Res 70:1208.

Lyngstadaas SP, Lundberg E, Ekdahl H, Andersson C, Gestrelius S (2001). Autocrine growth factors in human periodontal ligament cells cultured on enamel matrix derivative. J Clin Periodontol 28:181–188.

Machion L, Andia DC, Benatti BB, et al (2004). Locally delivered doxycycline as an adjunctive therapy to scaling and root planing in the treatment of smokers: A clinical study. J Periodontol 75:464–469.

Machtei EE, Cho MI, Dunford R, Norderyd J, Zambon JJ, Genco RJ (1994). Clinical, microbiological and histological factors which influence the success of regenerative periodontal therapy. J Periodontol 65:154–161.

Machtei EE, Schallhorn RG (1995). Successful regeneration of mandibular Class II furcation defects: An evidence-based treatment approach. Int J Periodontics Restorative Dent 15:146–167.

Machtei EE, Grossi SG, Dunford R, Zambon JJ, Genco RJ (1996). Long-term stability of Class II furcation defects treated with barrier membranes. J Periodontol 67:523–527.

Machtei EE, Dunford R, Hausmann E, et al (1997). Longitudinal study of prognostic factors in established periodontitis patients. J Clin Periodontol 24:102–109.

Machtei EE (2001). The effect of membrane exposure on the outcome of regenerative procedures in humans: A meta-analysis. J Periodontol 72:512–516.

Machtei EE, Oettinger-Barak O, Peled M (2003). Guided tissue regeneration in smokers: Effect of aggressive anti-infective therapy in class II furcation defects. J Periodontol 74:570–584.

Madianos PN, Papapanou P, Nannmark U, Dahlén G, Sandros J (1996). Porphyromonas gingivalis FDC381 multiplies and persists within human oral epithelial cells in vitro. Infect Immun 64:660–664.

Madinier I, Fosse T, Hitzig C, Charbit Y, Hannoun L (1999). Resistance profile survey of 50 periodontal strains of Actinobacillus actinomycetemcomitans. J Periodontol 70:888–892.

Magnusson I, Lindhe J, Yoneyama T, Liljenberg B (1984). Recolonization of a subgingival microbiota following scaling in deep pockets. J Clin Periodontol 11:193–207.

Magnusson I, Nyman S, Karring T, Egelberg J (1985). Connective tissue attachment formation following exclusion of gingival connective tissue and epithelium during healing. J Periodontal Res 20:201–208.

Magnusson I, Clark WB, McArthur WP, et al (1994). Treatment of subjects with refractory periodontal disease. J Clin Periodontol 21:628–637.

Magnusson I (1998). The use of locally delivered metronidazole in the treatment of periodontitis. Clinical results. J Clin Periodontol 25:959–963.

Maiden MF, Tanner A, McArdle S, Najpauer K, Goodson JM (1991). Tetracycline fiber therapy monitored by DNA probe and cultural methods. J Periodontal Res 26:452–459.

Mariotti A (2003). Efficacy of clinical root surface modifiers in the treatment of periodontal disease. A systematic review. Ann Periodontol 8:205–226.

Marsh PD (1994). Microbial ecology of dental plaque and its significance in health and disease. Adv Dent Res 8:263–271.

Masters DH, Hoskins SW (1964). Projection of cervical enamel into molar furcations. J Periodontol 35:49–53.

Matia JJ, Bissada NF, Maybury JE, Riccetti P (1986). Efficiency of scaling of the molar furcation area with and without surgical access. Int J Periodontics Restorative Dent 6:25–35.

Mayfield L, Söderholm G, Hallström H, et al (1998a). Guided tissue regeneration for the treatment of intraosseous defects using a bioabsorbable membrane. A controlled clinical study. J Clin Periodontol 25:585–595.

Mayfield L, Söderholm G, Norderyd O, Attström R (1998b). Root conditioning using EDTA gel as an adjunct to surgical therapy for the treatment of intraosseous periodontal defects. J Clin Periodontol 25:707–714.

McClain PK, Schallhorn RG (1993). Long-term assessment of combined osseous composite grafting, root conditioning, and guided tissue regeneration. Int J Periodontics Restorative Dent 13(1):9–27.

McClain K, Schallhorn G (2000). Focus on furcation defects—Guided tissue regeneration in combination with bone grafting. Periodontol 2000 22:190–212.

McGuire JR, Nunn ME (1999). Prognosis versus actual outcome. 4. The effectiveness of clinical parameters and IL-1 genotype in accurately predicting prognoses and tooth survival. J Periodontol 70:49–50.

McGuire MK, Cochran DL (2003). Evaluation of human recession defects treated with coronally advanced flaps and either enamel matrix derivative or connective tissue. 2. Histological evaluation. J Periodontol 74:1126–1135.

McGuire MK, Nunn M (2003). Evaluation of human recession defects treated with coronally advanced flaps and either enamel matrix derivative or connective tissue. 1. Comparison of clinical parameters. J Periodontol 74:1110–1125.

McNabb H, Mombelli A, Lang N (1992). Supragingival cleaning 3 times a week. The microbiological effect in moderately deep pockets. J Clin Periodontol 19:348–356.

Mengel R, Buns C, Steizel M, Flores-de-Jacoby L (1994). An in vitro study of oscillating instruments for root planing. J Clin Periodontol 21:513–518.

Meyer K, Lie T (1977). Root surface roughness in response to periodontal instrumentation studied by combined use of microroughness measurements and scanning electron microscopy. J Clin Periodontol 4:77–91.

Meyle J, Gonzalez JR, Bödeker RH, et al (2004). A randomized clinical trial comparing Emdogain and membrane treatment of buccal class II furcation involvement in mandibular molars. 2. Secondary outcomes. J Periodontol 75:1188–1195.

Michalowicz BS, Aeppli D, Kuba RK, et al (1991). A twin study of genetic variation in proportional radiographic alveolar bone height. J Dent Res 70:1431–1435.

Mombelli A, Nyman S, Brägger N, Wennström J, Lang NP (1995). Clinical and microbiological changes associated with an altered subgingival environment induced by periodontal pocket reduction. J Clin Periodontol 22:780–787.

Mombelli A, van Winkelhoff AJ (1997). The systemic use of antibiotics in periodontal therapy. In: Lang NP, Karring T, Lindhe J (eds). Proceedings of the 2nd European Workshop on Periodontology. Berlin: Quintessence, 1997: 38–77.

Mombelli A, Lehmann B, Tonetti M, Lang NP (1997). Clinical response to local delivery of tetracycline in relation to overall and local periodontal conditions. J Clin Periodontol 24:470–477.

Mombelli A, Schmid B, Rutar A, Lang NP (2002). Local antibiotic therapy guided by microbiological diagnosis. Treatment of *Porphyromonas gingivalis* and *Actinobacillus actinomycetemcomitans* persisting after mechanical therapy. J Clin Periodontol 29:743–749.

Mombelli A (2008). Antibiotics in periodontal therapy. In: Lindhe J, Lang NP (eds). Clinical Periodontology and Implant Dentistry, ed 5, vol 2. Oxford: Blackwell Munksgaard: 882–898.

Mongardini C, van Steenberghe D, Dekeyser C, Quirynen M (1999). One stage full- versus partial-mouth disinfection in the treatment of chronic adult or generalized early-onset periodontitis. 1. Long-term clinical observations. J Periodontol 70:632–645.

Moore J, Wilson M, Kieser JB (1986). The distribution of bacterial lipopolysaccharide (endotoxin) in relation to periodontally involved root surfaces. J Clin Periodontol 13:748–751.

Mörch T, Waerhaug J (1956). Quantitative evaluation of the effect of toothbrushing and toothpicking. J Periodontol 27:183.

Moskow BS, Lubarr A (1983). Histologic assessment of human periodontal defect after Durapatite ceramic implant. Report of a case. J Periodontol 54:455–462.

Mousquès T, Listgarten MA, Phillips RW (1980). Effect of scaling and root planing on the composition of the human subgingival microbial flora. J Periodontal Res 15:144–151.

Murakami S, Takayama S, Ikezawa K, et al (1999). Regeneration of periodontal tissues by basic fibroblast growth factor. J Periodontal Res 34:425–430.

Murphy KG, Gunsolley JC (2003). Guided tissue regeneration for the treatment of periodontal intrabony and furcation defects. A systematic review. Ann Periodontol 8:266–302.

Nabers CL, O'Leary TJ (1965). Autogenous bone transplants in the treatment of osseous defects. J Periodontol 36:5–14.

Nakib NM, Bissada NF, Simelink JW, Goldstine SN (1982). Endotoxin penetration into root cementum of periodontally healthy and diseased human teeth. J Periodontol 53:368–378.

Needleman I, Tucker R, Giedrys-Leeper E, Worthington H (2005). Guided tissue regeneration for periodontal intrabony defects—a Cochrane Systematic Review. Periodontol 2000 37:106–123.

Nevins M, Becker W, Kornman K (eds) (1989). Proceedings of the World Workshop in Clinical Periodontics. Chicago: American Academy of Periodontology.

Nevins M, Giannobile WV, McGuire MK, et al (2005). Platelet-derived growth factor stimulates bone fill and rate of attachment level gain: Results of a large multicenter randomized controlled trial. J Periodontol 76:2205–2215.

Nyman S, Rosling B, Lindhe J (1975). Effect of professional tooth-cleaning on healing after periodontal surgery. J Clin Periodontol 2:80–86.

Nyman S, Lindhe J, Rosling B (1977). Periodontal surgery in plaque-infected dentitions. J Clin Periodontol 4:240–249.

Nyman S, Karring T (1979). Regeneration of surgically removed buccal alveolar bone in dogs. J Periodontal Res 14:86–92.

Nyman S, Karring T, Lindhe J, Plantén S (1980). Healing following implantation of periodontitis-affected roots into gingival connective tissue. J Clin Periodontol 7:394–401.

Nyman S, Gottlow J, Karring T, Lindhe J (1982a). The regenerative potential of the periodontal ligament. An experimental study in the monkey. J Clin Periodontol 9:257–265.

Nyman S, Lindhe J, Karring T, Rylander H (1982b). New attachment following surgical treatment of human periodontal disease. J Clin Periodontol 9:290–296.

Nyman S, Sarhed G, Ericsson I, Gottlow J, Karring T (1986). Role of "diseased" root cementum in healing following treatment of periodontal disease. An experimental study in the dog. J Periodontal Res 21:496–503.

Nyman S, Gottlow J, Lindhe J, et al (1987). New attachment formation by guided tissue regeneration. J Periodontal Res 22:252–254.

Nyman S, Westfelt E, Sarhed G, Karring T (1988). Role of "diseased" root cementum in healing following treatment of periodontal disease. A clinical study. J Clin Periodontol 15:464–468.

Oda S, Nitta H, Setoguchi T, Izumi Y, Ishikawa I (2004). Current concepts and advances in manual and power-driven instrumentation. Periodontol 2000 36:45–58.

Offenbacher S, Katz V, Fertik G, et al (1996). Periodontal infection as a risk factor for preterm low birth weight. J Periodontol 67(suppl 10):1103–1113.

Offenbacher S, Jared HL, O'Reilly PG, et al (1998). Potential pathogenic mechanisms of periodontitis-associated pregnancy complications. Ann Periodontol 3:233–250.

Offenbacher S, Madianos PN, Champagne CME, et al (1999). Periodontitis-atherosclerosis syndrome: An expanded model of pathogenesis. J Periodontal Res 34:346–352.

Österberg T, Landt H (1976). Index for occlusal status. Tandläkartidningen 68:1216–1223.

Pack AR, Coxhead LJ, McDonald BW (1990). The prevalence of overhanging margins in posterior amalgam restorations and periodontal consequences. J Clin Periodontol 17:145–152.

Page RC, Martin J, Krall EA, Mancl L, Garcia R (2003). Longitudinal validation of a risk calculator for periodontal disease. J Clin Periodontol 30:819–827.

Paquette DW, Hanlon A, Lessem J, Williams RC (2004). Clinical relevance of adjunctive minocycline microspheres in patients with chronic periodontitis: Secondary analysis of a phase 3 trial. J Periodontol 75:531–536.

Park JB, Matsuura M, Han KY, et al (1995). Periodontal regeneration in class III furcation defects of beagle dogs using guided tissue regenerative therapy with platelet derived growth factor. J Periodontol 66:462–477.

Pattison AM (1996). The use of hand instruments in supportive periodontal treatment. Periodontol 2000 12:71–89.

Pavia MM, Nobile CG, Angelillo IF (2003). Meta-analysis of local tetracycline in treating chronic periodontitis. J Periodontol 74:916–932.

Pavicić MJ, van Winkelhoff AJ, Douqué NH, Steures RW, de Graaff J (1994). Microbiological and clinical effects of metronidazole and amoxicillin in *Actinobacillus actinomycetemcomitans*-associated periodontitis. A 2-year evaluation. J Clin Periodontol 21:107–112.

Persson GR, Persson RE (2008). Cardiovascular disease and periodontitis: An update on the associations and risk. J Clin Periodontol 35(8 suppl):362–379.

Pertuiset JH, Saglie FR, Lofthus J, Rezende M, Sanz M (1987). Recurrent periodontal disease and bacterial presence in the gingiva. J Periodontol 58:553–558.

Petersilka GJ, Ehmk B, Flemmig TF (2002). Antimicrobial effects of mechanical debridement. Periodontol 2000 28:56–71.

References

Petersilka GJ, Bell M, Mehl A, Hickel R, Flemmig TF (2003a). Root defects following air polishing. An in vitro study on the effects of working parameters. J Clin Periodontol 30:165–170.

Petersilka GJ, Steinmann D, Haberlein I, Heinecke A, Flemmig TF (2003b). Subgingival plaque removal in buccal and lingual sites using a novel low abrasive air-polishing powder. J Clin Periodontol 30:328–333.

Petersilka GJ, Tunkel J, Barakos K, Heinecke A, Häberlein I, Flemmig TF (2003c). Subgingival plaque removal at interdental sites using a low-abrasive air polishing powder. J Periodontol 74:307–311.

Pihlström B, Ortiz-Campos C, McHugh RB (1981). A randomized 4-year study of periodontal therapy. J Periodontol 52:227–242.

Pihlström B, McHugh R, Oliphant T, Ortiz-Campos C (1983). Comparison of surgical and nonsurgical treatment of periodontal disease. A review of current studies and additional results after 6½ years. J Clin Periodontol 10:524–541.

Pihlström B, Oliphant T, McHugh RB (1984). Molar and nonmolar teeth compared over 6½ years following two methods of periodontal therapy. J Periodontol 55:499–504.

Polimeni G, Xiropaidis AV, Wikesjö UME (2006). Biology and principles of periodontal wound healing/regeneration. Periodontol 2000 41:30–47.

Polson AM, Heijl LC (1978). Osseous repair in infrabony periodontal defects. J Clin Periodontol 5:13–23.

Pontoriero R, Lindhe J, Nyman S, Karring T, Rosenberg E, Sanavi F (1988). Guided tissue regeneration in degree II furcation-involved mandibular molars. A clinical study. J Clin Periodontol 15:247–254.

Pontoriero R, Lindhe J, Nyman S, Karring T, Rosenberg E, Sanavi F (1989). Guided tissue regeneration in the treatment of furcation defects in mandibular molars. A clinical study of degree III involvements. J Clin Periodontol 16:170–174.

Pontoriero R, Lindhe J (1995a). Guided tissue regeneration in the treatment of degree II furcations in maxillary molars. J Clin Periodontol 22:756–763.

Pontoriero R, Lindhe J (1995b). Guided tissue regeneration in the treatment of degree III furcation defects in maxillary molars. J Clin Periodontol 22:810–812.

Preber H, Bergstrom J, Linder LE (1992). Occurrence of periopathogens in smoker and non-smoker patients. J Clin Periodontol 19:667–671.

Prichard J (1957a). Regeneration of bone following periodontal therapy. Oral Surg 10:247.

Prichard JF (1957b). The intrabony technique as a predictable procedure. J Periodontol 28:202.

Quirynen M, Marechal M, Busscher HJ, Weerkamp AH, Darius PL, van Steenberghe D (1990). The influence of surface free energy and surface roughness on early plaque formation. An in vivo study in man. J Clin Periodontol 17:138–144.

Quirynen M, Bollen C, Vandekerckhove B, Dekeyser C, Papapanou W, Eyssen H (1995). Full- versus partial-mouth disinfection in the treatment of periodontal infections. Short-term clinical and microbiological observations. J Dent Res 74:1459–1467.

Quirynen M, Mongardini C, Pauwels M, Bollen C, Van Eldere J, Van Steenberghe D (1999). One-stage full- versus partial-mouth disinfection in the treatment of chronic adult or generalized early-onset periodontitis. J Periodontol 70:646–656.

Quirynen M, Mongardini C, De Soete M, et al (2000). The role of chlorhexidine in the one stage full-mouth disinfection treatment of patients with advanced adult periodontitis. Long-term clinical and microbiological observations. J Clin Periodontol 27:578–589.

Quirynen M, De Soete M, Dierickx K, van Steenberghe D (2001). The intraoral translocation of periodontopathogens jeopardises the outcome of periodontal therapy. A review of the literature. J Clin Periodontol 28:499–507.

Quirynen M, Teughels W, De Soete M, van Steenberghe D (2002). Topical antiseptics and antibiotics in the initial therapy of chronic adult periodontitis: Microbiological aspects. Periodontol 2000 28:72–90.

Quirynen M, De Soete M, Boschmans G, et al (2006). Benefit of "one-stage, full-mouth disinfection" is explained by disinfection and root planing within 24 hours: A randomized controlled trial. J Clin Periodontol 33:630–647.

Radvar M, Pourtaghi N, Kinane DF (1996). Comparison of 3 periodontal local antibiotic therapies in persistent periodontal pockets. J Periodontol 67:860–865.

Ramberg P, Axelsson P, Lindhe J (1995). Plaque formation at healthy and inflamed gingival sites in young individuals. J Clin Periodontol 22:85–88.

Ramberg P, Furuichi Y, Volpe AR, Gaffar A, Lindhe J (1996). The effects of antimicrobial mouthrinses on de novo plaque formation at sites with healthy and inflamed gingivae. J Clin Periodontol 23:7–11.

Ramfjord SP, Nissle RR, Schick RA, Cooper H (1968). Subgingival curettage versus surgical elimination of periodontal pockets. J Periodontol 39:167–175.

Ramfjord SP, Nissle R (1974). The modified Widman flap. J Periodontol 45:601–607.

Ramfjord SP, Knowles JW, Nissle RR, Schick RA, Burgett FG (1975). Results following three modalities of periodontal therapy. J Periodontol 46:522–526.

Ramfjord SP (1977). Present status of the modified Widman flap procedure. J Periodontol 48:558–565.

Ramfjord SP, Morrison EC, Burgett FG, et al (1982). Oral hygiene and maintenance of periodontal support. J Periodontol 53:26–30.

Ramfjord SP, Caffesse R, Morrison E, et al (1987). Four modalities of periodontal treatment compared over 5 years. J Clin Periodontol 14:445–452.

Rams T, Slots J (1996). Local delivery of antimicrobial agents in the periodontal pocket. Periodontol 2000 10:139–159.

Ramseier CA (2005). Potential impact of subject-based risk factor control on periodontitis. J Clin Periodontol 32(suppl 6):282–290.

Rateitschak KH, Wolf H, Hassel T (1989). Color Atlas of Dental Medicine, ed 2. New York: Thieme.

Rateitschak-Plüss EM, Schwarz J-P, Guggenheim R, Düggelin M, Rateitschak KH (1992). Non-surgical periodontal treatment: Where are the limits? A SEM study. J Clin Periodontol 19:240–244.

Ratka-Krüger P, Schacher B, Bürklin T, et al (2005). Non-surgical periodontal therapy with adjunctive topical doxycycline: A double-masked, randomized, controlled multicenter study. 2. Microbiological results. J Periodontol 76:66–74.

Reddy MS, Jeffcoat MK, Geurs NC, et al (2003). Efficacy of controlled-release subgingival chlorhexidine to enhance periodontal regeneration. J Periodontol 74:411–419.

Renvert S, Wikström M, Dahlén G, Slots J, Egelberg J (1990). On the inability of root debridement and periodontal surgery to eliminate *Actinobacillus actinomycetemcomitans* from periodontal pockets. J Clin Periodontol 17:351–355.

Renvert S, Persson GR (2004). Supportive periodontal therapy. Periodontol 2000 36:179–195.

Research, Science and Therapy Committee of the American Academy of Periodontology (2002). Lasers in periodontics (Academy Report). J Periodontol 73:1231-1239.

Reynolds MA, Aichelmann-Reidy ME, Branch-Mays GL, Gunsolley JC (2003). The efficacy of bone replacement grafts in the treatment of periodontal osseous defects. A systematic review. Ann Periodontol 8:227–265.

Reynolds MA, Aichelmann-Reidy ME (2005). The era of biologics and reparative medicine: A pivotal clinical trial of platelet-derived growth factor for periodontal regeneration. J Periodontol 76:2330–2332.

Ritz L, Hefti AF, Rateitschak KH (1991). An in vitro investigation on the loss of root substance in scaling with various instruments. J Clin Periodontol 18:643–647.

Robertson PB (1990). The residual calculus paradox. J Periodontol 61:65–66.

Robinson RE (1969). Osseous coagulum for bone induction. J Periodontol 40:503–510.

Roccuzzo M, Bunino M, Needleman I, Sanz M (2002). Periodontal plastic surgery for treatment of localized gingival recessions: A systematic review. J Clin Periodontol 29(suppl 3):178–194.

Rodrigues TL, Marchesan JT, Coletta RD, et al (2007). Effects of enamel matrix derivative and transforming growth factor-beta1 on human periodontal ligament fibroblasts. J Clin Periodontol 34:514–522.

Rodriguez-Ferrer HJ, Strahan JD, Newman HN (1980). Effect of gingival health of removing overhanging margins of interproximal subgingival amalgam restorations. J Clin Periodontol 7:457–462.

Rosén B, Olavi G, Badersten A, Rönström A, Söderholm G, Egelberg J (1999). Effect of different frequencies of preventive maintenance treatment on periodontal conditions. 5-Year observations in general dentistry patients. J Clin Periodontol 26:225–233.

Rosenberg MM (1988). Furcation involvement: Periodontic, endodontic and restorative interrelationships. In: Rosenberg MM, Kay HB, Keough BE, Holt RL (eds). Periodontal and Prosthetic Management for Advanced Cases. Chicago: Quintessence:249–251.

Rosling B, Nyman S, Lindhe J (1976a). The effect of systematic plaque control on bone regeneration in infrabony pockets. J Clin Periodontol 3:38–53.

Rosling B, Nyman S, Lindhe J, Jern B (1976b). The healing potential of the periodontal tissues following different techniques of periodontal surgery in plaque-free dentitions. A 2-year clinical study. J Clin Periodontol 3:233–250.

Rosling B, Wannfors B, Volpe AR, Furuichi Y, Ramberg P, Lindhe J (1997). The use of a triclosan/copolymer dentifrice may retard the progression of periodontitis. J Clin Periodontol 24:873–880.

Rosling B, Hellström M-K, Ramberg P, Socransky SS, Lindhe J (2001). The use of PVP-iodine as an adjunct to non-surgical treatment of chronic periodontitis. J Clin Periodontol 28:1023–1031.

Rossa C Jr, Marcantonio E Jr, Cirelli JA, Marcantonio RA, Spolidorio LC, Fogo JC (2000). Regeneration of Class III furcation defects with basic fibroblast growth factor (b-FGF) associated with GTR. A descriptive and histometric study in dogs. J Periodontol 71:775–784.

Rüdiger SG, Ehmke B, Hommens A, Karch H, Flemmig TF (2003). Guided tissue regeneration using a polylactic acid barricr. 1. Environmental effects on bacterial colonization. J Clin Periodontol 30:19–25.

Rudney JD, Chen R, Sedgewick GJ (2001). Intracellular Actinobacillus actinomycetemcomitans and Porphyromonas gingivalis in buccal epithelial cells collected from human subjects. Infect Immun 69:2700–2707.

Rühling A, Bernhardt O, Kocher T (2005). Subgingival debridement with a Teflon-coated sonic scaler insert in comparison to conventional instruments and assessment of substance removal on extracted teeth. Quintessence Int 36:446–452.

Rutherford RB, Ryan ME, Kennedy JE, Tucker MM, Charette MF (1993). Platelet-derived growth factor and dexamethasone combined with a collagen matrix induce regeneration of the periodontium in monkeys. J Clin Periodontol 20:537–544.

Ryder M, Pons B, Adams D, Beiswinger B (1999). Effects of smoking on local delivery of controlled-release doxycycline as compared to scaling and root planing. J Clin Periodontol 26:683-691.

Rylev M, Kilian M (2008). Prevalence and distribution of principal periodontal pathogens worldwide. J Clin Periodontol 35(8 suppl):346–361.

Saglie FR, Carranza F Jr, Newman M, Cheng L, Lewin K (1982a). Identification of tissue-invading bacteria in human periodontal disease. J Periodontal Res 17:452–455.

Saglie FR, Newman M, Carranza F, Pattison G (1982b). Bacterial invasion of gingiva in advanced periodontitis in humans. J Periodontol 53:217–222.

Salvi GE, Carollo-Bittel B, Lang NP (2008). Effects of diabetes mellitus on periodontal and peri-implant conditions: Update on associations and risks. J Clin Periodontol 35(8 suppl):398–409.

Sander L, Frandsen E, Arnbjerg D, Warrer K, Karring T (1994). Effect of local metronidazole application on periodontal healing following guided tissue regeneration. Clinical findings. J Periodontol 65:914–920.

Sandros J, Papapanou PN, Nannmark U, Dahlén G (1994). Porphyromonas gingivalis invades human pocket epithelium in vitro. J Periodontal Res 29:62–69.

Sanz M, Giovannoli L (2000). Focus on furcation defects: Guided tissue regeneration. Periodontol 2000 22:169–189.

Sanz M, Tonetti MS, Zabalegui I (2004). Treatment of intrabony defects with enamel matrix proteins or barrier membranes: Results from a multicenter practice-based clinical trial. J Periodontol 75:726–733.

Saxe SR, Greene JC, Bohannan HM, Vermillion JR (1967). Oral debris, calculus and periodontal disease in the beagle dog. Periodontics 5:217–225.

Saxton CA (1975). The Formation of Human Dental Plaque: A Study by Scanning Electron Microscopy [thesis]. London: Univ of London.

Saygun I, Kubar A, Özdemir A, Yapar M, Slots J (2004a). Herpes-viral-bacterial interrelationships in aggressive periodontitis. J Periodontal Res 39:207–212.

Saygun I, Yapar M, Özdemir A, Kubar A, Slots S (2004b). Human cytomegalovirus and Epstein-Barr virus type 1 in periodontal abscesses. Oral Microbiol Immunol 19:83–87.

Schroer M, Kri C, Wahö T, Hutchens L, Moriarty J, Bergenholtz B (1991). Closed versus open debridement of facial grade II molar furcation. J Clin Periodontol 18:323–329.

Schroers K (1994). Klinisch kontrollierte Studie zum Nachweis der Wirksamkeit von Bifluorid 12 bei der Behandlung überempfindlicher Zähne [unpublished report]. Cuxhaven, Germany: VOCO.

Schwarz F, Sculean A, Georg T, Reich E (2001). Periodontal treatment with an Er:YAG laser compared to scaling and root planing. A controlled clinical study. J Periodontol 72:361–367.

Schwarz F, Sculean A, Berakdar M, Georg T, Reich E, Becker J (2003). Periodontal treatment with an Er:YAG laser or scaling and root planing. A 2-year follow-up split-mouth study. J Periodontol 74:590–596.

References

Schwarz F, Aoki A, Becker J, Sculean A (2008). Laser application in non-surgical periodontal therapy: A systematic review. J Clin Periodontol 35(8 suppl):29–44.

Sculean A, Windisch P, Keglevich T, Gera I (2003). Histologic evaluation of human intrabony defects following non-surgical periodontal therapy with and without application of an enamel matrix protein derivative. J Periodontol 74:153–160.

Sculean A, Schwarz F, Berakdar M, et al (2004a). Non-surgical periodontal treatment with a new ultrasonic device (Vector ultrasonic system) or hand instruments. A prospective, controlled clinical study. J Clin Periodontol 31:428–433.

Sculean A, Schwarz F, Berakdar M, Windisch P, Arweiler NB, Romanos GE (2004b). Healing of intrabony defects following surgical treatment with or without an Er:YAG laser. A pilot study. J Clin Periodontol 31:604–608.

Sculean A, Schwarz F, Miliauskaite A, et al (2006). Treatment of intrabony defects with an enamel matrix protein derivative or bioabsorbable membrane: An 8-year follow-up split-mouth study. J Periodontol 77:1879–1886.

Sculean A, Pietruska M, Arweiler NB, Auschill TM, Nemcovsky C (2007). Four-year results of a prospective-controlled clinical study evaluating healing of intra-bony defects following treatment with an enamel matrix protein derivative alone or combined with a bioactive glass. J Clin Periodontol 34:507–513.

Sculean A, Nikolidakis D, Schwarz F (2008). Regeneration of periodontal tissues: Combinations of barrier membranes and grafting materials—Biological foundation and preclinical evidence: A systematic review. J Clin Periodontol 35(8 suppl):106–116.

Sherman PR, Hutchens LH Jr, Jewson LG, Moriarty JM, Greco GW, McFall WT Jr (1990). The effectiveness of subgingival scaling and root planing. 1. Clinical detection of residual calculus. J Periodontol 61:3–8.

Shiloah J, Patters M, Dean J, Bland P, Toledo G (1997). The survival rate of *Actinobacillus actinomycetemcomitans, Porphyromonas gingivalis* and *Bacteroides forsythus*. Following 4 randomized treatment modalities. J Periodontol 68:720–728.

Sigurdsson TJ, Lee MB, Kubota K, Turek TJ, Wozney JM, Wikesjö UME (1995). Periodontal repair in dogs: Recombinant human bone morphologic protein-2 significantly enhances periodontal regeneration. J Periodontol 66:131–138.

Slots J (2002). Interactions between herpesviruses and bacteria in human periodontal disease. In: Brogden KA, Guthmiller JM (eds). Polymicrobial Diseases. Washington, DC: ASM Press, 317–331.

Slots J, Ting M (2002). Systemic antibiotics in the treatment of periodontal disease. Periodontol 2000 28:106–176.

Slots J (2004). Systemic antibiotics in periodontics. J Periodontol 75:1553–1565.

Slots J (2005). Herpesviruses in periodontal diseases. Periodontol 2000 38:33–62.

Smith BA, Echeverri M, Caffesse RG (1987). Mucoperiosteal flaps with and without removal of the pocket epithelium. J Periodontol 58:78–85.

Smukler H, Tagger M (1976). Vital root amputation. A clinical and histological study. J Periodontol 47:324–330.

Socransky SS, Haffajee AD, Smith C, Dibart S (1991). Relation of counts of microbial species to clinical status at the sampled site. J Clin Periodontol 18:766–775.

Socransky SS, Haffajee AD, Cugini MA, Smith C, Kent RL Jr (1998). Microbial complexes in subgingival plaque. J Clin Periodontol 25:134–144.

Socransky SS, Haffajee AD, Smith C, Duff GW (2000). Microbiological parameters associated with IL-1 gene polymorphisms in periodontitis patients. J Clin Periodontol 27:810–818.

Socransky SS, Haffajee AD (2002). Dental biofilms: Difficult therapeutic targets. Periodontol 2000 28:12–55.

Socransky SS, Haffajee AD (2005). Periodontal microbial ecology. Periodontol 2000 28:135–187.

Söderholm G (1979). Effect of a Dental Care Program on Dental Health Conditions. A Study of Employees of a Swedish Shipyard [thesis]. Lund, Sweden: Univ of Lund.

Spahr A, Lyngstadaas SP, Boeckh C, Andersson C, Podbielski A, Haller B (2002). Effect of the enamel matrix derivative Emdogain on the growth of periodontal pathogens in vitro. J Clin Periodontol 29:62–72.

Spahr A, Haegewald S, Tsoulfidou F, et al (2005). Coverage of Miller class I and II recession defects using enamel matrix proteins versus coronally advanced flap technique: A 2-year report. J Periodontol 76:1871–1880.

Sreenivasan P, Meyer D, Fives-Taylor P (1993). Requirements for invasion of epithelial cells by *Actinobacillus actinomycetemcomitans*. Infect Immun 61:1239–1245.

Srisuwan T, Tilkon D, Wilson J, et al (2006). Molecular aspects of tissue engineering in the dental field. Periodontol 2000 41:88–108.

Stavropoulos A, Karring T (2004). Long-term stability of periodontal conditions achieved following guided tissue regeneration with bioresorbable membranes: Case series results after 6-7 years. J Clin Periodontol 31:939–944.

Stavropoulos A, Mardas N, Herrero F, Karring T (2004). Smoking affects the outcome of guided tissue regeneration with bioresorbable membranes: A retrospective analysis of intrabony defects. J Clin Periodontol 31:945–950.

Steed AM, Scott JB, Yukna RA (1995). Speed of calculus removal in furcation with ultrasonic diamond inserts [abstract 962]. J Dent Res 74(special issue):132.

Stoltenberg JL, Osborn JB, Pihlström BL, et al (1993). Association between cigarette smoking, bacterial pathogens, and periodontal status. J Periodontol 64:1225–1230.

Stoltze K, Stellfeld M (1992). Systemic absorption of metronidazole 25% dental gel. J Clin Periodontol 19:693–697.

Suomi JD, Greene JC, Vermillion JR, Doyle J, Chang JJ, Leatherwood EC (1971). The effect of controlled oral hygiene procedures on the progression of periodontal disease in adults: Results after third and final year. J Periodontol 42:152–160.

Svärdström G (2001). Furcation Involvements in Periodontitis Patients. Prevalence and Treatment Decisions [thesis]. Gothenburg: Gothenburg Univ.

Takayama S, Murakami S, Shimabukuro Y, Kitamura M, Okada H (2001). Periodontal regeneration by FGF-2 (bFGF) in primate models. J Dent Res 80:2075–2079.

Tal H, Panno JM, Vaidyanathan TK (1985). Scanning electron microscope evaluation of wear of dental curettes during standardized root planing. J Periodontol 56:532–536.

Tal H, Soldinger M, Dreiangel A, Pitaru S (1989). Periodontal response to long-term abuse of the gingival attachment by supracrestal amalgam restorations. J Clin Periodontol 16:654–659.

Tammaro S, Wennström JL, Bergenholtz G (2000). Root-dentin sensitivity following non-surgical peri-odontal treatment. J Clin Periodontol 27:690–697.

Theilade E (1986). The non-specific theory in microbial etiology of inflammatory periodontal diseases. J Clin Periodontol 13:905–911.

Tomasi C, Wennström JL (2004). Locally delivered doxycycline improves the healing following non-surgical periodontal therapy in smokers. J Clin Periodontol 31:589-595.

Tomasi C, Koutouzis T, Wennström JL (2008). Locally delivered doxycycline as an adjunct to mechanical debridement at retreatment of periodontal pockets. J Periodontol 79:431-439.

Tonetti M, Prato GP, Cortellini P (1993). Periodontal regeneration of human infrabony defects. 4. Determinants of the healing response. J Periodontol 64:934-940.

Tonetti MS, Prato GP, Cortellini P (1995). Effect of cigarette smoking on periodontal healing following GTR in infrabony defects. A preliminary retrospective study. J Clin Periodontol 22:229-234.

Tonetti MS, Prato GP, Cortellini P (1996). Factors affecting the healing response of intrabony defects following guided tissue regeneration and access flap surgery. J Clin Periodontol 23:548-556.

Tonetti M (1997). The topical use of antibiotics in periodontal pockets. In: Lang N, Karring T, Lindhe J (eds). Proceedings of the 2nd European Workshop on Periodontology. Chemicals in Periodontics. Berlin: Quintessence: 78-109.

Tonetti MS (1998). Cigarette smoking and periodontal diseases: Etiology and management of disease. Ann Periodontol 3:88-101.

Tonetti M, Lang NP, Cortellini P, et al (2002). Enamel matrix proteins in the regenerative therapy of deep intrabony pockets. J Clin Periodontol 29:317-325.

Tonetti MS, Cortellini P, Lang NP, et al (2004). Clinical outcomes following treatment of human intrabony defects with GTR/bone replacement material or access flap alone. A multicenter randomized controlled clinical trial. J Clin Periodontol 31:770-776.

Trombelli L, Heitz-Mayfield L, Needleman I, Moles D, Scabbia A (2002). A systematic review of graft materials and biological agents for periodontal intraosseous defects. J Clin Periodontol 29(suppl 3):117-135.

Trombelli L (2005). Which reconstructive procedures are effective for treating the periodontal intraosseous defect? Periodontol 2000 37:88-105.

Trombelli L, Minenna L, Farina R, Scabbia A (2005). Guided tissue regeneration in human gingival recessions: A 10-year follow-up study. J Clin Periodontol 32:16-20.

Trombelli L, Farina R (2008). Clinical outcomes with bioactive agents alone or in combination with grafting or guided tissue regeneration. J Clin Periodontol 35(8 suppl):117-135.

Tu YK, Tugnait A, Clerehugh V (2008). Is there a temporal trend in the reported treatment efficacy of periodontal regeneration? A meta-analysis of randomized-controlled trials. J Clin Periodontol 35:139-146.

Umeda M, Takeuchi Y, Noguchi K, Huang Y, Koshy G, Ishikawa I (2004). Effects of nonsurgical periodontal therapy on the microbiota. Periodontol 2000 36:98-120.

Van der Pauw M, Van den Bos T, Everts V, Beertsen W (2000). Enamel matrix–derived protein stimulates attachment of periodontal ligament fibroblasts and enhances alkaline phosphatase activity and transforming growth factor β1 release of periodontal ligament and gingival fibroblasts. J Periodontol 71:31-43.

Van der Weijden GA, Timmerman M, Danser M, Van der Velden U (1998). The role of automated toothbrushes: Advantages and limitations of automated toothbrushes. In: Lang NP, Attström R, Löe H (eds). Proceedings of the European Workshop on Mechanical Plaque Control. Berlin: Quintessence: 138-155.

Van der Weijden GA, Hioe KP (2005). A systematic review of the effectiveness of self-performed mechanical plaque removal in adults with gingivitis using a manual toothbrush. J Clin Periodontol 32(suppl 6):214-228 [comment: 32(suppl 6):291-293].

Van Steenberghe D, Rosling B, Söder PO, et al (1999). A 15-month evaluation of the effects of repeated subgingival minocycline in chronic adult periodontitis. J Periodontol 70:657-667.

Van Winkelhoff AJ, Rodenburg JP, Goene RJ, Abbas F, Winkel EG, de Graaff J (1989). Metronidazole plus amoxicillin in the treatment of Actinobacillus actinomycetemcomitans–associated periodontitis. J Clin Periodontol 16:128-131.

Van Winkelhoff AJ, Tijhof CJ, de Graaff J (1992). Microbiological and clinical results of metronidazole plus amoxicillin therapy in Actinobacillus actinomycetemcomitans–associated periodontitis. J Periodontol 63:52-57.

Van Winkelhoff A, Pavicić M, de Graaf J (1994). Antibiotics in periodontal therapy. In: Lang N, Karring T (eds). Proceedings of the 1st European Workshop on Periodontology, 1993. London: Quintessence: 258-273.

Van Winkelhoff AJ, Rams TE, Slots J (1996). Systemic antibiotic therapy in periodontics. Periodontol 2000 10:45-78.

Van Winkelhoff A, Gonzales DH, Winkel E, Dellemijn-Kippuw N, Vandenbroucke-Grauls C, Sanz M (2000). Antimicrobial resistance in the subgingival microflora in patients with adult periodontitis. J Clin Periodontol 27:79-86.

Van Winkelhoff AJ, Herrera D, Oteo A, Sanz M (2005). Antimicrobial profiles of periodontal pathogens isolated from periodontitis patients in the Netherlands and Spain. J Clin Periodontol 32:893-898.

Vandekerckhove BN, Bollen CM, Dekeyser C, Darius P, Quirynen M (1996). Full- versus partial-mouth disinfection in the treatment of periodontal infections. Long-term clinical observations of a pilot study. J Periodontol 67:1251-1259.

Vandekerckhove BNA, Quirynen M, van Steenberghe D (1998). The use of locally-delivered minocycline in the treatment of chronic periodontitis. A review of the literature. J Clin Periodontol 25:964-968.

Vertucci FJ, Williams RG (1974). Furcation canals in the human mandibular first molar. Oral Surg Oral Med Oral Pathol 38:308-314.

Wade WG, Moran J, Morgan JR, Newcombe R, Addy M (1992). The effects of antimicrobial acrylic strips on the subgingival microflora in chronic periodontitis. J Clin Periodontol 19:127-134.

Waerhaug J (1976). Subgingival plaque and loss of attachment in periodontosis as observed in autopsy material. J Periodontol 47:636-642.

Waerhaug J (1981a). Effect of toothbrushing on subgingival plaque formation. J Periodontol 52:30-34.

Waerhaug J (1981b). Healing of the dento-epithelial junction following the use of dental floss. J Clin Periodontol 8:144-150.

Walker CB, Gordon JM, McQuilkin SJ, Niebloom TA, Socransky SS (1981). Tetracycline: Levels achievable in gingival crevice fluid and in vitro effect on subgingival organisms. 2. Susceptibilities of periodontal bacteria. J Periodontol 52:613-616.

Walker C, Karpinia K (2002). Rationale for use of antibiotics in periodontics. J Periodontol 73:1188-1196.

Walmsley AD, Lea SC, Landini G, Moses AJ (2008). Advances in power driven pocket/root instrumentation. J Clin Periodontol 35(8 suppl):22-28.

Wang HL, Greenwell H, Fiorellini J, et al; Research, Science and Therapy Committee (2005). Periodontal regeneration. J Periodontol 76:1601-1622.

References

Weinstein P, Getz I (1978). Changing Human Behavior: Strategies for Preventive Dentistry. Chicago: Science Research Associates.

Wennström A, Wennström J, Lindhe J (1986). Healing following surgical and non-surgical treatment of juvenile periodontitis. A 5-year longitudinal study. J Clin Periodontol 13:869–882.

Wennström JL, Newman HN, MacNeill SR, et al (2001). Utilisation of locally delivered doxycycline in non-surgical treatment of chronic periodontitis. A comparative multi-centre trial of 2 treatment approaches. J Clin Periodontol 28:753–761.

Wennström JL, Lindhe J (2002). Some effects of enamel matrix proteins on wound healing in the dentogingival region. J Clin Periodontol 29:9–14.

Wennström JL, Tomasi C, Bertelle A, Dellasega E (2005). Full-mouth ultrasonic debridement versus quadrant scaling and root planing as an initial approach in the treatment of chronic periodontitis. J Clin Periodontol 32:851–859.

Westfelt E, Nyman S, Lindhe J, Socransky SS (1983a). Use of chlorhexidine as a plaque control measure following surgical treatment of periodontal disease. J Clin Periodontol 10:22–26.

Westfelt E, Nyman S, Socransky SS, Lindhe J (1983b). Significance of frequency of professional tooth cleaning for healing following periodontal surgery. J Clin Periodontol 10:148–156.

Widman L (1918). The operative treatment of pyorrhea alveolaris. A new surgical method. Sven Tandlak Tidskr [reviewed in Br Dent J 1920;1:293].

Wimmer G, Pihlstrom BL (2008). A critical assessment of adverse pregnancy outcome and periodontal disease. J Clin Periodontol 35(8 suppl):380–397.

Winkel EG, van Winkelhoff AJ, van der Velden U (1998). Additional clinical and microbiological effects of amoxicillin and metronidazole after initial periodontal therapy. J Clin Periodontol 25:857–864.

Winkel EG, van Winkelhoff AJ, Barendregt DS, van der Weijden GA, Timmerman MF, van der Velden U (1999). Clinical and microbiological effects of initial periodontal therapy in conjunction with amoxicillin and clavulanic acid in patients with adult periodontitis. A randomised double-blind, placebo-controlled study. J Clin Periodontol 26:461–468.

Winkel EG, van der Weijden GA, van Winkelhoff AJ, Timmerman M, van der Velden (2001). Metronidazole plus amoxicillin in the treatment of adult periodontitis patients. A double-blind placebo-controlled study. J Clin Periodontol 28:296–305.

World Health Organization (1994). WHO Oral Health Country Profile Programme 1994. Geneva: WHO.

Xajigeorgiou C, Sakellari D, Slini T, Baka A, Konstantinidis A (2006). Clinical and microbiological effects of different antimicrobials on generalized aggressive periodontitis. J Clin Periodontol 33:254–264.

Ximénez-Fyvie LA, Haffajee AD, Socransky SS (2000). Comparison of the microbiota of supra- and subgingival plaque in subjects in health and periodontitis. J Clin Periodontol 27:648–657.

Yukna RA, Scott JB, Aichelmann-Reidy ME, LeBlanc DM, Mayer ET (1997). Clinical evaluation of the speed and effectiveness of subgingival calculus removal on single-rooted teeth with diamond-coated ultrasonic tips. J Periodontol 68:436–442.

Zappa U, Smith B, Simona C, Graf H, Case D, Kim W (1991). Root substance removal by scaling and root planing. J Periodontol 62:50–754.

Zeichner-David M (2006). Regeneration of periodontal tissues: Cementogenesis revisited. Periodontol 2000 41:196–217.

LIST OF ABBREVIATIONS

ANUG—acute necrotizing ulcerative gingivitis
ANUP—acute necrotizing ulcerative periodontitis
APITN—Apical Periodontitis Index of Treatment
 Needs

BMP—bone morphogenetic protein

CAF—coronally advanced flap
CAL—clinical attachment level
CCITN—Community Caries Index of Treatment
 Needs
CEJ—cementoenamel junction
CEP—cervical enamel projection
CHX—chlorhexidine gluconate
CI—confidence interval
CPITN—Community Periodontal Index of Treat-
 ment Needs

DFDBA—demineralized freeze-dried bone allograft
DFS—decayed or filled surface
DS—decayed surface

EDTA—ethylenediaminetetraacetic acid
EMD—enamel matrix derivative
e-PTFE—expanded polytetrafluoroethylene

FDBA—freeze-dried bone allograft
FDI—Fédération Dentaire Internationale
FGF—fibroblast growth factor

GCF—gingival crevicular fluid
GTR—guided tissue regeneration

IGF—insulin-like growth factor
IL-1—interleukin 1

MPIC—mechanical and pharmacologic infection
 control

OFD—open flap debridement

PAL—probing attachment level
PCPC—professional chemical plaque control
PDGF—platelet-derived growth factor
PFRI—Plaque Formation Rate Index
PMNL—polymorphonuclear leukocyte
PM—periodontal maintenance
PMTC—professional mechanical toothcleaning
PRF—prognostic risk factor

RCT—randomized controlled trial
RF—risk factor
RI—risk indicator

TGF-β—transforming growth factor β

INDEX

Page numbers followed by "b" indicate boxes; "f" indicate figures; "t" indicate tables.